Fifth Edition

The Nursing Process

Assessing, Planning, Implementing, Evaluating

Helen Yura, Ph.D., R.N., F.A.A.N.
Eminent Professor and Graduate Program Director
School of Nursing
Old Dominion University
Norfolk, Virginia

Mary B. Walsh, M.S.N., R.N., F.A.A.N.
Associate Professor, Retired
School of Nursing
The Catholic University of America
Washington, D.C.

With a Foreword by Nellie Garzón, M.S.N., R.N.

APPLETON & LANGE
Norwalk, Connecticut/San Mateo, California

0-8385-7041-0

Copyright © 1988 by Appleton & Lange
A Publishing Division of Prentice Hall

Copyright © 1983, 1978 , 1973 by Appleton-Century-Crofts

Copyright © 1967 by The Catholic University of America Press, Inc.

88 89 90 91 / 10 9 8 7 6 5 4 3 2 1

Prentice-Hall of Australia, Pty. Ltd., Sydney
Prentice-Hall Canada, Inc.
Prentice-Hall Hispanoamericana, S.A., Mexico
Prentice-Hall of India Private Limited, New Delhi
Prentice-Hall International (UK) Limited, London
Prentice-Hall of Japan, Inc., Tokyo
Prentice-Hall of Southeast Asia (Pte.) Ltd., Singapore
Whitehall Books Ltd., Wellington, New Zealand
Editora Prentice-Hall do Brasil Ltda., Rio de Janeiro

Library of Congress Cataloging-in-Publication Data

Yura, Helen.
  The nursing process.

   "20th anniversary edition."
   Bibliography: p.
   Includes index.
   1. Nursing. I. Walsh, Mary B. II. Title. [DNLM:
1. Nursing Process. WY 100 Y95n]
RT41.Y87 1987   610.73   87-14472
ISBN 0-8385-7041-0

Production Editor: Karen W. Davis
Designer: M. Chandler Martylewski
Back cover photo: Kim Mosher

PRINTED IN THE UNITED STATES OF AMERICA

*To all professional nurses
who use the nursing process
in helping clients experience
human need fulfillment*

Contents

Foreword

It has been 20 years since Helen Yura and Mary Walsh wrote the first edition of the book "The Nursing Process: Assessing, Planning, Implementing, Evaluating". This fifth edition, marking the 20th anniversary, is not simply a launching of another updated version of their earlier work; rather, it represents a significant milestone in the troubled, yet challenging and exciting evolution of Nursing as it gains momentum towards establishing itself as a scientific discipline.

Since the time of Florence Nightingale, nurses have painstakingly grappled with questions for which definite and satisfactory answers remain elusive. What is Nursing? What is the nature of the practice of Nursing, as a profession, as an art, and as a science? Amidst controversies and debates from within and without, various outstanding nurse scholars and practitioners mainly in the United States set forth definitions, principles, declarations of beliefs, generalizations and dictums about the essence of Nursing and the use of the decision-making process, all of which, no doubt, have inexorably changed Nursing and nurses all over the world.

Yura and Walsh, in this book, articulate many of these thoughts and ideas on the nature of Nursing and the Nursing Process. They refine existing conceptualizations and offer an organized and systematic approach for the practice of Nursing as an applied Science and Art. Science besides being understood as an organized body of knowledge is also a process with a method of inquiry.

Furthermore, well-established scientific disciplines have a constantly growing body of knowledge, clearly stated principles and theories, and a well-defined method of inquiry. It follows then at this point in time that the crucial task for Nursing is not only to have definitions about its nature, but to have a method of inquiry within a conceptual framework.

This is what Yura and Walsh precisely offer us in this book. Using the human need theoretical framework, they present concrete illustrative examples of the application of the Nursing Process as the method of practice in a wide variety of client situations and settings in all-age groups. They clearly emphasize the Nursing Process as central to and the essence of nursing practice.

Another strength of this book is the scholarly form and style with which the authors elaborate on the Nursing Process as an efficient method of organizing thought processes for clinical analysis, judgment, and decision-making to maintain the integrity of human needs of individuals, families, and community.

Students, teachers, and practitioners alike should find immensely useful the specific case studies, and the taxonomy of nursing diagnoses within a human need framework compared to the NANDA list.

To further dwell on the merits of this book, allow me to quote K. Gibran in "The Prophet" when asked to speak on teaching, he said:

No man can reveal to you aught but that which already lies half asleep in the drawing of your knowledge.

The teacher who walks in the shadow of the temple, among his followers, gives not of his wisdom but rather of his faith and his loving kindness. . . .

Yura and Walsh certainly share with us through this book their faith, their dreams, and their knowledge to improve nursing practice and to revitalize our sense of purpose as nurses. They invite us—we who are in teaching, in research, and in service—to continue applying and adapting this method of the science and the art of Nursing in real situations in order to transform an obsolete task-oriented practice which leaves many nurses in a perpetual state of disillusionment and "stereotyped mediocrity."

Having been an alumni at the School of Nursing at The Catholic University of America, where Helen Yura and Mary B. Walsh were professors, I feel a sense of glowing pride and exhiliration for their work. I am convinced that it will be a provocative challenge for nurses in developing and developed countries to search for ways to construct a solid scientific and humanitarian foundation for the practice of Nursing.

Nelly Garzón A.
International Council of Nurses President

Preface

With this fifth edition of *The Nursing Process* we celebrate the 20th anniversary of the publication of the first edition. It is timely to look back at what we wrote in the first preface (1967) and the three that followed (1973, 1978, 1983). The preface for the first edition of *The Nursing Process* described the Continuing Education Series sponsored by The Catholic University of America School of Nursing where the nursing process was launched. "This is an opportunity for each nurse who is actively engaged in nursing to hear about trends and progress in nursing. . . ," we said. The nursing process as a process is now well developed and permeates almost every text and almost every action of most nurses. It has been propagated and accepted worldwide. The nursing process has become nursing's "public domain."

In the first edition we defined the elements of the nursing process: to "assess the *needs*, implement the plan of care, and evaluate the extent to which the plan of care has provided for meeting the *needs* of the patient." In subsequent prefaces we explained our view of the nursing process more fully and emphasized our philosophy and convictions about nursing. As early as 1973, theoretic content fundamental to and related to the nursing process was included. The term "client" was introduced to replace the term "patient" that we interpreted as a more sickness oriented term for the recipient of the nursing process. The preface to the third edition (1978) noted the enormous progress in the use of the nursing process as the core mode of nursing practice and the marked increase in publications bearing the nursing process label.

Developments for the fifth edition are no less phenomenal in terms of acceptance of the nursing process as *the* mode of nursing practice on both national and international levels. For the first time in the history of nursing, there is a generation of practitioners of nursing who know no other way to practice but by utilization of the nursing process. Perhaps the most far reaching adjunct to the nursing process is its application within a theoretic framework. Nursing's theoretic framework—human need theory—was included in the early editions and in the 1983 edition was the basis for the designation of nursing diagnoses. Three volumes of *Human Needs and the Nursing Process* (Volumes 1, 2, and 3) were published in 1978, 1981, and 1982 respectively. These volumes expanded upon the specific human needs.

For this fifth edition, Chapter 1 includes more detail about the early development of the nursing process and our role in developing and propagating the idea. The works of 16 nurse scholars are again presented with the added dimension of the conceptual/theoretic schemata developed by each one. This addition should be particularly useful for beginning nurse scholars who are learning and analyzing the works of these scholars. The major focus of Chapter 2 is human need theory. We have titled the chapter "Nursing's Human Need Theory" and rightly so. While we have drawn upon the works of Maslow, his predecessors and successors, and the international human need theorists, we have done something very different with the theory as the framework for the application of the nursing process. The theory has been developed further, with more specificity, so that its utility with the nursing process is enhanced. We put in writing what we believe has been operational for many years with the nursing process. The goal of human needs and the nursing process is optimal wellness for the client—as person, family/significant other(s), community—holistically supported and responded to by the nurse. A significant addition to human needs content is the set of definitions of 35 human needs with related descriptors to enhance the definitions. The theoretic schema of nursing's human needs is expanded from that presented in previous editions. Readers are asked to refer to the fourth edition for theoretic content related to the theories of general systems, decision-making, problem-solving, information, communication, and perception.

In Chapter 3, the components—assessing, planning, implementing, evaluating—are strengthened in their reflection of nursing's human need framework. Nursing diagnoses continue to be viewed in terms of human needs that are excessively met, unmet, or undergoing a disturbance in the pattern of fulfillment. Nurses designate those human needs that are met as well as those with fulfillment alterations and incorporate the level of fulfillment into the plan of care. All other components are reviewed and strengthened.

Chapter 4 follows the previously established pattern of the application of the nursing process. New nursing care plans are included. For the first time we have included a model nursing care plan developed with the human need framework for a person with the medical diagnosis of Alzheimer's disease. Readers will appreciate this all-encompassing model which can be individualized for use in contrast to the more limited standard nursing care plan. In addition selected nursing diagnoses are presented for the client with AIDS related complex (ARC).

Our expectations for the future of the nursing process are incorporated in Chapter 5. The very logical nursing process is ideal for computer application. If the nursing process were not developed it would have to be invented for use with computers.

End of chapter references identify those sources used for the development of the chapter content. The bibliography at the end of the text includes a limited number of more selected, recent and historical, references. Many of the bibliographic entries presented in the fourth edition are not repeated here. The appendices have been updated. Of particular interest to readers is the incorporation of an appendix that displays the diagnostic statements of Nursing's Human Need theory and those statements selected for research and clinical trial by the North American Nursing Diagnosis Association.

Our experiences in developing, defining, and writing about the nursing process and nursing's human need theory have provided us with professional fulfillment. It is our privilege to have shared this information with peers and colleagues. May readers and nurse scholars realize equivalent fulfillment as they explore the future using these two structures as guides.

Helen Yura
Mary B. Walsh

Acknowledgments

As with previous editions, and this fifth edition is no exception, we have many people to thank for participating in the development of the nursing process and for facilitating its publication. We are grateful to the thousands of nursing students and nursing school graduates who learned the use of the nursing process and who strive to enhance its application on a day-to-day basis. *Many* thanks are due the nursing faculty who have mastered, then shared with others the heritage of the nursing process. The faculty have fostered research related to the nursing process and to the theories encompassing the process—particularly human needs theory. The beneficiaries of this effort are the clients—the persons, the families/significant other(s), the community—who are the recipients of holistic, goal-directed nursing care.

Specifically, our thanks and respect go to Kathryn Caufield, Patricia Frensky Orfini, and Virginia Smith, all of whom were formerly at Old Dominion University in Norfolk, Virginia; and to Gaie Rubenfeld at Eastern Michigan University in Ypsilanti, Michigan, for their development of the nursing care plans in Chapter 4. Their ability to articulate the application of the nursing process within the human needs framework is exemplary. Their leadership in this application will be felt for generations to come. They also lent their expertise in critiquing the human needs definitions. Also critiquing the manuscript materials were: Loretta Brown, Dawn Crane, Kim Gillow, Christine Heine, Donna Johnson, Linda Lilley, Virginia McKenzie, Michele Musella, William Pheifer, Maryellen Remick, Brenda Scanelli, Pamala Stockho, and Sue Young. Their support, suggestions, and ideas strengthened the content considerably. Special recognition is given to the following who were Graduate Nursing Students at Old Dominion University: to Margaret Miller and Jeannette Theriault for their development of the model nursing care plan for the person with a medical diagnosis of Alzheimer's disease; and to Anne Laskin, Cynthia Loiacono, and Ellen Stammer for their contribution of nursing diagnoses for the client with AIDS-related complex (ARC). Their sensitivity to the human needs of the client and the client's caretaker is obvious in the models as is their ability to design the models within the human need theory/nursing process framework.

Most of all, we are grateful to Charles Bollinger who experienced a career goal change at the time this manuscript was in preparation. It was Charles Bollinger who said "yes" to the nursing process when we approached him about publishing the "new" second edition of *The Nursing Process*. We are ever grateful for his faith in the idea as well as in us. Thank you, Charlie! . . . . Special thanks go to Marion Kalstein Welch, the present editor, for her enthusiasm about the nursing process—its past, present, and future. Her interest and support are contagious and have energized us.

Finally, gratitude is extended to Karen W. Davis, who brought the manuscript from its submission to its completion with unmatched expertise, commitment to excellence, and personal interest. Special recognition goes to Helen Didion, who did the typing of this manuscript in a most efficient, accurate, and conscientious manner, and to Sue Cooke Hoebeke, who transformed the theoretic models in Chapter 2 from sketches into works of art.

Helen Yura
Mary B. Walsh

The Nursing Process
Past and Present

Nursing

Nursing is an encounter with a client as person, family, community in which the nurse observes, supports, communicates, ministers, teaches and cares; the nurse contributes to the maintenance of optimum wellness through the facilitation of human need fulfillment, and provides care during illness until clients are able to assume responsibility for the fulfillment of their own human needs; when necessary, the nurse provides compassionate care for clients who are dying.

Nursing Process

The nursing process is an orderly, systematic manner of determining the client's health status, specifying problems defined as alterations in human need fulfillment, making plans to solve them, initiating and implementing the plan, and evaluating the extent to which the plan was effective in promoting optimum wellness and resolving the problems identified.

The nursing process is the core and essence of nursing; it is central to all nursing actions; it is applicable in any setting and within any theoretic–conceptual reference. It is flexible and adaptable, adjustable to a number of variables, yet sufficiently structured to provide a base from which all systematic nursing actions can proceed. Phases, or steps, in the nursing process are identifiable. They may vary in label, size, intensity, and sequence; they can overlap, be examined and analyzed; and they are pursued deliberately by nurses as they care for clients. There is a basic theme that underlies the process: it is organized, systematic, and deliberate.

These statements about nursing and about the nursing process are familiar to all nurses today; these ideas form the substance of nursing whether the focus is research, education, administration, or practice. Indeed, the concepts of nurses assisting clients in human need fulfillment, and being concerned about maintenance of wellness as well as prevention of illness, all within the context of the nursing process, are second nature in 20th century nursing. Consumers of nursing services are better educated to expect the nurse to perform in the roles of advocate, supporter, and one who cares for and about the client. Nurses, too, are becoming more accountable in addressing these structures and processes of nursing.

However, the enunciation of nursing, what it is, and how it is performed was not always so clear. Many stormy decades have preceded the present status of nursing. Skies are not totally cloudless today, but there is a more logical, agreed upon base on which most nurses now function.

A review of significant events in Nursing Past (before 1967), a recognition of the important turning point in nursing in 1967 (the identification of the nursing process), and a description of the advances in nursing since 1967 will enable readers to better understand and more fully appreciate the growth and development of the very important profession of nursing. The growing pains have been excruciating. The well-developed, but still growing profession, has now reached a mature, self-confident adult status.

THE PAST—AND TRANSITION TO THE PRESENT

In the days of the early Christians, the practice of nursing was based on unselfishness and love of neighbor; there was concern for meeting the needs of each sick person. The actions of those who practiced nursing were directed toward helping the sick person get well so that he or she could lead a healthier and happier life. Persons who practiced nursing received little formal education. Most nursing behavior was learned by means of the apprenticeship system; the person who wanted to become a nurse accompanied an experienced practitioner, a role model, whose behavior was copied or imitated. Much nursing action imitated the actions of experienced practitioners.

As national changes resulted from upheavals in social and political structures, so were changes contributing to unrest and turmoil in the profession of nursing. History records many phases with high and low points through which nursing proceeded and survived. It was not until the days of Florence Nightingale (1820–1910) that nursing began to achieve some structure, some effort toward deliberate actions. In today's language, Florence Nightingale would have been called "militant." There was little establishment with which to disagree, yet she questioned traditions and customs that had been accepted for many years. She designed her own rules and ran a very "tight ship" to achieve what she judged necessary to provide the best care for clients. Despite her maverick nature, she was farsighted and set admirable goals, establishing some firm foundations on which nursing continues to rest today. She emphasized knowledge, suggesting that the preparation needed by the staff nurse is different from that needed by a supervisor or an administrator. She was concerned about just remuneration for nurses, although the 12-hour work day, the 7-day work week, and the 5-cent raise after a 6-month probationary period cannot compare with the work demands and pay of the 20th century. (See Figure 1–1 for a description of what was expected of the nurse during this era.) Regretfully, Florence Nightingale did not think kindly of male nurses, nor did she emphasize or even speak of the nursing process. Nevertheless, she deserves her title as the founder of modern nursing, having placed nursing on a respected and respectable level.[1]

In addition to caring for your 50 patients, each nurse will follow these regulations:

1. Daily sweep and mop the floors of your ward, dust the patient's furniture and window sills.
2. Maintain an even temperature in your ward by bringing in a scuttle of coal for the day's business.
3. Light is important to observe the patient's condition. Therefore, each day fill kerosene lamps, clean chimneys and trim wicks. Wash the windows once a week.
4. The nurse's notes are important in aiding the physician's work. Make your pens carefully; you may whittle nibs to your individual taste.
5. Each nurse on day duty will report every day at 7 A.M. and leave at 8 P.M. except on the Sabbath on which day you will be off from 12 noon to 2 P.M.
6. Graduate nurses in good standing with the director of nurses will be given an evening off each week for courting purposes or two evenings a week if you go regularly to church.
7. Each nurse should lay aside from each pay day a goodly sum of her earnings for her benefits during her declining years so that she will not become a burden. For example, if you earn $30 a month you should set aside $15.
8. Any nurse who smokes, uses liquor in any form, gets her hair done at a beauty shop, or frequents dance halls will give the director of nurses good reason to suspect her worth, intentions and integrity.
9. The nurse who performs her labors and serves her patients and doctors without fault for 5 years will be given an increase of 5 cents a day, providing there are no hospital debts outstanding.

Figure 1–1. "Nurses' Duties in 1887." *(Source unknown.)*

During the years between Florence Nightingale's efforts and the beginning of World War II, there was little progress in nursing. These years were known as *the era of maintenance* or *the era of little or no change.* World War I and the economic depression were among the reasons for this complacency in nursing. Other professions experienced similar lags in progress and merely maintained their status quo.

World War II was a propelling force behind many changes in the world. Technology increased during this era, and the health professions, especially nursing, felt the impact of this technological change. War casualties increased the need for physicians and nurses; the pressures of war and feelings of patriotism created different ways to cope with human needs; the relatively uncomplicated triad of *doctor–nurse–client* gave way to a multi-dimensional health team, the dimensions of which have continued to grow and expand.

The contributions of medical corpsmen during the war set the pattern for auxiliary personnel in the health professions. As knowledge grew and accumulated rapidly, it became apparent that more people were needed to cope with the consequent challenges. Advances in clinical medicine, such as early ambulation, changes and advances in the treatment of burns, and the discovery of new drugs, especially antibiotics, were forerunners of the changes that have occurred and are continuing in nursing.

The 15 years that followed V-J Day, 1945–1960, brought more areas of change more rapidly than did any other period in the history of nursing. Health care systems in the United States were viewed differently after the war. The public became more aware of what constitutes good health care, the population increased, and the economy changed and grew. There was a trend toward urbanization, an explosion of scientific knowledge, an acceleration of medical discoveries, new methods of therapy, new inventions and finally the recognition that it is just as important to keep people well as it is to treat illness. After World War II an effort was made to move more deliberately and more creatively; the impact of this movement continues to be felt with increasing intensity.

As knowledge increased and the economy changed, there were new developments in education. The GI Bill of Rights had a major impact; numerous veterans could now prepare for careers for which they, at one time, had never dreamed they could qualify. All schools, including nursing schools, were flooded with applicants for degrees. Education was changing the practice of nursing.

One theme heard frequently during the postwar era was, "The nurse must give total patient care." The person for whom the nurse cared was a "patient," and the nurse assumed responsibility for doing all things for the patient. Although other health team members were present, nurses were either reluctant to give up the idea of *total patient care* or perhaps did not know how to relinquish those aspects of care that were not nursing. The nurse was the constant presence in the health care arena and assumed the role of coordinator, or "traffic director," for all disciplines who were becoming part of the health care scene. The scene was usually the acute care facility, or the hospital. There were few options for the ill person, hence the ill person was usually hospitalized then returned to his or her own home. Because there was limited provision for recuperation between the hospital and home, hospital stays were longer to enable the patient to achieve some degree of stability before going home to "be on his or her own."

Gradually, emphasis shifted, and although the nurse continued to be aware of the totality of the individual client, the nurse's role was changing to include working cooperatively with other members of the health team who were also concerned with the client's care and welfare. Referral of clients to members of other disciplines became the nurse's responsibility. The concept of *total patient care* still prevailed but implementation of the concept became the responsibility of the entire health team, including the nurse. Communication was the critical factor responsible for cohesion and cooperation among all health team members.

The changes that were precipitated by the war resulted in a concerned nursing profession in the late 1940s. Health care personnel were struggling with the increased number of people who had been introduced into the health care system. Roles were defined to prevent duplication, yet each group tried to retain the essence of its own role as its members perceived it. The changes in nursing created turmoil that culminated, finally, in asking Esther Lucile Brown, a nonnurse, to provide an unbiased assessment of the status of the profession and to suggest ways in which it could move constructively. The report was presented by Brown in 1948 and became a major turning point in the lives of nurses and in nursing.[2] The groundwork provided by the recommendations of this report was the basis for many of the changes in nursing during the next 30 years.

As did Florence Nightingale, Esther Brown expressed her concern for adequate remuneration of nurses for quality service. Significantly, the discussion of remuneration seldom stood alone; it was usually coupled with mention of the responsibility for providing quality service. This concern is as true today as it was in the days of Florence Nightingale, and it is one of the major justifications for employing the nursing process. Through organized and deliberate nursing action, provision of quality care is more certain, and the means for evaluating the quality of care are provided.

Issues and Concerns

Criteria for a Profession

For many years there were discussions and debates about whether or not nursing is a profession. Several authors suggested criteria for a profession; those stated by Flexner were quoted frequently:

1. Professions are learned; they derive their essential characteristics from intelligence. The essence of learned professions is in the application of intelligence to the comprehension of problems.
2. Professions are result-oriented; their purposes are primarily objective, intellectual, and altruistic.
3. Professions have a code of honor.
4. Professions are made up of persons who have disciplined minds that are well stored with knowledge.[3]

More recently, in 1972, Schein suggested that it is difficult to precisely define certain professions because roles vary depending on the setting where the professional activity takes place. Other variables that impact on the definition of a profession are: (a) the profession is still evolving; and (b) various persons in society view it in different ways.[4]

Despite the problems that exist in trying to define a profession and to specify the criteria that should guide it, as well as to determine the priority or importance of each criterion, most people agree that multiple criteria should guide the specific definition that eventually is accepted. The following are examples of these multiple criteria as they might be used for nurses and nursing:

1. The professional activity is the person's full-time activity and principal income.
2. A strong motivation is the basis for the professional career choice.
3. A prolonged period of education and preparation provides the professional with a specialized body of knowledge and skills.
4. General principles, theories, or propositions are the bases for decisions made on behalf of the client.
5. The professional has a "service orientation;" that is, specific skills are used to help meet particular needs of clients. This particular expertise includes diagnostic skills, competency in performance, absence of self-interest.
6. A professional relationship and mutual trust exist between the client and the professional; actions on behalf of the client are based on the objective needs of the client and on an unbiased performance by the professional.

7. Autonomy of judgment is inherent in the performance of the professional. Strong ethical and professional standards guide the actions of the members of a profession to protect the client who is in a potentially vulnerable position, and enforcement of such standards is carried out by professional colleagues.
8. Professional associations are formed to protect the autonomy of the profession, and they establish rules or standards, such as criteria of admission, educational standards, licensing or other formal examinations, career lines within the profession, and areas of jurisdiction for the profession.
9. The knowledge of the professional is specific to one area of expertise and is not expected to extend beyond that area.
10. The service of the professional is made available to clients after the contact has been initiated by the client.

The ultimate criterion is the achievement of autonomy. This suggests the following:

1. The professional person has specialized preparations allowing for a better understanding than anyone else of what will benefit the client.
2. Decisions of the professional are subject only to colleagues for review and criticism.
3. Peer group associations control the establishment of professional standards and entry into the profession.[5]

Gail Stuart asked, "How professionalized is nursing?" and reviewed various criteria of professions; she summarized the thoughts about professionalism proposed by various authors.[6] Conclusions were reached by relating nursing to a summary of the characteristics of a profession:

1. Nursing has been a well-established occupation since the early part of the 19th century.
2. Personal commitment and self-sacrifice have characterized the roles played by nurses. Changing values are stimulating a closer examination of these roles today.
3. The American Nurses' Association has been the official professional organization for nurses since 1896; despite recognized difficulties in functioning, it continues to represent nurses and nursing.
4. Progress continues in the area of nursing education while coping with multiple levels of entry into nursing practice. There are encouraging trends indicating that the educational routes to professional nursing education may be more unified in the foreseeable future.

5. Nurses portray and give evidence of a strong inclination and orientation to provide a service for those in need.
6. The least progress has been made in establishing an autonomous base for practice. This limitation is due to the low status of what is primarily a female occupation, limited recognition by related disciplines and by the public, and a limited use of power.

To convince nurses, peers, colleagues in the health disciplines, and the public that nurses are professionals and nursing is a profession, the directions that should be taken are clear:

1. The knowledge base needs continued expansion to establish nursing science as a recognized body of knowledge.
2. Research endeavors need to be expanded, increased, and accelerated to enable the more rapid and more prolific accumulation of systematically gathered and analyzed data.
3. Autonomy and power need to be recognized and exercised to enhance the self-esteem of practitioners of nursing as well as to convince collaborators that nursing can identify independent functions and that nurses are capable of identifying and implementing functions and roles that are uniquely nursing.[7]

Ethics. During the latter part of the 1950s, attempts were made to define nursing functions in relation to professional activities. When nursing actions were discussed, a number of crucial questions were asked, such as: To what extent do the actions of the nurse affect people? How significant are the decisions and judgments of the nurse to the present and future welfare of the service consumer? How complex are these actions in terms of the nurse's education and experience? Is there ample and appropriate knowledge available to and used by the nurse as a basis for nursing action? Is there some check on the effectiveness of nursing actions? Does nursing performance improve with experience, and are the care plans modified according to available knowledge and experience? Are clients able to judge the effectiveness of a nursing action? They can judge it in terms of their own needs, but is this the only measure available to them? How does a specific act compare with similar actions of other nurses?[8]

Inherent within these criteria and questions is the pertinent observation that a code of ethics is both important and essential. The most recent revision of the Code for Nurses stresses self-determination of clients, the nurse's role as client advocate, and the requirement for quality assurance and peer review. There is, also, an International Code for Nurses that stresses the universality of nursing (see Appendix A).[9] Such a code is important because it meets one of the criteria for a profession. More important, however, is the availability of a code for the nurse to use in practice; the statements within the code are legitimate guidelines to direct the nurse–client relationship.

Nurses continue to be concerned that nursing meets the criteria for a profession; nursing actions are receiving increased emphasis, especially as these have an impact on the client. Nurses generally view nursing as a learned profession whose major concern is result-oriented activity for clients and pursuit of improved client care through the use of increased knowledge.

ANA Position Paper. One of the major events of the early 1960s was the publication of the *American Nurses' Association's First Position on Education for Nursing.*[10] The position paper was indicative of a major event in nursing. The position of the American Nurses' Association (ANA) was, and is, that the education of persons who practice nursing should take place in institutions of higher education: the professional nurse should be prepared in baccalaureate programs of nursing; the technical nurse, in associate degree programs; and the assistant in the health services, in preservice programs in vocational education institutions rather than in on-the-job training programs.

This position paper resulted from a study that covered more than a 10-year period, conducted by the ANA Committee on Current and Long-Term Goals and the ANA Committee on Education. The turmoil among nurses who reacted to the position paper has been long-lived. Some shortsighted nurses have failed to see the importance of educational preparation; others continue to approve the pursuit of education over a prolonged time. The reality of nursing is, however, that ". . . whether it suits us personally or not, education for nursing must be at least as encompassing and as rigorous as that for other professions."[11]

On October 31, 1985, the National League for Nursing (NLN) Board of Directors took formal action to support two levels of nursing practice: professional and associate. They issued a call for unity and urged a close working relationship between the NLN Councils and the ANA Cabinets in order to define the "scope and practice of nurses within these levels." The leadership of the profession recognized that educational advancement is the key to nursing taking its deserved position in the future; only if they are prepared can nurses participate in shaping the direction of nursing's role in the health care system for the present and the future.[12]

While the nursing leaders were setting directions for the profession, the rank and file of nurses were resisting change. A review of the *NEWS* items in the American Journal of Nursing over a 2-year period reveals the state of unrest that existed. For example, in 1985 and 1986 it was reported that the Georgia Nurses Association "endorsed career ladders for LPNs";[13] Kentucky agreed that after 1990, "a 'nurse' would have to hold a BSN and a 'practical nurse' would need an ADN";[14] Montana aimed "to retain the current titles: BSN and LPN."[15] Headlines heralded: "Arkansas Backs BSN";[16] Maine SNA Aims to Keep RN, LPN Licensure";[17] "Texas AD Nurses Vow to Keep Battling Move to Two Levels";[18] "West Virginia Legislature Bottles Two Bills Aimed at Entry Change."[19]

The titling issue and the entry level endeavors are highly emotional matters. The legal struggles are ongoing and there are major delaying tactics by those who oppose the B.S.N. entry level. Coalitions of nurses have organized to oppose the entry level despite efforts by nursing leaders to reach some areas of agreement that would not dilute the major intent of the effort. The struggle will continue, certainly; however, some reconciliation of the problems and the issues will surely be reached in the next decade.

Consultant Group on Nursing. Another significant event of nursing as a profession was the appointment in 1961, by the surgeon general of the United States Public Health Service, of the Consultant Group on Nursing that was to provide advice about nursing needs and problems in the United States. The group operated on the basis that nursing is an essential element in health care and that public understanding and support will be necessary to solve problems in nursing. Although the group was concerned with the increasing demand for nurses, the need for quality in nursing education, nursing service, and nursing research was constantly emphasized. The group identified needs and set goals for nursing during the 1970s.[20] The recommendations of this study led to the appointment of the National Commission for the Study of Nursing and Nursing Education. The appointed commissioners met for the first time in 1967. A comprehensive and in-depth study resulted from the efforts of the members of this commission; they pursued three areas: nursing roles and functions, nursing education, and professional growth and development. Specific recommendations related to increased research, altered educational patterns, and enhanced support for nursing are contained in the report.[21] The efforts of the consultant group and the commissioners further emphasized the importance of pursuing nursing in a systematic way, that deliberate goal-directed activity is the focus of nursing, and that evaluation of goal achievement is possible.

Growth and Change. Along with the movements toward independence that were occurring in society, nurses also began to think about independence in practice. Although these ideas did not fully develop until later decades, their germination can be traced to the 1960s. Throughout history nurses and nursing have been responsive and have responded to the environmental factors that existed around them and that impinged on their professional roles and their clients.

Many factors contributed to the turmoil and unrest of the 1960s. In the United States, the student and race riots, the assassinations of several leaders, the development of extremist groups, all had effects on nursing. Many of the changes in nursing education and in the practice of nursing were outgrowths of the social events of the day.

Nurses and nursing experienced reactions to the major events of the previous decades and despite the tragedies of the wars, health care practices advanced at an accelerated rate. The people changed; therefore, society changed. As growth in all areas of government, politics, legislation, and health care occurred, so too there was change and growth in nursing education and in nursing practice.

In nursing education, the number of baccalaureate and masters programs in nursing increased. More programs were offering a doctor of science in nursing degree. Continuing education programs were popular and "continuing education units" were defined to measure the level of education achieved. Staff education and development were established in health care agencies; nurses were employed as full-time educators to provide continuing education for the nursing staff.

Two events that have had an impact in the 1980s are significant enough to require elaboration, namely, the establishment of the Teaching Nursing Homes and of the National Research Center for Nursing.

In the 1980s, as the United States has faced a marked increase in the aging population, the Teaching Nursing Homes set a goal to help individuals cope with the health care needs of the aging. Funds from the Robert Wood Johnson Foundation and support from the American Academy of Nursing have enabled the nursing profession to establish 11 Teaching Nursing Home sites across the United States. Personnel in these 11 sites have pursued a 5-year pioneering effort to study and establish models of affiliation between university Schools of Nursing and nursing homes. Although each site pursues individual goals, the ultimate concerns are improving the quality of life of nursing home residents and improving the image of professional nursing in the nursing home. The successful endeavors of these professional nurses have set in motion a focus for nursing that will have long-range beneficial effects.

Professional nurses are demonstrating their concern about the care of older persons in various ways. One noteworthy effort is the applied research project that was funded by the W. K. Kellogg Foundation and sponsored by the American Nurses' Foundation, Inc.[22] Under the codirection of Dr. Mary P. Lodge and Dr. Robert Burmeister, the goal of this project was to improve the quality of care for the aged via improving the education and practice of the nurse administrator in long-term

care. The outcomes of this national effort were the development of the
following:

- A profile of nurse administrators in long-term care facilities.
- A tool for self-assessment of knowledge and skills that the nurse
  administrator needs to manage the services in a long-term care
  facility.
- A series of curriculum cluster modules to be offered through
  continuing education programs in selected graduate nursing
  programs for nurse administrators.

The long-range expectations are improved collaboration among nursing educators, practicing nurse administrators, and members of professional organizations to improve the practice of nurse leadership in long-
term care. At this time, the continuing education programs are in place
and nurse administrators are enrolling in the programs to benefit from
the self-assessment, career counseling, and self-instruction cluster
modules for learning. It is expected that the benefits of this endeavor
will be felt well into the 21st century.

As nurses have assumed a more scholarly stance in the world of
health care, research has become more significant and important. As
nurses have acquired advanced education, they have increased knowledge about the needs and problems of clients. It goes without saying
that nurses will be better able to solve their clinical problems through
research, and research is becoming an integral part of nursing functions. In April 1986, the National Center for Nursing Research was for-
mally opened. Funds for research that were previously distributed
through the Division of Nursing are now granted through the Research
Center. This is the most recent step in the systematic pursuit of solutions to clients' problems.

In nursing practice, hospitals employ large numbers of nurses in
many roles on all levels, from vice presidents for nursing to staff nurses.
Specialty units such as Intensive Care Units (ICU) and Coronary Care
Units (CCU) increase the demand for a special kind of expertise. As demands for nurses increase, so do demands by nurses for equitable
pay—compensation for the special expertise they bring to the clinical
settings. Some of the nurses who make the demands have resorted to
unionization to make their voices heard; some also have participated in
strikes to make their force felt. The hospitals have been challenged to
provide decent salaries, job benefits, and working conditions. These demands and events have resulted in innovative and attractive features of
hospital employment beginning in the 1970s.

The needs of clients were and continue to be the reason for nursing's existence; a review of clinical subjects in professional nursing
literature today reveal familiar topics: malnutrition; cancer; wound

care; dyspnea; diabetes; pressure sores. Occasionally a new problem appears; two of the most recent being herpes and acquired immune deficiency syndrome (AIDS). Technology continues and changes: cardiac catheterization, computer axial tomography (CAT), ventilators, pacemakers, and so forth all being examples of this.

In the 1980s, another challenge faces nursing in all settings: nurses are becoming fewer in number and not enough persons are prepared to fill the available professional nursing positions. Employers are faced with the need to attract qualified nurses by means of new and inviting benefits. The greatest needs for personnel continue to be in areas of specialization. As enrollments decrease in nursing educational programs, the profession becomes more determined to make adjustments, to make changes, to do whatever can be done to make the profession of nursing one that will be inviting to young, energetic, and enthusiastic learners.

New topics in the literature communicate a scenario about a new and different world of nursing than that of the early and mid-20th century. As the life of this century ebbs, and the 21st century approaches, new challenges face the professional nurse: Ethical dilemmas, malpractice insurance and lawsuits; nurses in politics; impairment due to chemical addiction. These are but a few of the issues and the responsibilities to which the nurse has become heir; other concerns will arise, to be sure.

As stress and "burnout" became common concerns in agencies where client care was provided, nurses sought alternatives to hospital nursing. Independent practice in various forms became a viable choice for many nurses. In an effort to produce more satisfaction for nurses and for clients, primary care became an option. The trend toward independent practice, which began as a concept during the 1960s, became a reality in the 1970s.[23,24] Although the role of the nursing practitioner grew during this period, not all practitioners performed nursing in a like manner. Some functioned independently as generalists. Others set up group practices, utilizing the special talents of several nurses. Still others functioned within the established health system and/or with a physician or group of physicians. Some practitioners pursued special programs to develop new skills and expertise; others relied on the knowledge and skills already acquired. An important positive result of this development in nursing was the emergence of nurses who perceived their role as nurse in a self-supporting way—a role not dependent on any other discipline or profession for viability, but sufficient unto itself to provide nursing for clients in the form of professional actions based on sound judgments.

Licensure. Licensure of the professional nurse was of concern, and its relation to continuing education was most complex. Several jurisdictions experimented with different plans. One plan provided continuing education units for each nurse and required a specific number of units for licensure renewal. An event that created much debate was the effort by the New York State Nurses' Association to require, by 1985, a baccalaureate degree for licensure as a professional nurse and an associate degree for licensure as a practical nurse.[25] The topic was deliberated at the ANA Biennial Convention in June 1976, and a suggestion was made that a national conference be called in which issues would be discussed and positions could be identified.[26] At the end of 1976 the American Nurses' Association launched a major study of credentialing in nursing—a study to be completed in a 22-month period so that the outcomes could be presented at the 1978 ANA Convention. The charge to the study group was to assess current credentialing mechanisms including certification, licensure, and accreditation of basic, graduate, continuing education, and organized nursing service programs.[27]

Credentialing. The Committee for the Study of Credentialing included representatives from the American Nurses' Association, the National League for Nursing, the National Council of State Boards of Nursing, and various nursing specialty organizations. These groups defined credentialing as "the process by which individuals or institutions, or one or more of their programs, are designated by a qualified agent as having met minimum standards at a specified time."[28]

The Committee functioned over a 2-year period (1977–1979) and addressed the major purpose of the credentialing mechanisms in nursing including accreditation, licensure, and certification; a wide range of problems and issues were identified. These credentialing variables continue to exist in the health care system and present a complex and complicated picture for the person who is examining or explaining the multiple factors that affect the operation of the health care system. Not to be taken facetiously, a critical question that the committee identified was "who credentials the credentialers who credential the credentialers?"[29] Thus, the circular nature of the complexity of the issues and problems was underlined.

The Committee specified 14 principles that it felt were basic to the premise that "credentialing exists to benefit and protect the public."[30] It identified the following major issues in nursing: definitions of nursing, entry into practice, educational mobility, control and cost of credentialing, accountability, and competence.[31] Position statements were developed for each of these issues; the mechanisms of credentialing were examined; and a model for credentialing for nursing was proposed. Fundamental to the model was the identified need for a structurally unified system and, to that end, the Committee recommended that there be established "a free-standing nursing credentialing center."[32] However, at the April, 1982 meeting of the Committee, the group was not yet ready to create such a credentialing center; in 1987, the Center remains a hope rather than a reality.

Although the vista of nursing continues to expand, nurses continue to disagree about some of the basics; for example, the assigning of appropriate labels for nurses in new roles—should nurses to be known as nurse practitioners? Nursing practitioners?[33] Independent practitioners? Generalists? Specialists? Primary nurses? Clinicians? Language and labels are important, and clarification of the terms used by nurses continue to be a challenge.[34]

It is now apparent that the events in nursing during the past decades set the stage and established the base for what would happen in nursing in later years. Moreover, the 1980s are proving to be exciting and challenging for nurses. Increased numbers of nurses are prepared at the doctoral level; research by nurses about nursing is becoming more evident, more visible, and more influential. The focus for exploration is client care and the quality thereof.

Improvement of the quality of life is a critical topic in client care. How can the economics of the United States provide for the health care needs of persons who want to stay well, or who want to recover from illness? Who will be the client advocates? Will nurses assume this advocacy as their territory or will other health team members share this role? From where will the financing come for education? For health care? For research? What will be the status of third-party payers and reimbursement to nurses for nursing?

Assertive nurses with better preparation and the capability to assume increased responsibilities are now being heard. Will their voices make a difference? Will pay scales be revised upward? Will Nurse Practice Acts be revised to enable *all* professional nurses to practice as professionals?

What will be the impact of the recently adopted National Commission Licensure Examination for Registered Nurses? Will it be a means of ensuring better client care? The new test plan became effective with the July 1982 State Board examination; it is structured to combine:

1. Nursing behaviors that have been grouped under the categories of assessing, analyzing, planning, implementing, and evaluating
2. Nursing systems that designate the extent of care required by the client and are labeled as wholly compensatory, partly compensatory, and supportive–educative
3. Levels of cognitive ability, namely, knowledge, comprehension, application, and analysis.[35]

The decade of the 1980s opened with several events that will be continuing themes in the years to follow. The potential for nursing in the future is limited only by what nurses are willing to risk. Exciting, highly stimulating, and enlightening opportunities lie ahead for those who are energetic and courageous. The satisfactions of setting the pace for the future of the nursing profession are there for any nurse who is willing to explore.

Frameworks for Nursing

Various theories from behavioral and biological sciences are being examined and tested as they are studied for their potential application in the performance of nursing. Concepts are being specified and enunciated to determine those data that will provide direction and logical explanations for the diverse and many parameters of nursing. In addition, nurses seem to want to precisely define, to specifically describe, to finish, to complete, to expect closure on such issues as the precise definition of nursing, nursing theories, conceptual frameworks, appropriate or acceptable philosophies.

In 1964 Wald and Leonard wrote about developing nursing practice theory.[36] Their astute observations and critical comments serve as a sound basis to examine the progress or lack of progress that has since occurred.

Two fundamental facts set the stage for deliberation:

1. Nurses have depended on social scientists for the direction and conduct of research about nursing. As a result, the studies that were done about nursing problems became social science problems.
2. While nurses were relying on social scientists to study problems in nursing, nurses were studying nurses. Virginia Henderson comments, ". . . no other discipline studies the workers rather than the work."[37]

Scientific theory begins with naming classes of events and this naming is usually in the form of concepts; further study includes investigation of the relationships among the concepts and their bearing on each other. Nursing practice theory development can begin in the same way, but the concepts that are identified to represent classes of nursing events should be derived, at least in part, from actual nursing experiences; they should then be tested by nurses and tested in the actual practice setting.

A number of impediments to the identification of theories of practice through research were identified. Although the "size and shape" of the problems have changed, the general contours of these obstacles are recognizable today:

1. The pattern of relationships that nurses maintain with interdisciplinary persons is "antithetical to the nurse scientist." The nurse's traditional role of carrying out the physician's orders after the physician has diagnosed and prescribed and of continued subordination to the medical profession makes for a role that is not consistent with that of a researcher who must observe, analyze, and conclude through the use of sound judgment.

2. The lack of self-esteem of nurses; they do not see themselves as rich sources of information. This sense of low esteem is reinforced by the attitude among the "pure scientists" that those of the applied fields are "second-class citizens."

3. Difficulty in developing a research attitude. The nature of nursing is such that nurses are often forced to act without sufficient time to reflect and to think, much less carry out research to validate that they are taking the best action possible.

4. A practice-oriented discipline's preparation is usually directed to making *no* mistakes; hence, there is no room for trying something that may prove to be less than best and no encouragement to examine one's practice in order to identify limitations or to determine mistakes so that practice can be improved.

5. Because a major thrust in nursing education is to care for the individual, nurses have difficulty generalizing. To do research, nurses will be required to shift their orientation and formulate those empirical generalizations that are a first step in the development of a theory of practice.

6. Limitations exist in research methodology. The ability to identify the problem in researchable terms, to develop relevant instruments for data collection, to ask the appropriate questions are a few of the areas where nurses have encountered difficulty.[38]

The trait of seeking closure has been identified by Dr. Frederick Suppe, a philosopher:

Nursing has a tendency to demand closure on conceptual and methodological issues. Good research demands the suspension of premature closure. One of the greatest benefits to the emerging nursing science that philosophy of science can offer is an appreciation of the merits of non-closure on methodological issues, and the development of a comfortableness with the absence of premature closure.[39]

Nurses are encouraged by Dr. Suppe's appreciation for nonclosure and they temper their thrust to specify all dimensions of theoretical and conceptual frameworks. They continually examine and pursue avenues that lead to the clarification of theoretical and conceptual frameworks—those that are consistent with specified philosophies of nursing. Studying philosophy of science is a benefit to nurse scholars; among other data it provides them with knowledge about the false starts experienced by those who have been developing knowledge about philosophy of science. Thus, nurses avoid the "unnecessary debate over the testability, value, and use of conceptual frameworks in the development of nursing theory."[40]

An inference drawn by examining some of the philosophy of science literature suggests the following:

- Identification of frameworks is an important endeavor.
- Orderly systematic definitions and labels are essential.
- Use of resources in other sciences is critical.
- Critique of resources is necessary to decide what is applicable to nursing situations.
- It is important to understand when one is using the theories proposed by other scientists and when one is using only the jargon, the terms of a theory without buying into the "metaphysics" or "epistemology" of the science.
- Scientists in related disciplines continue to discuss and deliberate their ideas about theory development and there is on-going research that proves, as well as disproves, elements of theories.[41]

One of the theories that has provided a rational framework for the care of clients is the theory of human needs. The maintenance and integrity of human needs are vital to the development of each individual, of each family, and of society. This maintenance and integrity of human needs is the territory of nursing.[42]

Human needs are the complex components of each person; they are challenging problems with which every human is confronted; they are motivators to act on behalf of oneself or others.[43] The existence of a need cannot be proved in a direct physical way. Inferences are drawn, and conclusions are reached about data that are available to the observer. Cues the observer can use include the satisfiers that persons use or will seek to meet their needs, or the symptoms of frustration experienced when their needs are not met or are not satisfied. Lederer suggests that a needs concept can be perceived and interpreted by:

1. The character of the need (universal, objective); that is, human requirements that make survival and development possible in a given society

2. The nature of the need (historical, subjective) determined according to social structure; that is, social practices determine what needs will be.[44]

A fundamental assumption in dealing with the idea of needs is that all humans have needs. The challenge is to identify what these needs are.

To begin with, the idea of *need* must be differentiated from *want* or *desire*. For example, a person who says "I need a car" is not stating a human need; rather this person has a *desire* for a car or *wants* a car to help meet a *need* for mobility, status, travel, and so forth.[45] Also, there should be a differentiation between human needs and basic human needs. Using this descriptive term *basic* is viewed by some authors as inappropriate. They suggest that there is insufficient scientific evidence to establish priority on the relative importance of needs. There is also a connotation of cultural insensitivity when using this term.[46]

Needs are universal; desires are temporal, spatial, or personal. Needs are theoretical constructs that cover human drives and frustrations; needs stand for general principles of human existence.[47] Jahoda has identified groups of needs that, when satisfied, or fulfilled, suggest a positive personality characteristic:

1. Affiliation, cognizance, inviolacy, recognition, autonomy. When these needs are satisfied, the person has self-awareness.
2. Achievement, dominance, recognition, sex. When these needs are satisfied, the person realizes growth, development, self-actualization, maturation.
3. Cognizance, order, nurturance, inviolacy. When these needs are satisfied, the person achieves integration, balance, a unifying outlook on life (often facilitated by a religious orientation).
4. Autonomy, inviolacy, recognition. When these needs are satisfied, the person is able to be autonomous, independent, and make decisions.
5. Cognizance, order, retention, sentience. When these needs are satisfied, the person has a correct perception of reality.
6. Aggression, acquisition, cognizance, achievement, construction, order, play, sex, autonomy, sentience. When these needs are satisfied, the person has mastery over environment, has adequate interpersonal relations involved with love, work, play, and adaptation and adjustment to situational requisites.[48]

In April 1978, the United Nations University initiated a project entitled "Goals, Processes, and Indicators of Development" as part of a larger program dealing with human and social development. A number of subprojects proceeded under the umbrella of the Goals, Processes and Indicators of Development (GPID) project in which 27 research institutions from all parts of the world participated. One of the several subprojects dealt with needs research. The persons involved in this subproject argued that the goal of development is to develop human beings, both materially and nonmaterially; to do this, the "image of human beings has to be rich, diverse, dynamic—and profoundly human."[49]

On May 27–29, 1978, at the International Institute for Environment and Society, Science Center, Berlin, the first of what is hoped will be many conferences was held. At this first conference, there were presentations by internationally recognized experts about the state of the art of research on human needs. Preliminary conclusions were presented and deliberated. The hope is that this first conference will serve as an impetus for further research and discussion on human needs.[50]

A report by Magi and Allander focused on the need for medical care; they studied the difference in this need as perceived by the lay person (client) and the physician. They presented a model that nurses can use to determine how clients' views of their needs differ from the nurse's perceptions of the same needs, and then to determine where, when, and whether a nurse is needed.[51]

The concept of need is analyzed by Magi and Allander. They suggest that: (a) statements about needs contain both factual and value components; (b) statements about needs have a suggestion about the end to be achieved (e.g., good health) and the change required to achieve that end (e.g., surgery); and (c) needs are relative to social forces and circumstances.[52]

Assessment of need is divided into those types of needs the assessor (nurse) believes should be cared for and those needs the client believes should be addressed. In terms of services Magi and Allander define need for care as the "type and amount of . . . service an assessor believes *ought* to be utilized for a particular health related condition" versus the "perceived need for . . . care" as that which the client believes he or she *ought* to have.[53] Values and norms of the assessor and the client are important here.

Despite similarities between the opinions of the client and the nurse regarding the needs and their intensity, there will also be differences. Some differences may be minimal but some may be great. Awareness of the differences is critical to enable clients to cope with and to meet their needs as they perceive them.

> In order to administer patient care, the nurse must identify the individual's needs for nursing services. Ever since nursing was first performed, the "nurse," by a process either wholly or partially conscious, viewed the patient and determined on the ba-

sis of intuition, experience, rote learning, knowledge or in some cases ignorance, what nursing acts were needed by the patient to relieve his distress.[54]

Analysis of this quote reveals some fascinating sources of reflection, especially since it was written in 1963:

1. There is awareness of the needs of the client, but they are addressed in terms of needs for nursing services rather than the human needs of the person who is the patient (the client).
2. Acknowledgment that nursing actions were based on intuition (ignorance) is humbling, yet neither surprising nor eye opening.
3. At least one component of the above quote suggests certain of the clients' discomforts could be relieved by nurse actions.

This report of Bonney and Rothberg developed the premise that chronically ill persons have needs that nursing can do something about; in order to identify those needs, it was necessary to develop some means by which these needs could not only be identified but also measured. To provide such an instrument, they developed a Nursing Evaluation Form as a means of establishing "nursing diagnosis and therapy." Their basic premise was that clients' needs (for nursing services) must be identified in order to establish staffing patterns.[55]

The tone of their writing suggests the holistic approach to client care, but the terms prevalent in the early 1960s were "total patient care" and "comprehensive patient care."[56] Although the exact words have changed, the idea remains the same and the message is clear regarding area of responsibility and sphere of activity.

Although the authors gave no indication of any theoretical framework or theoretical base for tool development or use, the instrument can be analyzed with postive conclusions in terms of its consistency with a human needs orientation. Areas were not labeled as human needs, but in light of the searches for data and in light of the continued development of human needs theory, these authors, in 1963, were approaching clients with an "instinctive" use of a human needs framework.[57]

It can be concluded that nursing is moving through developmental stages toward a nursing science. Advances have been made in specifying the philosophic and theoretic foundation on which nursing is based in diverse settings. Theories are being defined and tested; conceptual frameworks are being developed. Some efforts are being better accomplished than are others, but all are contributing to a data base for a science of nursing.

The Nursing Process

Over a 20-year period, from 1967 to 1987, the nursing process has experienced a happy birth, and healthy growth; it has now attained the comfortable state of full maturity. The fledgling idea that was introduced in 1967 has taken hold in the education and practice areas of nursing and is now recognized and appreciated by professional peers and colleagues. Nurses now recognize the value of this revolutionizing idea; all astute nurses are convinced of the worth of this orderly, systematic process.

Nursing Continuing Education Series in 1967

With a spirit of optimism in 1967, Helen Yura and Mary Walsh embarked on a successful voyage of discovering and promoting the nursing process. Eager to present this newborn idea to a clamoring profession, Yura and Walsh discussed and planned the 8-week Continuing Education Series at The Catholic University of America (CUA) School of Nursing. The thought of presenting this unique idea in an educational forum was stimulating and challenging. Deciding the format of the series was relatively easy. The nursing process clearly lends itself to a systematic, organized format. It comes as no surprise that the titles of the workshop sessions were: Assessing, Planning, Implementing, and Evaluating. Dr. Mary F. Liston, then Dean of the School of Nursing, encouraged, supported, and attended the series. The usual mechanics of planning the program were managed with no difficulty; calendars were set and space was scheduled for the important presentations on Thursday evenings from 7:30 to 9:30, March 2 through April 27, 1967.

The Presenters. In view of the significance of this 20-year milestone, it is important to recognize those faculty members who contributed to the initial program about the nursing process. The nine presenters were faculty members at the CUA School of Nursing. To the extent that their present locations are known, the "who and where" of the people who helped to make history in that spring series are presented in Table 1–1.

The Enrollees. An enthusiastic group of 45 professional nurses responded to the announcement about the Nursing Process Continuing Education Series. They eagerly participated in this historic series and can be recognized for their presence and contributions to this "once in a lifetime" endeavor. The names of the enrollees, their professional employment positions, and location of their employment in 1967 are recorded in Appendix 1–A at the end of this chapter.

TABLE 1–1. NAMES/TOPICS/PRESENT LOCATION OF 1967 FACULTY

Names	Topics	Present Location
Sister Kathleen Mary Black	Assessing patient needs	Deceased
Frances H. Harpine	Assessing patient needs	The Catholic University of America Nursing Faculty Washington, D.C.
Letha Hickox	Planning to meet patient needs	Unknown
M. Lucille Kinlein	Introduction	Teacher/Entrepreneur Maryland/Hawaii/Alaska
Joan Nettleton	Planning to meet patient needs	Unknown
Helen St. Denis	Evaluating the plan of care	The Catholic University of America Nursing Faculty Washington, D.C.
Mary B. Walsh	Application of the nursing process	The Catholic University of America Nursing Faculty Washington, D.C.
Mildred Wesolowski	Implementing a plan of care	Villanova University Nursing Faculty, Villanova, Pa.
Helen Yura	Application of the nursing process	Old Dominion University Nursing Faculty Norfolk, Va.

Publications

With a sixth sense communicating that something special had taken place at CUA in that spring semester, Yura and Walsh pursued the route of other continuing education courses that were presented at the CUA School of Nursing—that of publication. The 1967 series publication was different from the others, however, because it came off the press in the same year, 1967, that the series was held.[58]

1967 through 1973. After a record of seven printings of this important series, the CUA Press changed policies and was no longer able to publish professional nursing literature. Yura and Walsh acquired the copyrights of that initial text and gave some serious consideration to setting up an independent printing and mailing system, however, that dream was eventually abandoned. Steps were then taken to negotiate with Appleton-Century-Crofts for a new, up-to-date text about the nursing process. In 1973, the second edition of *The Nursing Process* was published by Appleton-Century-Crofts.[59] This was the first text completely written by Yura and Walsh. The 1967 report of the CUA Continuing Education Series was known as the first edition and Yura and Walsh were the editors of that publication; they are the authors of the 1973 and all later editions. The theoretical framework for the nursing process appeared in the 1973 text as did illustrations and diagrams to display relationships among components of the process. The steps of the process were elaborated upon; application of the nursing process to clinical situations was described; experiences of the authors were shared with the readers, and scholars recognized this 1973 text as very important to nursing.

1978 through 1987. New editions of the nursing process were written in 1978 and 1983. Appleton-Century-Crofts has published all editions and is the "proud parent" of this historic 20th anniversary edition. Mr. Charles Bollinger was the Senior Editor who supported this endeavor over many years. Marion Kalstein-Welch, the present editor, is as excited as are the authors and prospective readers about the "Anniversary Edition."

Outcomes

Over the 20-year period since the nursing process was introduced as the core and essence of nursing, the four steps or phases have become second nature to nurses everywhere. The logical and systematic process lends itself to problematic situations as well as various situations that are potentially problematic. The outcomes of this experience that began slowly in 1967 are worthwhile reflecting upon now, 20 years later:

- There were frequent requests for workshops and seminars to teach the nursing process. Nurses in the practice area recognized the value of the process and the authors received requests to present educational programs across the United States as well as in Britain, Sweden, and Finland. Other countries outside the United States, unable to present seminars and workshops in their own settings, sent nurses to the United States to learn the use of the nursing process. There was constant correspondence, consultation, and teaching activity over these 20 years.
- As nurses became more knowledgeable and efficient in the understanding and use of the nursing process, theoretical frameworks became the concern and focus. This thrust continues into the 1980s and shows signs of acceleration.
- Nurse educators include the nursing process as an essential component of the professional nursing curriculum. In fact, the majority of educators, scholars, and students cannot remember what structure guided the practice of nursing before the birth of the nursing process.

- Most nursing texts introduce the nursing topics by an initial presentation of the nursing process; whether in the form of one or two chapters, and/or as the structure for the entire text, it is obvious that the process is the glue that binds all nursing actions into a holistic unit.
- The nursing indexes listed nursing diagnosis as a separate label in 1976, before nursing process was recognized or acknowledged by the indexers. However, analysis of the ideas of influential nurse scholars (presented in this chapter) will show that some of them were talking about nursing process and nursing diagnosis in the 1950s. The mid-1960s was the propitious time, however, to define a precise process; nurses were maturing and nurse scholars were exerting leadership; the days of floundering and wondering about "what is nursing" were past. The readiness of the nursing profession to accept a process of nursing is evidenced by the positive response to the CUA series about the nursing process as well as the concurrent publication from the Western Interstate Commission on Higher Education (WICHE); this latter group defined the nursing process as ". . . that which goes on between a patient and nurse in a given setting; it incorporates the behaviors of patient and nurse and the resulting interaction. The steps in the process are: perception, communication, interpretation, intervention, and evaluation."[60]

Systematically addressing client problems by way of the nursing process is a series of deliberate actions directed toward the resolution of actual or potential problems. There is unquestionable merit to this more scientific and structured process of problem solving. However, the use of this orderly and definable activity does not preclude the use of intuition in making decisions and exercising judgment.

Intuition can be explained as the ability to know what to do in a complex situation without being able to explain why. It cannot be defined so precisely as one can define the nursing process; it does not bear rigorous scientific scrutiny. There is evidence, however, that intuition does exist and is a useful tool for the problem solver. Unconscious, implicit skills are associated with right brain intuitive skills while conscious, explicit skills are associated with left brain linear skills. Neither skill is sufficient alone, but a blend of the two can make a difference between mediocrity and excellence. A delightful blend of "seasoned intuition" and disciplined problem analysis will probably produce more qualitative solutions to problem situations.

Everyone has intuition; in the presence of spontaneity, flexibility, and open-minded receptivity to new ideas, intuition can be "tuned in" and insight into problems can thrive. The message for nursing process advocates is: use the analytical method of problem solving, as well as a healthy dose of intuition to assist in solving client's problems.[61]

The definition and phases of the nursing process have been used as bases for developing standards of practice, for establishing criteria for certification, for defining nursing for legal purposes in the Nurse Practice Acts of various jurisdictions, and for establishing the base for State Board of Nursing test item development. Nationally accredited baccalaureate programs employ the nursing process as an integral thread of the curriculum or as a framework for the curriculum structure. The focus of clinical nursing practice, clinical nursing research, and nursing education relies heavily on the systematic and orderly arrangement of the nursing process.

The 1973 edition of *The Nursing Process* was a forerunner in the presentation of theories that guide and support nursing. The theories that were identified at that time remain appropriate. As knowledge about specific theories has been acquired, that knowledge has been shared through professional publications and conferences. None of the theories is invalid or useless; rather, their use and validity have been enhanced and there has been increased recognition of the significance of these theories because of their increasing use in clinical practice.

Minor and Thompson report the use of the nursing process as a framework for a nurse internship program.[62] As specified by Kramer, they cite the four phases experienced by new employees in their first work experience: honeymoon, shock, recovery, and resolution phases.[63] Strengths and limitations of the nurses were noted, and roles of the clinical instructor, head nurse, and preceptor were identified. Four levels of performance were specified and expectations within each phase of the nursing process were outlined. Objectives for attaining Level I performance were cited according to the ability of the nurse to assess, plan, implement, and evaluate client care. This 4-year program has been effectively used to benefit newly employed staff nurses, to benefit continuing staff members, and ultimately to improve client care.

Prior to the mid-1960s, the term *nursing process* was seldom seen in the literature. Exceptions to this were references to a process inherent in the practice of nursing as reported by Peplau in 1952,[64] Hall in 1955,[65] Johnson in 1959,[66] Orlando in 1961,[67] and Wiedenbach in 1964.[68] Also influential in this period before 1965 were the ideas and definitions of nursing proposed by Gowan[69] and Kreuter.[70]

Donnelly and Sutterley stated, in 1986, that:

". . . The focus of assessment 20 or more years ago was to gather data for other health care providers to use in determining intervention. Nursing assessments in the not-so-distant past did not culminate in nursing diagnosis that led to plans, interventions, and evaluations. Assessments, in fact, were couched in obscure, indefinite language that told us what 'appeared' to be the signs or symptoms or what 'seemed' to be awry with clients' conditions. Nursing assessment leading to diagnosis, planning, and intervention results from nursing's growing body of knowledge and sense of autonomy in today's health care system. Assessment activities clearly indicate nursing's willingness to be directly accountable to consumers of health care. Assessment now serves as a foundation for nursing process and as the cornerstone for a professional nursing practice that helps clients to know more about their health."[71]

A plethora of assessment tools, instruments, devices, and mechanical means for gathering data about clients have appeared since 1967. Many were shared with professional members by publication. Many more were developed, used in specific situations, and have not been reported through publication. A recent report of instrument development is a good example of what can be done to design and test the instruments that are needed in the assessment phase of the nursing process. Leatt, et al. state that the care of each person should be individualized according to the person's needs, and one means of ensuring this is to provide valid and reliable mechanisms for the nurse to use in determining the client's needs.[72] They contend that assessment of client's needs is essential to the classification of clients according to the type of long-term care required. Before such a classification system can be developed, valid and reliable instruments for assessment are needed. They define assessment as the "systematic evaluation and determination of a set of selected attributes of a patient with particular reference to health characteristics."[73] Of significance is the recognition that the assessment of long-term clients "must be multidimensional because of the complexities in health states of patients who are chronically ill." Also important is the identification of variables that are used as indicators of health of chronically ill persons, namely, functional level, disease category, health risk factors, and health indexes.[74] Means for measuring each and all of these variables are numerous but continue to be examined, criticized, and revised. Obviously there will be continued work in this area.

Rather useful is the conceptual framework used for this reported study. Health, or the lack of it, was viewed in a multifaceted way with biological, sociological, and psychological dimensions. The concept of health was assumed to be subjective, relative, and dynamic; it is a state that is subject to modification by invasion of pathogens, by the functional ability, adaptability, and reserve capacity of a person.[75]

Four factors were used as a basic framework, essential to the concept of health in long-term clients: demographic characteristics, physical status, psychosocial status, and self-care practices. Extensive testing for reliability and validity produced an instrument that can assist the nurse in classifying clients according to the types of care they need. Although commendable strides were made by this group, continued and further testing is necessary to improve the tool, and ultimately to improve all aspects of the client care process.

Planning, implementing, and evaluating were emphasized to a greater extent in the early 1970s than they had been previously. Phaneuf's work and other publications about nursing audit emphasized evaluation[76] as did the study by Wandelt and Stewart.[77] Little and Carnevali[78] stressed planning as did Mayer.[79] These authors have contributed valuable data to strengthen and underline the nursing process—its value, its significance, its importance, and the necessity of its existence in the performance of nursing.

Nursing Diagnosis

In the 1950s, there were indications in the literature that the term *nursing diagnosis* would best describe what nurses were able to do, and actually *were* doing, in practice. When nurses were challenged about their ability to diagnose, the issue was sidestepped and a number of substitute labels were adopted. Nurses usually included conditional words that softened the significance of their observations. For example, the nurse recorded or said, "The patient appears to be anxious" or "The patient appears to be sleeping." How justifiable would it have been to record "The patient appears to be bleeding"? Patient care records of that decade give evidence of the skirting of the issues and the "game playing" that nurses did to avoid offending persons who believed that nurses could not diagnose the problems or the needs of clients. There is little or no evidence in the literature of the time to suggest that nurses were able to say they were diagnosing the needs of clients, but analysis of records about what nurses were doing confirms that nursing diagnoses were being made.

The literature published in the next decade presents a changing picture about the use of "nursing diagnoses." The mid-1960s were critical years—the turning point for nurses to be heard as they asserted their beliefs about nursing diagnoses. Those authors whose ideas were historic and who published trailblazing articles in the early 1960s included Wilda Chambers[80] and Nori Komorita;[81] they were among the earliest authors to draw criticism about the use of "nursing diagnosis." Myra Levine participated in the activity of endorsing the identification of diagnoses by nurses; she felt that a change in the label would be influential in a positive way. At a clinical conference in Washington, D.C., in 1964, Levine suggested that the term "trophicognosis" be adopted and used instead of nursing diagnosis (trophic = nourishment, gnosis = knowledge).[82] Despite the fascinating possibilities with the use of such a term, there was no ground swell toward its use.

As the nursing process was born and developed in the mid and later 1960s, the term *nursing diagnosis* became more prevalent in the nursing literature. Durand and Prince presented a significant article "Nursing diagnosis—process and decision."[83] A series of articles by Kelly and Hammond provided a sound basis for clinical inference in nursing that continues to provide substantive data for practice today.[84–90]

In addition to the nursing literature, the medical literature also addressed the concept of diagnosis. King suggested that ". . . although diagnosis ordinarily has medical connotations, this is not essential, for the term involves activities by no means unique to medicine. Although we may think of diagnosis as the identification of disease, such usage is far too narrow."[91] How prophetic were these words. Despite continued biases on the part of some of the health discipline personnel, the word *diagnosis* is being used by increasingly large numbers of nurses. With increasing frequency, conference titles and advertisements suggest that the word *diagnosis* is the domain of many persons, including chaplains, plumbers, auto mechanics, and others.

In the early 1970s, a core of interested persons organized and initiated an effort that has been proceeding with marked momentum, namely, the classification of nursing diagnoses. Gebbie and Lavin spearheaded this movement and were responsible for organizing the First National Conference of this group in St. Louis from October 1–5, 1973.[92] Succeeding conferences were held March 4–7, 1975; April 5–9, 1978. Since 1980, the conferences are held biennially. In addition to the National Conferences that are held, numerous efforts are directed toward the increase of knowledge about nursing diagnosis and the increased and improved use of diagnoses in the practice setting. Audiences and participants from nursing education, nursing practice, and nursing research are engaged in regional conferences, annual educational and research programs, special professional programs, classroom endeavors involving deliberations and dialogues, term paper productions, clinical practice using the suggested diagnoses, and nursing research studies to validate and verify the observations, judgments, priorities, and decisions being made about nursing diagnosis.

In the fall of 1982, bylaws were accepted for the North American Nursing Diagnosis Association (NANDA) and the first meeting of the Board of Directors of this newborn organization was held on August 22–

23, 1983 in Boston; Marjory Gordon presided. History was made at the Sixth Conference on the Classification of Nursing Diagnosis in April 1984, when "A Janus View" of nursing diagnosis enabled participants to reflect upon the past of nursing diagnosis, examine the present status of nursing diagnosis activity, and set directions for the future. Readers are referred to Appendix E at the end of the book for a presentation of nursing diagnoses specified by Nursing's Human Need Theory (developed in Chapter 2) and those selected for clinical trial and research by NANDA in 1986.

Momentum is gathering for defining and testing nursing diagnoses; nurses are showing interest and ability to refine and develop this important part of the nursing process. The professional literature contains many reports of experiences with nursing diagnosis in a variety of nursing settings.[93] Besides diagnosis validation studies, a number of other studies are needed; such as studies in (1) development of new diagnoses; (2) taxonomy testing and developing; (3) testing interventions for specific diagnoses; (4) use of computers to facilitate nursing diagnoses; (5) cost of nursing services using nursing diagnoses; (6) diagnostic reasoning; and (7) implementation of nursing diagnoses in education and practice.[94] Beginning in 1987, NANDA will give yearly awards for endeavors in nursing diagnosis research. A solid base of activity is obviously moving this area of nursing into a worthwhile arena that will enhance client care well into the 21st century.

The conclusions reached about data collected and analyzed in client assessment are the nursing diagnoses. Nursing diagnoses are defined in various ways, although a review of several definitions reveals certain common elements. Roy defines nursing diagnosis as a summary statement or a conclusion based on data gathered in the assessment process.[95] McCain considers it to be an identification of the client's functional disabilities or symptoms, as well as an identification of the client's most important functional abilities.[96] Aspinall sees it as a process of clinical inferences from observed changes in a client's physical or psychological condition.[97] Gordon defines a diagnostic category with three components: health problem, or state of the client; etiology of the problem; and signs and symptoms of the problem. She refers to this as the PES syndrome—the problem, etiology, and signs/symptoms.[98]

Discussions among nurses usually identify what a nursing diagnosis is and what it is not in order to differentiate and relate this term to some of the more familiar jargon and activities in nursing. Nursing diagnosis is identified as the end product of the assessment process; it is a statement of conclusion, either tentative or definitive, drawn by the nurse after having assessed the client's status, that is, after having collected and made some judgment about the data. The nursing diagnosis is an expression of the status of the client, identifying assets and strengths as well as disturbances and weaknesses. It is a "statement of a patient problem arrived at by making inferences about the collected data. The problem is one that can be alleviated by nursing intervention."[99] Nursing diagnosis is neither the same as the goals set for the client nor the term to be used synonymously with nursing intervention; however, it forms the basis for setting goals and for planning interventions.

"A nursing diagnosis describes a combination of signs and symptoms that indicate an actual or potential health problem nurses are licensed to treat and capable of treating."[100] Dossey and Guzzetta reported the effectiveness of establishing nursing diagnoses for a client whose medical diagnosis and care were being studied and deliberated by the medical team. A dramatic change in client satisfaction occurred when the nurses specified nursing diagnoses and planned care accordingly. The client was better able to cope with the temporary uncertainty of the medical plan and the nurses were more patient with the client and more fulfilled in their rendering of care.[101] To determine the nursing diagnoses, three steps were followed: (a) signs and symptoms of the client were identified and the actual or potential problems of the client were cited; (b) the causes of the problems were identified; (c) the diagnostic statement was formulated.[102] Guidelines for writing the nursing diagnoses are:

1. Keep the process simple.
2. Cite problems that the nurse can do something about.
3. Make clear and concise the statements of problems and diagnoses.
4. Describe the etiology clearly and concisely.
5. Differentiate the problem and the etiology clearly.
6. Use the diagnostic statement as the basis for the next step in client care, i.e., planning.[103]

The importance of identifying and using clients' strengths was pointed out by Popkess.[104] For many years nurses focused on the problems of clients to determine the care needed. Emphasis today includes the use of clients' strengths or assets to help them cope. For example, a supportive wife can be a major factor in the recovery of her spouse; a feeding or mobility problem of a client can be greatly alleviated, if a wife is willing and able to assist her husband. To identify the strengths of a client, Popkess suggests the nurse can examine a list of nursing diagnoses that are stated as problems and restate them in a positive way if the client data indicate they are strengths.[105]

For many nurses who are dealing with the health maintenance of clients, or whose client goals are to remain well, a negative or problem-focused diagnosis is not appropriate. Marjory Gordon defines nursing diagnosis as a description of the client's "actual or potential health problems which nurses by virtue of their education and experience are capable and licensed to treat."[105a] Inclusion of the term "potential health problem" in an attempt to focus on health promotion strategies, falls somewhat short of the positive or neutral diagnosis, according to Stolte.[106] Assuming a problem can develop, and developing health care plans around "actual or potential problems" continues to belabor the negative and gives insufficient emphasis to the strengths and assets of the client. Stolte presents a plea for positive diagnoses and suggests the following diagnoses as examples:

1. Successful, rapid convalescence related to philosophy of positive thinking.
2. Joy related to birth of a healthy baby.
3. Adaptive coping with chronic illness related to adequate family support mechanisms.
4. Developing self-awareness related to trust and respect among group members.[107]

A nursing diagnosis is not a medical diagnosis. A nursing diagnosis is a client problem amenable to nursing intervention; whereas, a medical diagnosis is a client problem amenable to medical intervention. It will be necessary for a period of time to use the adjectives *nursing* and *medical* with the word *diagnosis* until both professions become familiar and comfortable with the distinction between the two terms.

From a legal standpoint, a number of jurisdictions are now including the term *nursing diagnosis* in the definition of nursing in the Nurse Practice Acts. In at least one state, the legal definition of nursing states that the professional nurse "diagnoses and treats human responses to actual and potential health problems."[108]

Bernzweig, a member of the New York bar, states:

. . . nursing diagnosis is an established and independent function of the professional nurse and calls for the utmost in intelligent judgment and sensitivity on her part. . . . Good nursing diagnosis is one of the keys to the successful practice of nursing and is therefore a skill all nurses should learn.[109]

Examination of the entries in the *International Nursing Index* reveal a significant history about nursing process and nursing diagnosis; it also raises a number of questions and suggests ideas for further exploration. Until 1969, a majority of publications were listed under the general heading of "Nursing" and seven other labels: Nursing Audit, Nursing Care, Nursing Homes, Nursing—Practical, Nursing—Private Duty, Nursing Records, and Nursing—Team. Staff Nursing was added in 1974. Three labels were added in 1978: Nursing Services—Hospital, Nursing Services, and Nursing Staff—Hospital. Supervisory Nursing was added in 1979; Nursing Theory was added in 1986.

Until 1976 there was no entry label for nursing process or nursing diagnosis. Since then, there has been an initial surge of articles followed by a decline in the number of publications under these labels, as illlustrated in Figure 1–2. The label "Nursing Diagnosis" was listed from 1976 through 1979; entries included Nursing Process and Nursing Assessment Information. In 1980, and in following years, the *Index* referred readers who sought articles about nursing diagnosis to the Nursing Assessment listings.

Questions and suggestions for exploration include: In the years prior to 1976, how many of the Nursing Diagnosis articles were listed in the general category of "Nursing"? Beginning in 1980, how many of the

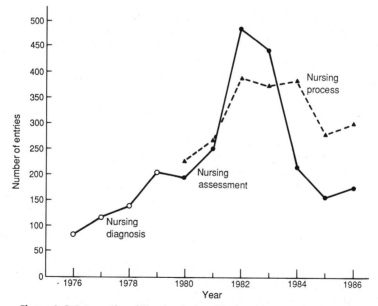

Figure 1–2. International Nursing Index: Nursing Diagnosis/Assessment/ Process. Entries by year: O = Nursing Diagnosis; ● = Nursing Assessment; ▲ = Nursing Process. *(From International Nursing Index, Annual Cumulations. Philadelphia: American Journal of Nursing Co., 1976– 1986.)*

Nursing Assessment articles focused on nursing diagnosis? On nursing process? In all years prior to 1980, how many of the articles classified as "Nursing" included data about nursing process, yet were not labeled as such?

The ultimate goal of this effort to define and classify nursing diagnoses is to standardize labels and to facilitate communication (a) among nurses and (b) between nurses and those persons in other disciplines. To achieve this ultimate goal, research data are needed by persons in practice and in education. It is hoped that when the profession has agreed on the nomenclature, then the next steps of planning, the implementation of plans, the establishment of outcome criteria, and their evaluation can be better realized.

Criteria to Evaluate Theories

Ideas about nursing science, nursing theory, and nursing concepts are appearing in the professional nursing literature with increasing frequency. As a result, some standard or frame of reference is necessary to guide the readers' thought processes. Several authors have suggested criteria for appraising or evaluating the various ideas that are being proposed. A few of the groups of criteria available follow.

Stevens suggests that a person's judgment about a theory can be based on: (a) personal taste, i.e., personal preference, or (b) clearly defined criteria that, when applied equally by different people, enable all to arrive at a similar conclusion: the theory is good, mediocre, or poor.[110]

I. Internal criticism
   a. Clarity—is the theory understandable?
   b. Consistency—is the content consistent in use of terms, principles, method, and interpretation?
   c. Level of theory development—at what level of development is this theory?[111]
II. External criticism
   a. Adequacy—does the theory account for the subject matter with which it deals?
   b. Utility—is the theory useful to the practitioner, educator, researcher, administrator?
   c. Significance—does the theory address essential issues in nursing and contribute to the development of nursing knowledge?
   d. Discrimination—do these ideas differentiate nursing from other health care disciplines; are boundaries of nursing evident?
   e. Scope—is the theory stated in broad or in limited dimensions?

f. Complexity—is there a balance between complexity and parsimony that allows for adequate addressing of the essential components of the theory?[112]

King has published her ideas about nursing theory in two texts written a decade apart. The second text enunciates a theory of goal attainment that was derived from an explicitly identified conceptual framework.[113] The first text was a presentation of a conceptual frame of reference for nursing as this was being developed by King to identify a theory of nursing.[114] It was in the latter book that she presented the following ten criteria to evaluate theory; these criteria were selected from various theorists in the philosophic and behavioral sciences:

1. What are the terms of the theory?
2. Are the terms defined so they are understandable?
3. Are characteristics of a science evident (i.e., certainty, structure, generalizations)?
4. Are the terms universal or specific?
5. Have research findings been reported to verify the concepts or test the hypotheses?
6. Are the following components present: assumptions, defined concepts, model, rules of correspondence?
7. Is the theory generalizable?
8. What specific events are explained by the theory?
9. Is the theory limited by time and place?
10. Does the theory add to the understanding of nursing?[115]

Research and theory development are linked in an inextricable manner. Through research, ideas are explored in a systematic manner; hypotheses are tested; and conclusions are reached that assist the practitioner in explaining and predicting events in nursing. Torres and Yura presented these ideas and then specified the following criteria that a nursing theory should meet[116]:

1. Assumptions and terms are defined.
2. Boundaries and limitations are explicit.
3. It is internally consistent, and interrelationships are logical.
4. It is congruent with empirical data.
5. The theory can generate hypotheses.
6. Generalizations exist that go beyond the data.
7. Data can be collected to prove or disprove the theory; it is verifiable.
8. Past events can be explained by the theory and future ones can be predicted.
9. Propositions can be derived from the data.[117]

Ellis suggests that the nursing theories that are important provide enlightenment about the client, rather than focus primarily on nurses, addressing who or why certain persons enter nursing, for example.[118] Characteristics that make theory important for nursing include the following:

1. Scope—is the theory broad enough to cover and include a number of concepts; does it provide a framework for examining numerous phenomena?
2. Complexity—are multiple variables of phenomena addressed; are relationships among variables considered?
3. Testability—is the theory recognized as a construct that is subject to change?
4. Usefulness—does the theory have potential for guiding practice; will it be useful for the practitioner?
5. Implicit values—does the theory recognize implicit values that are made explicit in theory enunciation?
6. General information—is the theory capable of generating multiple hypotheses; does the theory stimulate ideas that will lead to the derivation of new data?
7. Terminology—are the terms used in the theory clear, unambiguous, and understood by the practitioner; can the terms be used in a practical and meaningful way by the nurse?[119]

Ellis concludes by suggesting that theoretical formulations for nursing will be needed because these pertain, in particular, to individuals. Theories that address groups and communities may be the starting point for theory development, but it is the phenomena about the individual that will contribute the most qualitative data to theories about nursing. Ellis also recognizes the existence of patterning and order in human nature and advises that these be considered when devising studies about the individual. In working with a human subject, one has an established base of knowledge about human structure, human processes, and human needs; these provide the starting point for the identification of complex variables within a broad scope that are useful, can be tested, and contain implicit values that can be readily stated in explicit terms.[120]

Throughout recent history, there have been milestones in the development of nursing as a profession, and certain persons stand out as do their struggles and efforts to define and to demonstrate what nursing is and what it should be. In the remaining section of this chapter their contribution to nursing will be described through their writings. The ideas of these nurses will be summarized and acknowledged in terms of what they have contributed to the advancement of nursing in general and to the nursing process in particular.

PROGRESS AND PEOPLE IN NURSING

The profession of nursing has experienced significant progress, especially during the past 20 years. Prior to the 1960s, a limited number of persons were leaders in moving the profession of nursing to its present heights. The number of outstanding persons increased dramatically in the 1960s and the 1970s. Their pronouncements about nursing, what it is, how it is defined, and how theory and science guide and direct nursing activities continue to be influential today. Presently, in the 1980s, nursing is assuming an adult, mature role in setting directions and performing a qualitative service for clients. The following is an identification of the progress and the people who have made nursing what it is today.

The Progress—A Successful Journey

1. The latter part of the 19th century was under the influence and leadership of Florence Nightingale.
2. Through the first half of the 20th century, Virginia Henderson was an outstanding leader, writer, practitioner, educator, and researcher.
3. Sister Olivia Gowan was among the foremost educators in the 1930s and 1940s. For a number of years, especially in the 1940s and the 1950s, there was emphasis on the need to define nursing. Although a few nurses were able to put together a statement that a majority of nurses could support, most definitions were limited to citing the functions of nurses in particular settings. As a result of such diversity, there was no one statement accepted by all professional nurses that defined nursing. One of the earliest definitions of nursing was presented in 1944 by Sister Olivia Gowan. She was a farsighted pioneer in nursing education and she viewed nursing in its broadest sense, as being both an art and a science involving the total patient; promoting spiritual, mental, and physical health; stressing health education and health preservation; ministering to the sick; caring for the patient's environment; and giving health service to the family, the community, and the individual.[121] This definition appeared in print long before it was fashionable to define nursing, and the comprehensive definition of nursing given by Sister Olivia was, for many years, most accepted and often quoted. (Long recognized as an outstanding leader in nursing, Sister Olivia died in April 1977.)
4. Frances Reiter Kreuter, another respected leader in nursing, expressed her vision of the nurse as that of a mother surrogate.[122] Not all nurses agree with this interpretation of their role, but if one analyzes Erikson's identification of the developmental phases of childhood and the role of the parent in each phase, the term *parent*

surrogate can become more acceptable. For example, a basic tenet in teaching a child is to gain his or her trust; so too, trust in the nurse is the basis for the client care he or she provides. Children learn independence gradually; the parent teaches them and helps them to become independent as they grow and develop. Developing initiative is fostered and encouraged by the parent so that children can progress to the limit of their abilities.[123] These findings can be applied to the roles of nurse and client, in which Kreuter saw the nurse as protecting the client, teaching, performing those acts of self-care the client cannot do unaided, and providing comfort and encouragement. Although she called these "ministrations," they can also be viewed as nursing actions—ministering to basic needs, administering, observing, teaching, supervising or guiding, and planning with and communicating with the client. Kreuter also discussed direct care, in which the nurse gives direct physical care, and indirect care, in which the nurse engages in activities that do not bring him or her into immediate contact with the client.[124] Some nurses agree with these concepts in their entirety; some agree with them partially; nevertheless, Kreuter made major contributions to the development of concepts of nursing through her numerous and thought-provoking ideas.

5. The influence of these pioneers continues to be felt to the present day. In addition, increased numbers of nurses became visible and their writings became more prolific. The acceleration of ideas, research, stimulation, and challenge began as a rumble in the 1950s with the ideas and efforts of Hildegard Peplau and Lydia Hall.

6. This rumble increased in intensity into the 1960s when it became a low-level roar. The thoughts and writings of the following nurses were influencing the direction of nursing: F. Abdellah, D. Johnson, M. Levine, I. Orlando, J. Travelbee, and E. Wiedenbach. Along with the pioneer efforts of these nurse authors, several nonnurses were collaborating with nurses in various intellectual and research endeavors, namely Dickoff and James, philosophers, and Kelly and Hammond, psychologists. The discussions and stimulation that were pursued with these resource persons provided a base and a framework for continued anc continuing scientific development.

7. Momentum accelerated in the 1970s when exciting advances were made in nursing. The increased number of nurse authors was paving the road for (a) the development of conceptual frameworks, (b) the designation of nursing diagnoses, and (c) the recognition of the nursing process as the core and essence of nursing. The ideas of the following nurse authors were publicized in the 1970s: I. King, B. Neuman, D. Orem, M. Rogers, Sr. Callista Roy, J. Paterson, and L. Zderad. Nurses who were discussing and writing about nursing di-

agnoses in particular were K. Gebbie, M. Gordon, P. Kritek, and M. A. Lavin.

8. Reflecting on events in the 1980s and reviewing the professional literature today (through 1986) reveals a significant story:

    a. There have been no new initiatives relative to the development of theoretic–conceptual frameworks that have been proposed, presented, and/or published in this decade. Since 1980, the energies of nurse educators, practitioners of clinical nursing, and nurse researchers have been directed to the application of one or several of the theoretic–conceptual structures proposed in the 1960s and 1970s.

    b. Proposed nursing diagnoses are being tested and validated in a variety of clinical settings. In some instances, the diagnoses proposed by NANDA are selected and validated. In other instances, the NANDA diagnoses are adapted/adjusted/altered to better accommodate a specific clinical area. Clinical validation of these revised diagnoses are pursued, then the results are presented in public forums and find their way into appropriate professional literature.

    c. There is extensive use of the systematic processes of research and of nursing process as nurses seek answers to the numerous dilemmas that are faced in health care. While they seek new knowledge through research and they seek solutions to problems by means of the nursing process, both processes are critical means to assist professional nurses in the delivery of qualitative care for the client.

    d. A subject that has received much attention during past decades is a "definition of nursing." While not *one* definition has been identified as *the* definition of nursing, a number of nurse scholars have presented statements that are acceptable definitions. Table 1–2 illustrates a cluster of 17 definitions of nursing that are available in the literature and that are used in various settings to define "what is nursing."

The People—Influential Nurse Scholars

Florence Nightingale

Florence Nightingale (1820–1910) has been long remembered for the treatise entitled *Notes on Nursing* that she authored in the mid-1800s. She did not speak of the nursing process by name but spoke of the elements of nursing that are included today in the nursing process. Among the areas she wrote about are the following:

1. Knowledge is an essential ingredient in nursing. The nurse must know about the client, must have knowledge of the envi-

TABLE 1–2. DEFINITIONS OF NURSING

Nurse Authors	Date Published	Nursing Defined
Sister M. Olivia Gowan	1944	Nursing in its broadest sense may be defined as an art and a science which involves the whole patient—body, mind, and spirit; promotes his or her intellectual, mental, and physical health by teaching and by example; stresses health education and health preservation, as well as ministration to the sick; involves the care of the patients' environment—social and spiritual as well as physical; and gives health service to the family and the community as well as to the individual.
Virginia Henderson	1964	The unique function of the nurse is to assist the individual, sick or well, in the performance of those activities contributing to health or its recovery (or to peaceful death) that the client would perform unaided if he or she had the necessary strength, will, or knowledge.
Dorothy E. Johnson	1961	The achievement and maintenance of a stable state is nursing's distinctive contribution to patient welfare and the specific purpose of nursing care.
Imogene King	1971	Nursing is a process of human interactions between nurse and client whereby each perceives the other and the situation; and through communication, they set goals, explore means, and agree on means to achieve goals.
Frances Reiter Kreuter	1957	The nurse is viewed as a mother surrogate; she ministers to basic needs, administers, observes, teaches, supervises or guides, plans with and communicates with the client. Nursing involves protecting the client, teaching, performing those acts of self-care the client cannot do unaided, and provides comfort and encouragement.
Myra Levine	1967	Nursing can fulfill its conservation function in four major areas of care: conservation of patient energy, conservation of structural integrity, conservation of personal integrity, conservation of social integrity.
Betty Neuman	1980	Nursing is a unique profession concerned with all the variables affecting an individual's response to stressors.
Dorothea Orem	1971	Nursing is a personal, family, and community service within the health field. Its dimension of concern for human life and well-being is shared with other health services.

(continued)

TABLE 1–2 *(continued)*

Nurse Authors	Date Published	Nursing Defined
		Nursing differs from these services because of the nature of its contributed effort. Provisions for making nursing available in a social group should consider both its shared and its unique dimension.
Ida Jean Orlando Pelletier	1961	The purpose of nursing is to supply the help a patient requires in order for his or her needs to be met.
Hildegard Peplau	1952	Nursing is a significant, therapeutic, interpersonal process. It functions cooperatively with other human processes that make health possible for individuals in communities. Nursing is an educative instrument, a maturing force, that aims to promote forward movement of personality in the direction of creative, constructive, productive, personal, and community living.
Martha Rogers	1970	Professional practice in nursing seeks to promote symphonic interaction between man and environment, to strengthen the adherence and integrity of the human field, and to direct and redirect patterning of the human and environmental fields for realization of maximum health potential.
Sister Callista Roy	1970	Nursing is concerned with man as a total being at some point along the health-illness continuum. The goal of nursing is to bring about an adaptive state in the four adaptive modes of adaptation: physiological needs, self-concept, role function, and interdependence.
Social Policy Statement (ANA)	1980	Nursing is the diagnosis and treatment of human responses to actual or potential health problems.
Joyce Travelbee	1966	Nursing is an interpersonal process whereby the professional nurse practitioner assists an individual or family in preventing and coping with the experience of illness and suffering and, if necessary, assists the individual or family in finding meaning in these experiences.
Ernestine Wiedenbach	1964	The purpose for clinical nursing is to facilitate the efforts of individuals to overcome the obstacles which currently interfere with their ability to respond capably to demands made of them by their condition, environment, situation, and time.

(continued)

TABLE 1–2 *(continued)*

Nurse Authors	Date Published	Nursing Defined
Helen Yura & Mary Walsh	1967, 1987 (revised)	Nursing is an encounter with a client as person, family, or community in which the nurse observes, supports, communicates, ministers, teaches, and cares; the nurse contributes to the maintenance of optimum wellness through the facilitation of human need fulfillment, and provides care during illness until clients are able to assume responsibility for the fulfillment of their own human needs; when necessary, the nurse provides compassionate care for clients who are dying.
Loretta Zderad & Josephine Paterson	1976	Nursing is always an interhuman act, a living human act, an experience lived between human beings, a transactional relationship, an intersubjective transaction.

ronment, and must know what are the potential and actual alterations that the client can experience. This knowledge is distinct from medical knowledge.[125]

2. Observation of the client is a major skill used by the nurse. It is important to note changes that have occurred or that are occurring in the state of the client and to be knowledgeable about what the changes mean.

3. Putting the client in the best state possible for nature to act was the thrust of Nightingale's ideas. Rather than telling the nurses that they were responsible for curing the client, Nightingale proposed that nature was the primary healer of the ill; nurses were to be adjuncts in the curative, healing process.[126]

4. Along with the intellectual skills to be used by the nurse, there were activities of nursing care for which nurses were accountable and responsible. These included responsibility for proper nutrition of the client, administration of medications, concern for cleanliness, and a multitude of activities that dealt primarily with the physiologic human needs.

Although Nightingale did not classify activities according to the nursing process, the components she spoke about were a sound base for the nursing process as it was developed in the 1960s. She encouraged the use of intellectual and technical skills. Observation of the client was emphasized as a means of data gathering. Accountability for actions was addressed, and there was recognition that the nurse supported the client in the process of a recovery from illness while other factors in the environment and in nature were enhancing the health state of the client.[127]

This base for nursing was a sound foundation for these past 100 years—a base provided by a forward-looking "lady with the lamp," Florence Nightingale.

Virginia Henderson

Virginia Henderson's contributions to nursing spanned a long period of time. Her writings first appeared in 1939 when she collaborated with Bertha Harmer on the fourth edition of the *Textbook of the Principles and Practice of Nursing*.[128] Although a wide variety of contributions to nursing can be attributed to the efforts and writings of Virginia Henderson, the following are specific to the development of the nursing process:

1. Because of her firm conviction that nursing must be defined in order for the public and the professionals to know what nurses do, Henderson set about defining the functions of nursing. Her definition has been accepted by nurses and others since it was published in 1955.
2. Sequential to defining what nursing is, Henderson specified 14 components of basic nursing care. They remain comprehensive, complete, and consistent with various hierarchies and levels of human need.
3. With emphasis on the need for the educational preparation of nurses, Henderson continues to plead for the development of the intellectual ability of nurses and for the use of technical skills. She encourages nurses to "get inside the skin" of clients in order to relate to and understand their needs.
4. Consistent with the use of intellectual and technical skills, Henderson also stresses the use of interpersonal skills by the nurse. Their use as well as the nurse's use of the client's strengths will permit independence for the client as soon as possible.

Prominent features of Virginia Henderson's ideas include her clear and complete definition of nursing with the specification of 14 components of care. Although differing from many other nurse authors, Henderson includes the concepts of all phases of the nursing process in her discussions about nursing. Outstanding is her identification of the intellectual, interpersonal, and technical skills needed to perform nursing functions.[129]

Lydia Hall

Lydia Hall is remembered not for her concern about those persons whose needs result from an acute illness but for her concern for those recovering from an acute illness who need support services to help

them resume normal lives in the post-acute phase of life. Three components—care, core, and cure—present the essence of Hall's ideas[130]:

1. Care is the exclusive domain of nursing and represents the nurturing, caring, and comforting component of professional activities. This component is concerned with the basic needs of
   persons, and the nurse relies on his or her intellectual skills to
   direct the technologies required for client comfort. As these
   needs are being stabilized, the nurse's interpersonal skills are
   used as an integral part of care delivery.
2. Core is the component of nursing that involves the total health
   team. All disciplines contribute to the fulfillment of needs of the
   client. The nurse's role is to assist clients to muster their own
   energies through encouragement and motivation; to help them
   achieve a higher level of functioning by recognizing their
   strengths and potential.
3. Cure is the component in which the nurse is an advocate for the
   client as the total health team pursues health or maximum
   functioning as the client goal. The client is encouraged to progress and is guided in the identification of increasingly higher
   goals to be met.

The interrelationship of these three components is the essence of
the philosophy of the Loeb Center for Nursing and Rehabilitation where
Lydia Hall was the first director. Although her ideas and pleas for qual-
ity patient care were pronounced in the late 1950s and early 1960s,
Lydia Hall's philosophy continues to be the basis of client care at the
Loeb Center.[131]

Hildegard Peplau

Although Hildegard Peplau could not foresee the impact that *Interpersonal Relations in Nursing* would have on nursing, she and many other
nurses have been witness to the recognition of her text as a classic in
the area of psychiatric nursing. When the text was published, the
boundaries of tradition were pushed into the background, and Dr.
Peplau became known for her recognition of the value and worth of
nurses and nursing.

Nurses were seen as vital and essential components in the nurse–
client relationship. The nurse and client were seen as individuals and
separate entities in the situation where the client experienced some
need. Each was perceived as a whole person, and there was strong emphasis on growth and development. The importance and necessity of
maturity was stressed. Needs were identified in relation to emotional
maturity. Having identified initial needs in the nurse–client encounter,

these are to be met and then outgrown; more mature needs arise and are subsequently met.

Nursing is perceived as a purposeful act and a service where health is the primary goal of nursing. When a person is ill or in need of health services and a nurse responds to that need, nursing occurs; this becomes the basis for a human relationship.

Hildegard Peplau recognized nursing as a process that "demands certain steps, actions, operations, or performances that occur between an individual who does the nursing and the person who is nursed."[132] It is a therapeutic, interpersonal process in which nurse and client share in the solution of problems.

Four overlapping phases of nurse–client relationships can be identified as:

1. Orientation—the client seeks assistance on the basis of a felt need. While supporting the client in the phase, the nurse may function as a resource person, a counselor, a surrogate, or a technical expert.
2. Identification—first impressions held by the client are clarified and the client begins to understand what the situation can offer as help. Preconceptions and expectations are discussed and clarified.
3. Exploitation—full use is made by the client of all the services available.
4. Resolution—old ties and dependencies are relinquished and the client gradually becomes free of identification with the helping persons. Ability to stand alone is strengthened.

Research and systematic study are stressed by Dr. Peplau. She suggests that observation, communication, and recording are interlocking elements of interpersonal relations that make it possible for nurses to study what is happening with the client.[133]

Ida Jean Orlando Pelletier

Ida Jean Orlando is among those nurses who dared to present a creative way to define and analyze nursing. Her publication *The Dynamic Nurse Patient Relationship* created reaction and interaction among nurses when it appeared in 1961.[134] Her ideas have been further developed since that time, and numerous persons have explored with Orlando the way that her ideas can contribute to the improvement of quality care.

As the title of her text suggests, Orlando's orientation is in the behavioral science area; her clinical specialty is psychiatric nursing. She views nursing as an interaction with an ill person who is experiencing a need. Unless the client has a need that cannot be met unassisted, there is no requirement for nursing.

Her efforts to identify the process of nursing began in the mid-1950s as a funded project under a National Institutes of Mental Health Grant. The nursing process was identified as an interactive process that comprises "the behavior of the patient, the reaction of the nurse, and the nursing actions designed for the patients' benefit."[135] More recent interpretations of these elements have been translated into the following: perception and observation, validation, thoughts and feelings, say and do.

The concept of client need forms the basis for nursing intervention according to Orlando's ideas. She defines need as "a requirement of the patient which, if supplied, relieves or diminishes immediate distress or improves the immediate sense of well being." This need concept is based on the premise that the person who requires nursing is ill and that a physician has identified the illness. The "dynamic" facet of her idea suggests that the requirements for nursing change; the interaction concept she is speaking of applies to the *present*. This emphasis is intended to avoid the performance of nursing in an automatic way. Deliberate actions are to be emphasized; instinctive or automatic actions are to be avoided. Orlando suggests that a dynamic process of nursing focusing on the ever changing status of the client will prevent an instinctive and less than thoughtful performance by nurses.

The Nursing Theories Conference Group has presented a comparison between Orlando's process of nursing and the four phases of the nursing process presented in this text. The client's behavior and nursing reaction are aligned with and related to the assessment phase of the nursing process. If a client need is identified, this can be perceived as the diagnosis; the nurse should continue to relate to the client only if such a finding is established. Nursing action as described by Orlando incorporates the planning and implementation phases of the nursing process. There is emphasis on the participation of the client throughout the process; also, the validation by and with the client is reiterated and stressed. Written goals, prioritization of plans, and the means to resolve the clients' needs are integral parts of the nurse's actions on behalf of the client.[136]

The degree of success of the nurse's actions is measured by changes in the client's behavior. Whether the client improves or not, the nurse is responsible for validating with the client whether his or her actions were effective or not. Continuous referral to the client for input and feedback makes the Orlando process a very client-centered and client-oriented process.

Limitations of this process that have been identified are the focus on the ill person as well as limitation to the conscious person. Nurses who have discussed Orlando's ideas express concern about the practicality of using this framework with a client who is unconscious or who is so acutely ill as to be unable to validate the nurse's perceptions and observations.

Despite these limitations, Orlando deserves credit for her courage in presenting a process in nursing before any other had been clearly identified. Also worthy of note is the provision of safeguards for the client by focusing on deliberate actions rather than automatic or instinctive actions.

Ernestine Wiedenbach

Ernestine Wiedenbach is among those pioneers in nursing who have explored the dimensions of nursing theory and nursing concepts; she has provided the ideas and motivation that can lead to a framework of nursing.

Although her practice of nursing began in the 1920s, Wiedenbach provided the philosophers Dickoff and James with stimulating dialogues about nursing during the 1960s.[137] Nurses were challenged by that dialogue, and verbal and written reactions between nurses and philosophers arose in response.

Outcomes of Wiedenbach's deliberations with Dickoff and James included the identification of three factors that are inherent in her prescriptive or situation-producing nursing theory: (a) the central purpose; (b) the prescription for fulfilling the central purpose; and (c) the realities in the situation that influence the fulfillment of the central purpose.[138]

According to Wiedenbach, the concepts of nurturing and caring are central to nursing. She sees nursing as a helping service that is rendered with compassion, skill, and understanding. To bring her beliefs and ideas to professional peers, she wrote *Clinical Nursing, A Helping Art* in the early 1960s.[139]

Wiedenbach emphasizes that the nurse possesses certain beliefs and values, and that he or she behaves in accordance with those beliefs when delivering client care. Essential components for a nursing philosophy are reverence for the gift of life; respect for the dignity, worth, autonomy, and individuality of each person; and a resolution to act consistent with one's beliefs. Respect for a person, according to Wiedenbach, includes the following:

1. Each human is endowed with unique potential.
2. Each human strives toward self-direction and relative independence.
3. Each human requires stimulation to realize self-worth.
4. Whatever individuals do represents their best judgment at the time.[140]

Seven levels of awareness are identified by Wiedenbach: sensation, perception, assumption, realization, insight, design, and decision. The first three levels consist of an activating situation. That is, with these levels of sensation, perception, and assumption, the nurse focuses attention on the stimulus, and nursing actions become automatic and involuntary. Realization, insight, design, and decision—the other levels of awareness—are perceived as voluntary. In the activating situation, with a focus on the stimulus rather than on the client, the nurse acts intuitively or instinctively. There is no validation with the client. In the voluntary situation, the nurse validates with the client (realization), involves the client in mutual planning and goal setting (insight), establishes a plan of action to deal with the client's problems (design), and determines what he or she can do to help the client (decision).

According to the Nursing Theories Conference Group, Wiedenbach's ideas would be difficult to validate or to test by means of research.[141] However, there is value in analyzing her ideas; she presents some fundamental beliefs that can be used when planning and implementing client care. There is an orderliness to her presentations about nursing and a quality to her beliefs that deserve attention. The following paragraph briefly summarizes Wiedenbach's beliefs about nursing.

Nursing is a deliberate blend of thoughts, feelings, and overt actions practiced in relation to an individual in need of help, triggered by a behavioral stimulus from the individual, rooted in an explicit philosophy, and directed toward fulfillment of a specific purpose. She suggested that clinical nursing comprises four interlocking yet distinct components: philosophy (the way), purpose (the why), practice (the what), art (the how). The nurse is responsible for: (a) identifying the client's need for help; (b) ministering the help needed; (c) validating that the help given was indeed the help that was needed, and (d) coordinating the resources for help available to the client.[142]

Dorothy Johnson

Dorothy Johnson has been making significant contributions to the nursing literature for more than two decades. In the late 1950s and early 1960s, she presented her ideas about the science of nursing.[143,144] In the early 1960s she discussed nursing education.[145] Clinical specialist roles were her focus in the mid-1960s[146]; theory development was the thrust in the mid-1970s.[147] More recently she presented a behavioral systems model.[148]

Johnson views the human person as a behavioral system. She defines a system that functions as a whole by virtue of the interdependence of its parts. She suggests that nursing science consists of (a) descriptions and explanations of disorders in the behavioral system, and (b) theoretical bases for preventing and controlling these disorders.[149]

Fundamental to the "whole" behavioral system are four assumptions that are necessary in order to understand the nature and operation of the whole behavioral system:

1. There is organization, interaction, interdependency, and integration of parts and elements.
2. Each system tends to achieve a balance among the various forces operating within and on it. Individuals continuously strive to maintain a behavioral system balance and a steady state via automatic adjustment and adaptation to the "natural" forces that impinge on the individual.
3. The behavioral system is essential to man; it serves a useful purpose in social life and within the individual.
4. The balance of a behavioral system reflects adjustments and adaptations that are successful to some degree and extent.

The central idea of Dorothy Johnson's model is that each person's life forms an integrated and organized functional unit that is a system. Within this system, seven subsystems are identified: affiliative, achievement, aggressive/protective, dependency, eliminative, ingestive, sexual. Grubbs has used the Johnson model in practice and has added an eighth subsystem: the restorative.[150] Each of the subsystems has a structure that includes a goal (purpose), a set (what is the need, what is the usual behavior?), a choice (what are the alternatives, the choices?), and an action (the implementation of acts). The functional requirements or sustenal imperatives of the whole system include: (a) a protection from noxious stimuli, from unnecessary threats, from threats to clients; (b) nurturance to cope with environmental stimuli, to support growth and development of behaviors, to encourage effective behavior, to discourage ineffective behavior; (c) stimulation to bring forth new behavior, to increase an actual behavior, to increase appropriate behavior, to increase motivation.[151]

To achieve the purposes for which this behavioral system exists, Johnson specifies a nursing process that includes assessing (first- and second-level assessing), diagnosing, intervening, and evaluating. First-level assessment includes a general examination of the clients' behaviors to determine if a problem exists. Second-level assessing enables an in-depth analysis of the data identified in the first-level assessment. Diagnosing includes clustering of those behaviors that are healthy versus those that are not. Intervention includes choices of restricting, defending, inhibiting, or facilitating. Evaluating includes examination of outcomes achieved and measured against goals set in the diagnosing phase.

Imogene M. King

Imogene King is among those nurse authors who had the courage to present her beliefs and ideas in the early 1970s. In *Toward a Theory for Nursing*, published in 1971, she presented a number of components that continue to provide a base for a model of nursing.[152] For 10 years, King discussed her ideas, encouraged and directed research and the systematic study of the conceptual components of her ideas, and published progress reports and results of various efforts. She published a new text in 1981: *A Theory for Nursing*.[153] (Examination of the titles of the two texts alone suggests the progress that Dr. King made in pursuing her beliefs and convictions about nursing.)

The theory of general systems was influential in Dr. King's idea development. She also relied upon the sciences of philosophy, psychology, and sociology. She asked: What changes in society and in education are affecting nursing? What are the constants in nursing? What are the goals of nursing? What are the practice dimensions of nursing? Pursuit of these questions enabled King to arrive at a framework that has proved valuable to a number of nursing educators, practitioners, and researchers.

A distinctive definition of nursing by King states that nursing is a process of action, reaction, interaction, and transaction.[154] She suggests that this process takes place in a nursing situation that includes a nurse and a client involved in establishing a relationship in order to cope with a health state or to make changes that are necessary to improve the health state. The goal of nursing is to help persons maintain health so that they can perform their roles. The boundaries of nursing are the promotion of health for individuals and groups, maintenance and restoration of health, care of the sick and injured, and care of the dying.[155] In order to achieve this goal, the nurse operates on the belief that each human is an open system who interacts with the environment. The open systems are defined by King as social systems (society), interpersonal systems (groups), and personal systems (individuals). These are conceived as dynamic and interacting; they provide the conceptual base for the performance of nursing. With the base established for a conceptual framework and theory for nursing, King's ideas can continue to be explored and studied, and the potential is excellent for continued data collection, validation, and verification of these ideas.

Dorothea E. Orem

Dorothea Orem has expended effort since the late 1950s to "give form and structure to knowledge that describes and explains nursing."[156] It is a tribute to Orem that a number of nurses in practice and a number of nursing education programs use her ideas and scholarly productions as a base, a foundation, and a framework for their own efforts. Although the adaptation of Orem's ideas may vary with the person or groups who interpret and use her concepts, the essence of her theory is retained.

In the 1980 edition of *Nursing: Concepts of Practice*, she calls her ideas the theory that is used by nurses to guide their endeavors. She presents three main subjects: (a) the domain and boundaries of nursing, (b) the object of nursing, and (c) the need for nurses to be able to "think nursing."[157]

The domain of nursing practice is defined according to the persons or groups who can be helped through nursing.[158] Also, the domain is defined according to the activities in which the nurse engages when he or she renders nursing care. Five areas of activities for nursing practice are:

1. Establish and maintain nurse–client relationships.
2. Determine if the person can be helped by nursing.
3. Respond to the client's requirements and needs for nursing.
4. Provide help to the client and family through nursing.
5. Coordinate and integrate nursing with other services needed by the client.[159]

The object of nursing can be defined according to the special concerns of nursing as identified by Orem: "the individual's need for self-care action and the provision and management of it on a continuous basis in order to sustain life and health, recover from disease or injury, and cope with their effects."[160]

In order to explain relationships Orem specifies three constructs: (a) self-care deficits indicate the client's needs for nursing, (b) self-care involves systematized and deliberate actions that are necessary for the client, and (c) a nursing system is the result of nursing practice that can provide the necessary help for clients. These three constructs of self-care deficits, self-care, and nursing systems form the essence of Orem's ideas. Each is developed further in her textbook presentations. Also, each of the constructs is analyzed and elaborated by persons who subscribe to her ideas.

Self-care requisites are perceived as developmental, universal, or health deviation requisites.[161] To accomplish these requisites, Orem refers to the human ability of self-care agency.[162] When nurses enter the client situation to provide nursing, special abilities are needed; these are called nursing agency.[163]

Nursing systems are based on the belief that nurses or clients, or both, can meet the needs of the client. The variation of these nursing systems are (a) wholly compensatory systems—when the client is unable to carry out self-care actions and the nurse becomes totally responsible; (b) partly compensatory systems—when the nurse and the client are mutually engaged in client care; (c) supportive-educative systems—when the client needs assistance in activities such as decision making or acquisition of knowledge in order to be self-responsible.

Orem discusses the dimensions of nursing practice, including its social, interpersonal, and technological aspects. Her perception of the nursing process is directly related to her beliefs and philosophy about what nursing is and for what nursing is responsible. She summarizes the three steps of the nursing process as determining why a person needs nursing; designing a system of nursing for the person when there is a need for nursing; and initiating, conducting, and controlling nursing actions as these relate to the needs of the person.[164] Orem emphasizes that these steps of the nursing process are the technological components of nursing and must be coordinated with the interpersonal and social components of each situation.[165]

The framework, the theory, and the ideas proposed by Orem have been provocative, constructive, and thoughtful. It can be predicted that further exploration and application of her ideas will be realized.

Martha E. Rogers

Martha Rogers has exerted a profound influence on the profession of nursing through her writing, research, teaching, and dialogues with students and nurses. Her ideas have been stimulating, challenging, and motivating. A comparison of Rogers's early and late writings reveals a growth and development in her concepts about nursing. Improvement of initial concepts is a hallmark of her later work. (She labels some of her early works as "naive meanderings.") Several assumptions, stated by Rogers, are fundamental to the development of nursing science:

1. Man is a unified whole possessing self-integrity and manifesting characteristics that are more than and different from the sum of the parts.[166]
2. Man and environment are continuously exchanging matter and energy with one another.[167]
3. The life process evolves irreversibly and unidirectionally along the space–time continuum.[168]
4. Pattern and organization identify man and reflect man's innovative wholeness.[169]
5. Man is characterized by the capacity for abstraction and imagery, language and thought, sensation and emotion.[170]

Beliefs that are central to her ideas include the following: (a) man is unique; (b) man and environment evolve as a unified whole; (c) man and environment are involved in a continuous interactive process for both are open systems; (d) self-regulation is an expression of wholeness; (e) human beings are more than and different from the sum of their parts; (f) human beings are characterized by mass, structure, function, and feelings.

Dr. Rogers's statement, "a conceptual frame of reference is an indispensable prerequisite to the ordering of knowledges and to the formulation of meaningful propositions," is a defense of the struggle in nursing to identify conceptual frameworks. With this as a rationale, the identification of these "abstract structures" can move nursing toward the science it hopes to become. Rogers suggests that the "translation of scientific nursing knowledge into humanitarian practice carries with it the potential for health services" that are much broader than those presently provided.[171]

In addition to the assumptions and beliefs proposed by Rogers, she also suggests some dimensions of man and of nursing that can be identified as homeodynamic principles; two of these are the principles of reciprocy and helicy. Reciprocy is based on the belief that man and environment are inseparable; the relation between the two is one of constant mutual interaction and mutual change. Helicy postulates that human life proceeds in one direction, evolves in sequential stages, and is unitary in nature; continuous interactive change describes the concept of this principle.[172]

As a dimension of nursing, Rogers emphasizes nursing practice in all settings and stresses the responsibility of nurses to care for all people, sick or well. The aim of nursing is to help people achieve maximum health potential; nursing's goals include the maintenance and promotion of health, prevention of disease, nursing diagnosis, intervention, and rehabilitation.

Joyce Travelbee

Joyce Travelbee's personal beliefs and experiences as an existentialist and as a lay Carmelite had profound influences on her ideas about nursing. Her writings and publications reflect a rich background in psychiatric nursing practice and education. (The untimely death of Joyce Travelbee in the early 1970s was truly a loss to the profession of nursing.) According to Travelbee, the purpose of nursing is the establishment of an "interpersonal process, whereby the professional nurse practitioner assists the individual, family, or community to prevent or to cope with the experience of illness and suffering and, if necessary, to find meaning in these experiences."[173] Nursing therefore is a service, initiated to effect a change in the client (or the recipient of the service). In this human-to-human relationship the needs for nursing are met by the nurse who combines a disciplined, intellectual approach to the client's problems with a therapeutic use of self. Travelbee described the therapeutic use of self as the ability to consciously use one's personality (talents) to structure nursing intervention. She specified two major functions of nursing: (a) to assist individuals, families, and communities to prevent or to cope with the stress of illness and suffering, and (b) to assist individuals, families, and communities to find meaning in illness and suffering.[174] Underlying these two functions is the responsibility of the nurse to help the client experience hope so that illness and suffering can be tolerated and managed.

Despite Travelbee's focus and emphasis on the individuality and uniqueness of each person, the following phases can be experienced generally in the establishment of the human-to-human relationship:

1. The original encounter
2. Emerging identity
3. Empathy
4. Sympathy
5. Rapport

To accomplish the necessary relationships and to proceed through these five phases, the nurse observes, develops inferences and value judgments, interprets, makes decisions, derives a plan of action, and evaluates.[175]

Analysis of these ideas suggests a firm philosophical base from which the nurse can proceed using the phases of the interpersonal relationship or the process of nursing, or both, as proposed by Travelbee. The *why* of nursing is emphasized by Travelbee, yet she speaks to the *how* of nursing with sufficient attention to accomplish both. She attempts to link the emotional and intellectual capabilities of the nurse and stresses the uniqueness and individuality of the client. Her perception of the nurse and the client includes concepts of change, coping, and caring. Travelbee admonishes nurses to use a sense of values to guide their actions, yet these personal values should not be imposed on the client.

Sister Callista Roy

Sister Callista Roy has been prominent in the world of nursing through her activities as an educator, writer, lecturer, and theorist. Her energy and involvement in a multitude of professional endeavors makes her name readily recognized in professional circles. The following components are distinctly recognized as Roy's ideas:

1. Each human is viewed as a complete entity in constant interchange with the environment.
2. The interchange that occurs is affected by four modes of adaptation:
   a. Physiological needs—man adapts to changes to maintain physiologic integrity

    b. Self-concept—adaptation to change to maintain psychological integrity

    c. Role function—adaptation to change through social interaction (family, groups, community, and society)

    d. Interdependence—adaptation to change to enable need fulfillment on higher levels of love, belonging and establishment of unity among significant persons.[176]

3. The nurse's use of decision making and the value of good judgment are components of Roy's ideas. These are implemented through the use of the nursing process that Roy defines as first- and second-level assessment, nursing diagnosis, implementation, and evaluation.[177]

4. Various stimuli impinge on persons as they strive to adapt to ever changing environments. Some of these stimuli are in the immediate environment (focal); some are more remote but evident to the person (contextual); and some are a part of that person because of heritage or culture (residual).[178]

The main thrust of Sister Callista Roy's ideas point to the need for persons to adapt. The nurse uses the nursing process within the framework of the four modes (physiologic needs, self-concept, role function, interdependence) to determine how effectively the client is adapting (are maladaptive behaviors evident?). The nurse is responsible for manipulating the various stimuli (focal, contextual, residual) or assisting the client in such manipulation to promote or ensure adaptation.

Loretta Zderad and Josephine Paterson

Clinical nursing and clinical theorizing are fundamental to the ideas of Loretta Zderad and Josephine Paterson; these nurse authors believe the two are inextricably linked to each other. Clinical nursing has been described as an experience lived between human beings.[179] It involves a mode of being, is an act of doing something, and is a response to a human situation. With humanistic nursing as their base, Zderad and Paterson propose that the "stuff" of nursing includes man needing and man helping.[180] To describe the components of these nursing situations, their goal has been to define and to describe the phenomena nursing comprises.

One phenomenon in nursing is nursing itself.[181] Paterson defines the act of nursing as the "intersubjective transactional relation, the dialogue experienced, lived in concert between persons where comfort and nurturance produce mutual human unfolding."[182] Important values that underlie various clinical nursing situations include "comfort, nurturance, clinical, empathy, and all-at-once."[183] Attributes of the person that influence the nursing actions of Zderad and Paterson include their perception of each person as unique with the person's own potential and limitations; each person related to other persons in some way—in time and in space; and each person becoming, and his or her individuality being actualized through his or her relationships with other persons.

The impetus for clinical theorizing according to Zderad and Paterson is a "personal professional need to find answers."[184] Sharing questions about the nature of nursing with professional colleagues and searching for answers in the practice, research, and teaching settings are essential for theory development. Further requirements include an inquiring attitude on the part of the nurse; development of skills in clinical judgment and in a priority setting; a sense of intelligent and imaginative freedom and responsibility that enables the nurse to see clinical realities in a creative light; and a constant awareness of the need to theorize.[185]

Zderad and Paterson use an existential phenomenological approach to theorizing. This implies an openness to all possibilities in the clinical situation and the identification of experience as the starting point for theory development. Approximately 30 phenomena were identified as essential to nursing by a group of registered nurses with whom Zderad and Paterson were associated.[186]

Their experience with theory development has convinced Zderad and Paterson that theory is an "articulated vision of experience."[187] They perceive humanistic nursing as a metatheory—a systematized body of knowledge formulated to make something else possible. They emphasize clinical nursing as the site of phenomena through the nurse's experience, through the client's behavior, and through a "presence" that is a phenomenon basic to the total process of nursing.[188] Zderad and Paterson propose that development of theorizing methods can shape the growth of nursing science methodology. They ask, "Will our theory support the evolvement of nursing as a fully human response to a human need?"[189]

Myra Estrin Levine

Myra Levine has been active in many areas of nursing for a number of years. She has been a practitioner, author, educator, and innovator. In 1969, and again in 1973, Dr. Levine wrote about clinical nursing.[190,191] In her work, she presents her views on nursing and the nurse–patient relationship. She sees nursing as "a human interaction."[192] This interaction, which arises through communication (i.e., a system of exchange between persons) represents a dependency on fellow humans and, hence, is the essence of nursing.

While relying on and drawing from several experts in other sciences, Dr. Levine focused on the holistic nature of man and the integrated network of man's needs, thus the need for nurses to use a holistic approach to nursing.[193] The views of Paul Tillich, theologian, about the "multidimensional unity of life in man" were basic to Dr. Levine's ideas.[194] Also important were the works of Claude Bernard, Walter Cannon, and Charles Darwin; these authorities provided a physiologic and environmental base for the holistic approach. Erik Erikson's ideas provided a psychosocial dimension.[195]

Nursing interventions were identified as being therapeutic or supportive and were based on four conservation principles:

1. Conservation of energy—balancing the patient's energy input and energy output
2. Conservation of structural integrity—protecting the patient from environmental threats and trauma as well as promoting healing when assaults do occur
3. Conservation of personal integrity—promoting self-respect and self-esteem in patients, as well as respecting the rights, beliefs, and values of each person
4. Conservation of social integrity—strengthening personal and social ties with other persons and with groups; these ties are important in a more limited family sense, but are significant, too, in contributing positively to the social structure in society.

The nursing process was used freely and empirically by Dr. Levine. She was one of the very early advocates of the term *nursing diagnosis.*[196] While trying to provide an alternative to this emotionally charged term, Dr. Levine suggested *trophicognosis* at the 1965 ANA clinical conference.[197] Although it is a legitimate term according to derivation, it has not been readily used by nurses.

The Nursing Theories Conference Group reviewed the strengths of Dr. Levine's ideas. Besides the contributions she has made toward the development of a science of nursing, the Group reported a limitation in her ideas, namely, her focus on the individual, on illness, and on the dependency of the individual. They question the applicability of such ideas with the present trend toward family, groups, and communities as well as health promotion and disease/illness prevention.[198]

Betty Neuman

The model proposed by Betty Neuman is known as a health care systems model that can be used by all health care personnel. It is a total person approach to the problems of clients. The aim of this model is to reduce stress factors and adverse conditions that do affect or could affect the optimal functioning of the system in any given situation. Neuman suggests that this model enables the care giver, i.e., the nurse, to assist persons, families, and groups to attain and maintain the maximum level of total wellness through purposeful interventions.

The following assumptions are fundamental to Betty Neuman's model:[199]

1. Each person is unique but also a composite of "knowns."
2. Of the many stressors a person experiences, each one is different in its potential to disturb the equilibrium of a person or the person's normal line of defense.
3. Each person has a normal line of defense against stressors, i.e., a normal range of response to stressors.
4. Each person also possesses a flexible line of defense that consists of the relationship among the variables that are exerted on an individual.
5. The interrelationship of variables determines the person's reaction to stressors and whether the flexible and the normal lines of defense can be or will be penetrated.
6. Each person has an internal set of resistance factors that attempt to return the person to normal lines of defense.
7. When the flexible line of defense can no longer protect against the stressors, the normal line of defense is penetrated.
8. Four variables are always present, whether a person is sick or well: physiologic, psychologic, sociocultural, and developmental. These are the dynamic composites of each individual.
9. Primary prevention is the intervention that occurs when a stressor is either suspected or identified; a reaction has not yet occurred. This is the phase when general knowledge is needed to perform a client assessment in an attempt to identify the risk factors that are associated with stressors or to strengthen the flexible line of defense.
10. Secondary prevention is that activity that relates to an analysis of symptomatology identified in an attempt to rank the priorities and identify the intervention needed. The actions occurring along the lines of resistance designate the treatment.
11. Tertiary prevention refers to those interventions aimed at helping the client to adapt, stabilize, be reeducated, and maintain the desired state of wellness. The overall purpose is the prevention of any penetration of the line of defense. Reconstitution is the thrust at this point in the wellness-seeking activity and in the effort to establish at least the same level of normal defense that existed prior to penetration owing to stressors or perhaps to achieve a higher state of wellness than existed previously.

COMMENTS

The "Past of Nursing" is a rich heritage. The development of the nursing process in the 1960s and the focus on nursing diagnosis in the 1970s have provided a solid base for a scholarly profession. It is from this heritage that "Nursing's Present" is fashioned. Valiant efforts are recorded to describe and prescribe nursing's knowledge base and to focus on theoretical frameworks for the nursing process. The core of "Nursing Present" is presented in Chapters 2 through 4. Nursing's human need theory is developed in Chapter 2.

REFERENCES

1. Nightingale, F. *Notes on nursing. What it is and what it is not* (facsimile of 1859 edition). Philadelphia: Lippincott, 1946.
2. Brown, E.L. *Nursing for the future.* New York: Russell Sage Foundation, 1948.
3. Flexner, A. *Universities.* New York: Oxford University Press, 1930, pp. 29–31.
4. Schein, F.H. *Professional education—Some new directions.* New York: McGraw-Hill, 1972, pp. 7–14.
5. *Ibid*, pp. 9–10.
6. Stuart, G.W. How professionalized is nursing? *Image*, 1981, *13*(1), 18–23.
7. *Ibid*, p. 23.
8. Coladarci, A.P. What about that word profession? *American Journal of Nursing*, 1963, *63*, 116–118.
9. American Nurses' Association. Code for Nurses with Interpretive Statements. Kansas City, Mo.: American Nurses' Association, 1985.
10. American Nurses' Association's First Position on Education for Nursing. *American Journal of Nursing*, 1965, *65*, 106–111.
11. Nayer, D.D. The ANA position paper. *Imprint*, 1976, *23*, 23ff.
12. Kinder J.S. Letter to NLN Members, from NLN President, Nov. 6, 1985.
13. News. *American Journal of Nursing.* February, 1985, *85*(2), 202.
14. *Ibid*.
15. *Ibid*, p. 196.
16. *Ibid*.
17. *Ibid*, p. 195.
18. News. *American Journal of Nursing.* July, 1986, *85*(7), 852.
19. *Ibid*, p. 853.
20. U.S. Department of Health, Education, and Welfare, Public Health Service. *Toward quality in nursing. Needs and goals. Report of the Surgeon General's consultant group in nursing.* Washington, D.C.: US Government Printing Office, 1963.
21. Lysaught, J.P. *An abstract for action.* New York: McGraw-Hill, 1970, pp. 81–147.

22. Lodge, M.P. & Pietraschke, F. *Professional education and practice of Nurse Administrators/Directors of Nursing in long-term care*. Kansas City, Mo.: American Nurses' Foundation, Inc., 1986.

23. Mauksch, I.G., & Young, P.R. Nurse-physician interaction in a family medical care center. *Nursing Outlook*, 1974, *22*, 113–119.

24. Kinlein, M.L. Independent nurse practitioner. *Nursing Outlook*, 1972, *20*, 22–24.

25. Two New York nurses debate the NYSNA 1985 proposal. *American Journal of Nursing*, 1976, *76*, 930–935.

26. ANA Convention '76. *American Journal of Nursing*. 1976, *76*, 1127.

27. Study of credentialing launched. *American Journal of Nursing*. 1976, *76*, 1893–1895.

28. *The study of credentialing in nursing: A new approach*. Kansas City, Mo.: American Nurses' Association, 1979, p. x.

29. *Ibid*, p. 41.

30. *Ibid*, p. 43.

31. *Ibid*, p. 20.

32. *Ibid*, p. 77.

33. Ozimek, D., & Yura, H. *Who is the nurse practitioner?* New York: National League for Nursing, 1975.

34. Bloch, D. Some crucial terms in nursing—What do they really mean? *Nursing Outlook*, 1974, *22*, 689–694.

35. American Nurses' Association. New RN examination based on nursing process. *The American Nurse*, 1982, *14*(3), 1.

36. Wald, F.S., & Leonard, R.C. Towards development of nursing practice theory. *Nursing Research*, 1964, *13*, 309–313.

37. Henderson, V. Research in nursing practice—When? *Nursing Research*, 1956, *4*, 99.

38. Wald & Leonard, *op cit.*, p. 311.

39. Suppe, F. Implications of recent developments in philosophy of science for nursing theory, in Fifth Biennial Eastern Conference on Nursing Research. Baltimore, University of Maryland, April 15–17, 1982, pp. 9–16.

40. *Ibid*, p. 14.

41. *Ibid*, p. 15.

42. Yura, H., & Walsh, M.B. *The nursing process* (3rd ed.). New York: Appleton-Century-Crofts, 1978, p. 76.

43. Lederer, K. (Ed.). *Human needs*. Cambridge, Mass.: Oelgeschlager, Gunn & Hain, 1980, pp. 2–3.

44. *Ibid*, p. 6.

45. Klineberg, O. Human needs: A social-psychological approach. In K. Lederer (Ed.): *Human needs*. Cambridge, Mass.: Oelgeschlager, Gunn & Hain, 1980, pp. 28–29.

46. *Ibid*, p. 6.

47. *Ibid*, p. 8.

48. Jahoda, M. *Current concepts of positive mental health*. New York: Basic Books, 1958.

49. Lederer, *op cit.*, pp. ix, x.

50. *Ibid*, pp. vi, vii.

51. Magi, N., & Allander, E. Towards a theory of perceived and medically defined need. *Sociology of Health and Illness*, 1981, *3*(1), 49–71.
52. *Ibid*, p. 50.
53. *Ibid*, p. 61.
54. Bonney, V., & Rothberg, J. *Nursing diagnosis and therapy—An instrument for evaluation and measurement*. New York: The League Exchange, National League for Nursing, 1963.
55. *Ibid*, p. 3.
56. *Ibid*, p. 6.
57. *Ibid*, pp. 8–15.
58. Yura, H., & Walsh, M.B. (Eds.). *The nursing process* (1st ed.). Washington, D.C.: The Catholic University of America Press, 1967.
59. Yura, H., & Walsh, M.B. *The nursing process* (2nd ed.). New York: Appleton-Century-Crofts, 1973.
60. Western Interstate Commission on Higher Education. Defining Clinical Content, Graduate Nursing Programs, Medical and Surgical Nursing, 1967, p. 6.
61. Buffington P.W. Intuitively speaking. *Sky*, Delta Airlines, 1986, *15*(4), pp. 127–132.
62. Minor, M.A., & Thompson. L. Nurse internship program based on nursing process. *Supervisor Nurse*, 1981, *12*(1), 28–32.
63. Kramer, M. *Reality shock*. St. Louis: Mosby, 1974.
64. Peplau, H.E. *Interpersonal relations in nursing*. New York: Putnam, 1952.
65. Hall, L.E. Quality of nursing care. Address at meeting of Department of Baccalaureate and Higher Degree Programs of the New Jersey League for Nursing. February 7, 1955. Seton Hall University, Newark, New Jersey. *Public Health News*, New Jersey State Department of Health, June 1955.
66. Johnson, D.E. A philosophy of nursing. *Nursing Outlook*, 1959, *7*, 198–200.
67. Orlando, I.J. *The dynamic nurse-patient relationship*. New York: Putnam, 1961, p. 26.
68. Wiedenbach, E. *Clinical nursing, A helping art*. New York: Springer, 1964.
69. Gowan, M.O. Administration of college and university programs in nursing, from the viewpoint of nurse education. *Proceedings of the Workshop on Administration of College Programs in Nursing*. Washington, D.C.: The Catholic University of America Press, 1944, p. 10.
70. Kreuter, F.R. What is good nursing care? *Nursing Outlook*, 1957, *5*, 302–304.
71. Donnelly G.F., & Sutterley D.C. From the editors. *Topics in Clinical Nursing*, April, 1986, *8*(1), v.
72. Leatt, P., Bay, K.S., & Stinson, S.M. An instrument for assessing and classifying patients by type of care. *Nursing Research*, 1981, *30*(3), 145–150.
73. *Ibid*, p. 145.
74. *Ibid*.
75. *Ibid*, p. 146.
76. Phaneuf, M.C. *The nursing audit* (2nd ed.). New York: Appleton-Century-Crofts, 1976.
77. Wandelt, M.A., & Stewart, D.S. *Slater nursing competencies rating scale*. New York: Appleton-Century-Crofts, 1975.

78. Little, D.E., & Carnevali, D.I. *Nursing care planning* (2nd ed.). Philadelphia: Lippincott, 1976.
79. Mayer, M.G. *A systematic approach to the nursing care plan.* New York: Appleton-Century-Crofts, 1972.
80. Chambers, W. Nursing diagnosis. *American Journal of Nursing*, 1962, *62*, 102–104.
81. Komorita, N.I. Nursing diagnosis. *American Journal of Nursing*, 1963, *63*, 83–86.
82. Levine, M.E. Trophicognosis: An alternative to nursing diagnosis. In *ANA Regional Clinical Conference.* New York: Appleton-Century-Crofts, 1965, pp. 55–70.
83. Durand, M., & Prince, R. Nursing diagnosis: Process and decision. *Nursing Forum*, 1966, *5*(4), 50–64.
84. Kelly, K.J. An approach to the study of clinical inference in nursing. *Nursing Research*, 1964, *13*, 314–322.
85. Kelly, K.J. Clinical inference in nursing—A nurse's viewpoint. *Nursing Research*, 1966, *15*, 23–26.
86. Hammond, K.R. Clinical inference in nursing—A psychologist's viewpoint. *Nursing Research*, 1966, *15*, 27–38.
87. Hammond, K.R., Kelly, K.J., Schneider, R.J., & Vancini, M. Clinical inference in nursing: Analyzing cognitive tasks representative of nursing problems. *Nursing Research*, 1966, *15*, 134–138.
88. Hammond, K.R., Kelly, K.J., Schneider, R.J., & Vancini, M. Clinical inference in nursing: Information units used. *Nursing Research*, 1966, *15*, 236–243.
89. Hammond, K.R., Kelly, K.J., Castellan, N.J., Jr., Schneider, R.J., & Vancini, M. Clinical inference in nursing: Use of information-seeking strategies. *Nursing Research*, 1966, *15*, 330–336.
90. Hammond, K.R., Kelly, K.J., Schneider, R.J., & Vancini, M. Clinical inference in nursing: Revising judgments. *Nursing Research*, 1967, *16*, 38–45.
91. King, L.S. What is a diagnosis? *Journal of the American Medical Association*, 1967, *202*, 154–157.
92. Gebbie, K., & Lavin, M.A. *Classification of nursing diagnoses.* St. Louis: Mosby, 1975, pp. 28–29.
93. Symposium on Nursing Diagnosis. *Nursing Clinics of North America*, December, 1985, *20*(4), 609–808.
94. McCloskey J.C. Research column: Nursing diagnosis research studies are of interest. *Nursing Diagnosis Newsletter*, Fall, 1986, *13*(2), 2–3.
95. Roy, C. A diagnostic classification system for nursing. *Nursing Outlook*, 1975, *23*, 90–94.
96. McCain, F. Nursing by assessment, not intuition. *American Journal of Nursing*, 1965, *65*, 82–84.
97. Aspinall, M.J. Nursing diagnosis—The weak link. *Nursing Outlook*, 1976, *24*, 433–436.
98. Gordon, M. Nursing diagnoses and the diagnostic process. *American Journal of Nursing*, 1976, *76*, 1298–1300.
99. Mundinger, M.O., & Jauron, G.D. Developing a nursing diagnosis. *Nursing Outlook*, 1975, *23*, 96.

100. Dossey, B., & Guzzetta, C.E. Nursing diagnosis. *Nursing 81*, 1981, *11*, 34–38.
101. *Ibid.*
102. *Ibid.*
103. *Ibid.*
104. Popkess, S.A. Diagnosing your patient's strengths. *Nursing 81*, 1981, *11*(7), pp. 34–37.
105. *Ibid.*
105a. Gordon, *op cit*, p. 1299.
106. Stolte K. A complimentary view of nursing diagnosis. *Public Health Nursing*, March, 1986, *3*(1), 23–28.
107. *Ibid.*
108. Mundinger & Jauron, *op cit.*
109. Gebbie & Lavin, *op cit.*
110. Stevens, B.J. *Nursing theory—Analysis, application, evaluation.* Boston: Little, Brown, 1979.
111. *Ibid*, pp. 50–60.
112. *Ibid*, pp. 60–66.
113. King, I.M. *A theory for nursing.* New York: Wiley, 1981.
114. King, I.M. *Toward a theory for nursing.* New York: Wiley, 1971.
115. *Ibid*, p. 18.
116. Torres, G., & Yura, H. The meaning and functions of concepts and theories within education and nursing. In *Faculty-curriculum development.* New York: National League for Nursing, 1975, pp. 1–8.
117. *Ibid*, pp. 5–6.
118. Ellis, R. Characteristics of significant theories. *Nursing Research*, 1968, *17*(3), 217–222.
119. *Ibid*, pp. 219–222.
120. *Ibid*, p. 222.
121. Gowan, *op cit.*
122. Kreuter, *op cit.*
123. Erikson, E.H. *Childhood and society* (2nd ed.). New York: Norton, 1963, pp. 247–251.
124. Kreuter, *op cit.*
125. Nightingale, *op cit*, p. 3.
126. *Ibid*, pp. 74–75.
127. *Ibid.*
128. Harmer, B., & Henderson, V. *Textbook of the principles and practice of nursing* (4th ed.). New York: Macmillan, 1939.
129. Henderson, V. *The nature of nursing.* New York: Macmillan, 1966.
130. Hall, *op cit.*
131. Hall, L.E. A center for nursing. *Nursing Outlook*, 1963, *11*, 805–806.
132. Peplau, *op cit*, p. 5.
133. *Ibid.*
134. Orlando, I. J. *The dynamic nurse-patient relationship.* New York: Putnam, 1961.
135. *Ibid*, p. 25.

136. Crane, M.D. Ida Jean Orlando. In J.B. George, Chairperson, the Nursing Theories Conference Group, *Nursing theories*. Englewood Cliffs, N.J.: Prentice-Hall, 1980, pp. 123–137.

137. Dickoff, J., James, P., & Wiedenbach, E. Theory in a practice discipline. *Nursing Research*, 1968, *17*(6), 545–554.

138. Bennett, A.M., & Foster, P.C. Ernestine Wiedenbach. In J.B. George, Chairperson, the Nursing Theories Conference Group. *Nursing theories*. Englewood Cliffs, N.J.: Prentice-Hall, 1980, pp. 138–149.

139. Wiedenbach, E. *Clinical nursing—A helping art.* New York, Springer, 1964.

140. *Ibid*, p. 17.

141. Bennett & Foster, *op cit*, p. 147.

142. Wiedenbach, *op cit*, p. 31.

143. Johnson, D.E. The nature of a science of nursing. *Nursing Outlook*, 1959, *7*, 291–294.

144. Johnson, D.E. The significance of nursing care. *American Journal of Nursing*, 1961, *61,* 63–66.

145. Johnson, D.E.: Patterns in professional nursing education. *Nursing Outlook*, 1961, *9*, 608–611.

146. Johnson, D.E., Wilcox, J.A., & Moidel, H.C. The clinical specialist as a practitioner. *American Journal of Nursing*, 1967, *67*, 2298–2303.

147. Johnson, D.E. Development of theory. *Nursing Research*, 1974, *23*, 372–377.

148. Johnson, D.E. The behavioral system model for nursing. In J.P. Riehl & C. Roy (Eds.), *Conceptual models for nursing practice* (2nd ed.). New York: Appleton-Century-Crofts, 1980, pp. 207–216.

149. *Ibid*, pp. 207–209.

150. Grubbs, J. An interpretation of the Johnson behavioral system model for nursing practice. In J.P. Riehl & C. Roy (Eds.), *Conceptual models for nursing practice* (2nd ed.). New York: Appleton-Century-Crofts, 1980, pp. 216–254.

151. *Ibid*, pp. 231–233.

152. King, I.M. *Toward a theory for nursing.* New York: Wiley, 1971.

153. King, I.M. *A theory for nursing.* New York: Wiley, 1981.

154. *Ibid*, p. 2.

155. *Ibid*, p. 4.

156. Orem, D.E. *Nursing: Concepts of practice* (2nd ed.). New York: McGraw-Hill, 1980, p. vii.

157. *Ibid*.

158. *Ibid*, p. 25.

159. *Ibid*.

160. *Ibid*, p. 6.

161. *Ibid*, p. 52.

162. *Ibid*, p. 83.

163. *Ibid*, p. 87.

164. *Ibid*, p. 202.

165. *Ibid*.

166. Rogers, M.E. *An introduction to the theoretical basis of nursing.* Philadelphia: Davis, 1970, p. 47.

167. *Ibid*, p. 54.
168. *Ibid*, p. 59.
169. *Ibid*, p. 65.
170. *Ibid*, p. 73.
171. *Ibid*, p. 132.
172. *Ibid*, pp. 96–109.
173. Travelbee, J. *Interpersonal aspects of nursing* (2nd ed.). Philadelphia: Davis, 1971, p. 7.
174. *Ibid*, pp. 12–13.
175. *Ibid*, pp. 130–155.
176. Roy, C. The Roy adaptation model. In J.P. Riehl & C. Roy (Eds.), *Conceptual models for nursing practice* (2nd ed.). New York: Appleton-Century-Crofts, 1980, pp. 185–186.
177. *Ibid*, p. 187.
178. *Ibid*, p. 181.
179. Paterson, J.G., & Zderad, L.T. *Humanistic nursing*. New York: Wiley, 1976, p. 3.
180. *Ibid*, p. 12.
181. Paterson, J.G. The tortuous way toward nursing theory. In *Theory development, what, why, how?* New York: National League for Nursing, 1978, p. 51.
182. *Ibid*.
183. *Ibid*.
184. Zderad, L.T. From here-and-now to theory: Reflections on "how." In *Theory development, what, why, how?* New York: National League for Nursing, 1978, p. 38.
185. *Ibid*, p. 39.
186. Paterson, *op cit*, p. 65.
187. Zderad, *op cit*, p. 45.
188. *Ibid*, p. 40.
189. *Ibid*, p. 48.
190. Levine, M.E. *Introduction to clinical nursing*. Philadelphia: Davis, 1969.
191. Levine, M.E. *Introduction to clinical nursing* (2nd ed.). Philadelphia: Davis, 1973.
192. *Ibid*, p. 1.
193. *Ibid*, p. 12.
194. *Ibid*, p. 6.
195. *Ibid*, pp. 6–12.
196. *Ibid*, pp. 26–30.
197. Levine, M.E. Trophicognosis: An alternative to nursing diagnosis. In *ANA Regional Clinical Conference*. New York: Appleton-Century-Crofts, 1965.
198. Esposito, C.H., & Leonard, M.K. Myra Estrin Levine. In J.B. George, Chairperson, the Nursing Theories Conference Group. *Nursing Theories*. Englewood Cliffs, N.J.: Prentice-Hall, 1980, p. 162.
199. Neuman, B. The Betty Neuman health-care systems model: A total person approach to patient problems. In J.P. Riehl & C. Roy (Eds.), *Conceptual models for nursing practice* (2nd ed.). New York: Appleton-Century-Crofts, 1980, pp. 119–134.

APPENDIX 1–A

FORTY-FIVE ENROLLEES IN 1967 CONTINUING EDUCATION SERIES AT THE CATHO-LIC UNIVERSITY SCHOOL OF NURSING

Name	Employment Position	Employment Location
Abram, Joyce, R.N. B.S.N.	Supervisor	Public Health Department Washington, D.C.
Beans, Jeannette, R.N.	Staff Nurse	Frederick Memorial Hospital Frederick, Md.
Bevard, Faye, R.N.	Instructor	Frederick County Board of Education Frederick, Md.
Calhoun, Virginia, R.N.	Head Nurse	Frederick Memorial Hospital Frederick, Md.
Chaney, Linda, R.N.	Staff Nurse	Union Memorial Hospital Baltimore, Md.
Coblentz, Janice, R.N.	Supervisor	Frederick Memorial Hospital Frederick, Md.
Colicchio, Gregorine, R.N.	Supervisor	Hadley Memorial Hospital Washington, D.C.
Conroy, Colleen, R.N.	Instructor	Johns Hopkins Hospital Baltimore, Md.
Covabey, Phyllis, R.N.	Instructor	Frederick Memorial Hospital Frederick, Md.
Daneker, Barbara, R.N.	Head Nurse	Union Memorial Hospital Baltimore, Md.
Demyen, Ruby, R.N.	Instructor	Hadley Memorial Hospital Washington, D.C.
Dillon, Edith, R.N.	Staff Nurse	Union Memorial Hospital Baltimore, Md.
Dobson, Frances, R.N.	Head Nurse	Veterans' Administration Hospital Washington, D.C.
Erdmanis, Shirley, R.N.	Supervisor	Union Memorial Hospital Baltimore, Md.
Galbraith, Jane, R.N.	Staff Nurse	Hadley Memorial Hospital Washington, D.C.
Gil, Anna, R.N.	Staff Nurse	Hadley Memorial Hospital Washington, D.C.
Habbert, Frieda, R.N.	Instructor	Perkins State Hospital Jessup, Md.
Hale, Christine, R.N., B.S.N.	Instructor	Frederick Memorial Hospital Frederick, Md.
Harler, Leonor, R.N.	Head Nurse	DeWitt Army Hospital Fort Belvoir, Va.

(continued)

FORTY-FIVE ENROLLEES IN 1967 CONTINUING EDUCATION SERIES AT THE CATHO-LIC UNIVERSITY SCHOOL OF NURSING *(continued)*

Name	Employment Position	Employment Location
Hawkins, Zella, R.N.	Head Nurse	Veteran's Administration Hospital Washington, D.C.
Hensen, Donna, R.N., B.S.N.	Instructor	Perkins State Hospital Jessup, Md.
Heyde, Helen, R.N.	Assistant Director Nursing Service	Union Memorial Hospital Baltimore, Md.
Jackson, Irene, R.N., B.S.N.	Instructor	Washington County Hospital School of Nursing Hagerstown, Md.
Jewell, Sr. Margaret Charles, R.N., B.S.N.	Supervisor	U.S. Soldiers' Home Hospital Washington, D.C.
Jones, Chrystie, R.N.	Supervisor	Freedmen's Hospital Washington, D.C.
Kemerer, Agnes, R.N., B.S.N.	Instructor	Washington County Hospital School of Nursing Hagerstown, Md.
Kisner, Ruth E., R.N.	Head Nurse	Frederick Memorial Hospital Frederick, Md.
Ledbetter, Ruth, R.N., B.S.N.	Supervisor	St. Elizabeth's Hospital Washington, D.C.
Mackey, Helen, R.N.	Head Nurse	Union Memorial Hospital Baltimore, Md.
MacDonald, Martha, R.N.	Supervisor	St. Agnes Hospital Baltimore, Md.
Marchall, Martha, R.N., B.S.N.	Supervisor	Visiting Nurse Association Washington, D.C.
McCarthy, Margaret, R.N., B.S.N.	Instructor	Frederick Memorial Hospital Frederick, Md.
Miller, Judith, R.N.	Assistant Head Nurse	Union Memorial Hospital Baltimore, Md.
Mossbury, Doris, R.N.	Instructor	Federick Memorial Hospital Frederick, Md.
Pensing, Sr. Mary Bernard, R.N., B.S.N.	Supervisor	U.S. Soldiers' Home Hospital Washington, D.C.
Poynek, Doris, R.N.	Staff Nurse	Visiting Nurse Association Washington, D.C.
Rickert, Elizabeth, R.N., B.S.N.	Instructor	Johns Hopkins School of Nursing Baltimore, Md.
Riley, Florence, R.N.	Head Nurse	Sibley Memorial Hospital Washington, D.C.

(continued)

FORTY-FIVE ENROLLEES IN 1967 CONTINUING EDUCATION SERIES AT THE CATHO-LIC UNIVERSITY SCHOOL OF NURSING *(continued)*

Name	Employment Position	Employment Location
Roberts, Betty, R.N., B.S.N.	Supervisor	St. Elizabeth's Hospital Washington, D.C.
Roche, Joan, R.N., M.S.N.	Head Nurse	Washington Hospital Center Washington, D.C.
Savage, Elizabeth, R.N.	Staff Nurse	Washington Hospital Center Washington, D.C.
Schuh, Mary C., R.N.	Supervisor	St. Agnes Hospital Baltimore, Md.
Row, Emma, R.N.	Charge Nurse	Washington Hospital Center Washington, D.C.
Welling, Patricia, R.N.	Staff Nurse	Washington Hospital Center Washington, D.C.
Winters, Sr. M. Patricia, R.N., B.S.N.	Supervisor	U.S. Soldiers' Home Hospital Washington, D.C.

Nursing's Human Need Theory

The nursing process is a designated series of actions intended to fulfill the purposes of nursing—to maintain the client's wellness—and, if this state changes, to provide the amount and quality of nursing care the situation demands to direct the client back to wellness, and if wellness cannot be achieved, then to contribute to the client's quality of life, maximizing his or her resources as long as life is a reality. Inherent in these purposes is the fulfillment and maintenance of the integrity of the human needs of the client as well as those of the family and the community. To fulfill these purposes, the idea of the nursing process and the development of its human need theoretical framework must be considered.

Many different theories from various disciplines are related to the nursing process. These include general systems, perception, information, communication, decision, and problem-solving theories. Only human need theory will be developed in this chapter, thus its title, Nursing's Human Need Theory. The reader is referred to the fourth edition of this text for treatises on the forementioned theories. Human need theory gives credence to the nurse's as well as the client's actions, providing a framework within which the nursing process can be analyzed and applied. In addition, this theory provides the broader framework or roots for much of the work of nurse scholars, whose efforts are directed toward the identification and development of nursing theory.

In the system of nursing, which comprises the nurse as a person and the client (person, family, or community) in interaction with each other to enhance the state of health from any point on the wellness–illness continuum, human needs and their satisfaction are the tangible focus for the human service called nursing (Fig. 2–1). Human need theory provides the theoretical substance and the knowledge base for the application of the nursing process and defines the territory for the practice of client-centered nursing. It is believed that the *preservation of, the fostering of, the maintenance of, and the facilitation of the integrity of all the human needs of the person(s) is the territory of nursing.*

The works of Maslow, Montagu, Alderfer, Combs et al., McHale and McHale, Klineberg, Mallmann, and Galtung provide the theoretical substance for the understanding of human needs and the motivation inherent in meeting these needs.[1–3,19,21] The earlier works of such persons as H. A. Murray, Bronislaw Malinowski, Laurence Kubie, G. L. Freeman, and Ralph Linton are acknowledged for their contributions to the development of human need theory.[4–8] Nursing's human need theoretic framework is grounded in these works.

Proponents of human need theory view the person as an integrated, organized whole who is motivated toward meeting human needs. A human need is viewed as an internal tension that results from an alteration in some state of the system. This tension expresses itself in goal-directed behavior of the person that continues until goal satisfaction (freedom from tension) is achieved.[9] A basic or vital human need is one that must be satisfied if the person or the group is to survive.[10] The

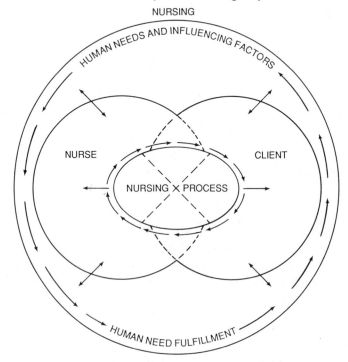

Figure 2–1. Human need theory framework for the interacting elements of the nursing system: nurse–client and the nursing process.

family, the neighborhood, the community, the state, the nation, and the family of nations are developed to assure the meeting of these human needs and to perpetuate humanity and its diversity. The nurse's role encompasses completely basic or vital human needs and their satisfaction for the nurse and the client, although the fulfillment of one or a selection of human needs poses problems for the client due to biologic, intellectual, emotional, social, spiritual, economic, environmental, pathophysiologic, and psychopathological affronts.

Preconditions to assure health and humanness include physical, chemical, biologic, psychological, interpersonal, and cultural conditions that either do or do not supply people with the basic necessities and rights that allow them to develop their strength and humanity to the degree that facilitates their assumption of self-responsibility. Maslow believes that the actualization of a person's full and real potential is further conditioned by the presence of parents and other persons who satisfy basic human needs, by ecologic and cultural factors fostering health, and by the situation in the world at large.[11] Health with all of its values, truth, goodness, and beauty is viewed as an attainable, real state.

A person is motivated by human needs for air, food, water, sleep, movement or activity, for safety and escape from danger, protection and care, freedom from pain, for gregariousness and affection, interdependence, love relationships, for respect, standing in relation to others, status with the consequent self-respect, and by the need for self-fulfillment and realization of the full potential of the individual (self-actualization). Self-actualization is confined to the adult. In addition, a person has cognitive needs for knowledge, curiosity, and understanding (philosophic, theologic, and ethical and value system). A person has aesthetic needs—beauty, symmetry, simplicity, completion, order—as well as the need to express and act out, and for motor accomplishment, related to these aesthetic needs.[12,13]

Maslow emphasizes the holism of the person when he states that most drives cannot be isolated or localized somatically, or considered as if they were the only things happening. "The typical drive or need or desire is not and probably never will be related to a specific, isolated, localized somatic base. The typical desire is much more obviously a need of the whole person."[14] From anthropological evidence, he concludes that "fundamental or ultimate desires of all human beings do not differ as much as do their conscious everyday desires."[15]

It is believed that it is normal for an act or conscious wish to have more than one motivation. Maslow believes that fundamental goals or needs, rather than a listing of drives, provide a framework for the construction of motivational life. "Human motivation rarely actualizes itself in behavior except in relation to the situation and to other people."[16]

Of course, consideration must be given to the person as an integrated whole in addition to the person's character structure. When *successfully* facing and experiencing a great joy, or a creative moment, or a problem, threat, or emergency, a person is considered to be most unified or most completely integrated. If the threat is overwhelming however, or if the person feels weak or helpless, disintegration rather than integration may occur.[17]

A person is motivated to gratify basic or vital human needs—to seek what is required for need fulfillment. A five-level hierarchical structure is used by Maslow to designate human needs with consideration given (from first to fifth level) to physical needs, safety needs, belonging and love needs, esteem needs, and finally to self-actualization. This contrasts with both the two-structure hierarchy specified by Montagu, namely, vital basic human needs and nonvital basic human needs, and the singular basic need approach proposed by Combs and colleagues. Listings of human needs and their categories having implications not only for the person but relating to the family as a household unit, the community, the state, the nation, and the countries of the world have been specified by such international human needs scholars as McHale and McHale, Mallmann, Nudler, Galtung, and Klineberg.[18,19]

Any number of fundamental physical needs may be delineated, with varied degrees of specificity stated. Generally, physical needs relate to air, food, fluids, sleep, rest, sex, exercise and activity, elimination, stimulation, excitement, and maternal response. These needs are relatively independent of each other and have a localized somatic base. These are comparable to the vital human needs delineated by Montagu, which include the need to inhale air, ingest food, take in liquid, rest, be active, sleep, urinate, defecate, and escape from danger, as well as a craving for internal equilibrium. Sex is not viewed as a vital basic need because a person can survive in perfect health without its satisfaction. But it is clearly a need that must be satisfied by some members if the group is to survive.[20,21]

The physical needs and the consuming behavior involved with their fulfillment serve as channels for other needs as well. These physical needs are viewed as the most influential of all needs in that if a person were lacking in food, safety, love, and esteem, that person would most probably hunger for food to a greater extent and more strongly than anything else. This is supported by Montagu in his explanation of basic human needs and their vital sequences. The physiological tension of oxygen hunger results in the need or urge to take in air, which leads to the act of breathing, resulting in oxygenation of tissues. This restores equilibrium, homeostasis. Or, the physiological tension of fright results in the urge or need to escape, which leads to the act of escaping from danger and results in relaxation. A person is dominated by physical needs; if these are unsatisfied, all other needs may seem nonexistent or be relegated to low priority. If a person is overcome by severe fluid loss and is thirsty or starving, all human capacity is directed toward restoration of normal fluid balance with effective replacement of affected electrolytes and toward obtaining food. Of these two needs, the need for water may, at times, be more pressing. The nurse will readily acknowledge these human states from personal or client experiences.[22,23]

Gratification and deprivation are important concepts in motivation theory. Higher needs emerge when physical or vital basic human needs are reasonably well satisfied. This is the reason for the organization of needs in a hierarchy, beginning first with the powerful physical or vital human needs.

Need fulfillment dominates human activity to the extent that the behavior of the person is organized only in relation to unsatisfied needs. For example, if sleep deprivation occurs and restful sleep ensues, the need becomes relatively unimportant in the dynamics of the person. Maslow points out that it is precisely those persons in whom a certain need has always been met or satisfied who are best equipped to withstand deprivation of that particular need at some future time. Persons who have been deprived in the past will respond differently to current need satisfaction than the person who has never been deprived.[24]

Safety needs emerge when physical needs are gratified. Safety needs include security, stability, dependency, protection, freedom from fear and anxiety, and structure. Montagu's specification of the need to escape from danger may be equated with the safety needs expressed by Maslow—freedom from fear. Safety needs incorporate the need for structure, law, order, limits, and the strength of a protecting person. These basic human needs encompass a person's current outlook of the world and philosophy of living, including an idea of what is in the future. In times of threat or danger, self-preservation and the need to assure safety and protection become paramount. At times, every other need appears to be less important. If a person is held at gunpoint by someone seemingly intent on causing fatal injury or if an infant is disturbed, dropped suddenly, hurt, startled, or handled roughly, little thought in these intense moments will be given to food, sleep, rest, and so forth. The reaction of infants to threat or danger is spontaneous, total, uninhibited, and, therefore, more obvious than in adults, who are expected to cover up this response.[25,26]

Human beings need undisrupted routine and rhythm. They thrive in a predictable, lawful, peaceful, and orderly world. They flourish early in life within the encompassing nurturing and protective function of parents and normal family settings. Disruptions within the family relationships due to quarreling, physical assault, separation, abandonment, divorce, or death may be especially devastating. Children, particularly, may respond with terror when confronted with new, unfamiliar, strange, and unmanageable stimuli and situations. All of us can recall the response of the child who becomes lost in a department store. The impact of hospitalization on children is well known to nurses. This impact is particularly devastating (perhaps even irreversible) if parents are either restricted by health agency policy, in terms of visiting hours, from participation in protecting, caring, and comforting, or separated by structures or partitions, room dividers, or lack of space, so that what is familiar, safe, and known from the child's viewpoint is restricted from view. This situation may be duplicated for aged persons who can no longer manage their affairs and are moved to unfamiliar environments. As will be noted later, this situation could contribute to the lack of fulfillment of love and belonging needs as well. Loss of the parental role of protection, new tasks, being confronted with strangers, uncontrollable objects, illness, and death are threats to the need for safety.[27]

Safety needs are expressed when a person seeks a peaceful, smoothly running, stable, good social system that provides a safe environment for its members—one protected from dangerous insects and animals, harmful organisms, odors, chemicals, and related substances, extremes of temperature, humidity level; one free from environmental, technical and criminal injury, and murder. This implies protection from a breakdown of authority. Safety needs are also expressed in a person's desire for a job with tenure and protection, an employment contract, desire for a saving's account, varying kinds of insurance, and a sound, reliable retirement plan. Safety needs dominate and are socially urgent during emergencies, wars, disease and injury (particularly brain injury), crime waves, kidnapping, hostage holding, strikes, mass rallies, protests and marches, and natural disasters, and during a breakdown of authority at the local, state, national, or international level. With any threat of chaos, human beings will regress from attempting to meet the highest level needs to meeting the suddenly more powerful safety, belonging, and love needs.[28]

Love and belonging needs emerge when physical and safety needs are reasonably gratified. These needs are expressed through a person's need for parents, a wife, husband, children, friends, colleagues, acquaintances. The absence of these is keenly and deeply felt. We strive for affectionate relationships, for a place within our culture, group, family. We will intensely strive to achieve these goals. Montagu's second category of nonvital human needs can be equated with love and belonging needs. He believes that if the person and the group are to survive, the need to be with others and the need for expression must be met. The fulfillment of these two needs is strategic if the person is to develop and maintain adequate mental health. The nonvital basic needs originate in the same kind of physiologic states as do the vital basic needs. Thus, the physiologic tension of the feeling of nondependency or aloneness leads to the need to be with others which, in turn, leads to the act of physical contact or association, which results in a feeling of security or interdependency. A person whose need for love and belonging is unmet can feel lonely, separated, ostracized, rejected, friendless, abandoned, and restless. This need is thwarted for children (sometimes with disastrous personal results) when the family moves too often, as well as from the disorientation of the general overmobility brought on by technological advances and industrialization. It is also thwarted for adults and children without roots, in a situation where their origin is despised, or when cut off from family, friends, neighbors (such as often imposed through institutionalization, and segregation in an intensive care, coronary care, or communicable disease unit), or when one is a transient, an orphan, a foreigner, a displaced person, or a newcomer rather than a native.[29,30]

Love and belonging needs are expressed through our desire for tenderness, affection, contact, intimacy, togetherness, and face-to-face encounters. They are expressed in the need to overcome feelings of alienation, aloneness, and strangeness brought on by the scattering of family, friends, and significant others. Maslow and Montagu believe that the thwarting of love and belonging need satisfaction is the core reason for maladjustments and severe psychopathology. Maslow points out that love is not synonymous with sex since sex may be viewed as strictly a physical need. In the true sense, sex behavior is multidetermined and multidimensional when viewed in relation to love and affection needs. Love needs involve both giving *and* receiving love.[31]

Esteem needs emerge with the fulfillment of love and belonging needs. A person has needs for a stable, firmly based wholesome self-evaluation and for respect and esteem of self as well as esteem for others. There is a desire for strength, achievement, adequacy, mastery, and competence. There is a need for a feeling of confidence in the face of the world, for independence, for freedom. A person has a desire for reputation or prestige (esteem from others), status, fame, dominance, recognition, attention, dignity, and appreciation. Fulfillment of esteem needs results in self-confidence; feelings of worth, strength, capability, usefulness, adequacy; and a willingness to be a contributor to society. Need deprivation results in feelings of inferiority, helplessness, weakness, and discouragement; when serious, it leads to compensatory and neurotic behavior. The respect sought by a person that results in a healthy self-esteem is the deserved respect from others rather than external fame, celebrity, and unwarranted flattery. Maslow states that it is helpful to distinguish the actual competence and achievement that comes naturally and easily based on the person's inner nature, constitution and biological destiny from that based on sheer determination, will power, and responsibility alone.[32]

Self-actualization completes the hierarchy of needs, as designated by Maslow, and means that the person is self-fulfilled. As noted earlier, self-actualization is confined to adults. Young persons grow toward self-actualization. Even if all needs are satisfied, discontent and restlessness soon develop again unless the person is doing that which he or she is suited to do. A person must be true to his nature (he must be what he can be). He must fulfill his purpose in the world. A person has a desire for self-fulfillment. Self-actualization emerges after prior satisfaction of physical, safety, love, and esteem needs.[33]

From Montagu's point of view, all needs are dependent and must be satisfied by some object(s) in a manner in which they are structured. The requirements of these needs are such that they enjoin the manner in which they must be satisfied if the person is to function as a *healthy whole*. Man's biologic nature—what man is—determines the direction that his development as a person must take. It gives a biologic validation to the principles of cooperation and love in human life. In this view, the values for human life are biologically determined and are not matters of opinion. Acting against these inherent values can disorder our lives as persons, as groups, and as nations in the world of human beings.[34] Maslow sketches a profile of the self-actualized person:

1. Healthy, polite, versatile, expressive, lets go when wishes to, can drop controls, inhibitions, and defenses when deemed desirable, can relate interpersonally on a deeper level.
2. Has self-control, can avoid hurting others, can have fun or give up fun.
3. Thinks of the present and the future, has a large array of responses and can move toward full humanness.
4. Efficient and superior in perception of and relations with reality, can see concealed or confused realities more swiftly and more accurately than others.
5. Superior in the ability to reason, to perceive truth, to make conclusions, to be logically and cognitively efficient, can discriminate between good and evil, means and ends.
6. Accepts self, others, nature; is natural, simple, and spontaneous.
7. Strongly focuses on external problems, is not a problem to self or generally concerned with self, has a mission in life, a task to fulfill, i.e., some outside problem that uses one's energies.
8. Displays a quality of detachment, of a desire for privacy, autonomy, independence of the culture and the physical and social environment, has the capacity for fresh appreciation of the

basic things of life, has a philosophical, nonhostile sense of humor.

9. Capable of intense peak or even mystic experiences (problem centering, intense concentration, self-forgetfulness, intense enjoyment of music, art, and sensations).

10. Able to feel an identification, sympathy, and affection for the human beings of the world (in spite of occasional anger, disgust, or impatience), has a democratic character, and a desire to be of genuine help to the human beings of the world.[35]

Characteristics of basic or vital human needs demonstrate a fixed order in the hierarchy of needs and the existence of unconscious degrees of relative satisfaction of these needs. Each need represents but one functioning aspect of the whole person. There is a cultural specificity and generality of basic human needs. People in different cultures have more similarities than differences. Differences tend to be superficial rather than basic or vital and are more related to the individual's conscious motivational intent.[36] People have always met the demands of their basic needs and of those needs derived from them by organizing into cooperative groups, using artifacts, and developing knowledge, values, and ethics. "Man's institutions are based fundamentally on the satisfaction of his basic needs, though the structure of his institutions is made up of those derived needs which rise out of the cooperative process of satisfying the basic needs."[37] It is well known that persons in different human and cultural groups "learn to make the same responses to their basic needs in a large variety of ways."[38] Basic human needs cease to play an active determining role as soon as they are gratified, i.e., a basically satisfied person no longer has needs for air, food, safety, love, and esteem. Higher needs (after long gratification) may become independent of both their powerful prerequisites and their own proper satisfaction. For example, an adult whose love needs were satisfied in early and past years becomes more independent than average with regard to safety, belonging, and love gratification. It takes a strong, healthy, autonomous person to withstand the loss of love and popularity.[39] When a person has satisfied higher level needs and values, that person becomes autonomous and is no longer dependent on lower need gratification.[40]

According to Maslow the arrangement of basic or vital human needs in a hierarchy is based on their state of power or strength. For example, safety needs are stronger than love needs because safety needs dominate when both are thwarted; physical needs are stronger than safety and esteem needs. Additional conclusions regarding the hierarchy indicate that the higher the level of need, the more specifically human it is, the less imperative for survival, the longer gratification can be postponed, the easier it is for the need to disappear permanently, and the greater the survival and growth value for the person. When the person lives at the higher need level, there is greater biological efficiency, longevity, and health; thus pursuit and gratification represent growth toward health and away from psychopathology. More preconditions and greater complexity of life require more outside conditions for higher need fulfillment. In addition, the value that is placed on higher needs is greater than that placed on lower needs when both are gratified. Satisfaction of higher needs is closer to self-actualization than is lower need satisfaction.[41]

A human being needs love. Once satisfied, this person proceeds to develop in his or her own unique style, using these universal necessities to his or her own personal purpose. This person's development proceeds from within, rather than from without, toward self-fulfillment and self-actualization.[42]

Clayton Alderfer developed and tested an alternative to Maslow's theory and to a simple frustration hypothesis of the problem of relating need-satisfaction to strength of desires.[43] His alternative theory is based on a conceptualization of three human needs—existence, relatedness, and growth (ERG). Alderfer did not assume the prerequisite of lower level satisfaction as a prerequisite for the emergence of higher-order needs as did Maslow. He did include propositions relating to the impact of higher-order frustration to strength of lower-order needs. Empirical tests of differential predictions among Maslow's theory, the simple frustration hypothesis, and ERG theory were conducted by a questionnaire study of 110 employees at several job levels at a bank. The results supported the ERG theory more than Maslow's or the simple frustration hypothesis. The simple frustration hypothesis read—"for any need, frustration results in increased desire, while satisfaction results in decreased desire."[44] Frustration and satisfaction were used to refer to opposite ends of the same continuum by Alderfer. ERG theory assumed that human beings strive to obtain their material existence needs, maintain interpersonal relatedness with significant others, and seek opportunities for their unique personal development and growth.[45] Existence needs include all the various forms of material and physiological desires with hunger and thirst representing deficiencies. Alderfer pointed out that a basic characteristic of existence needs is that "they only can be divided among people in such a way that one person's gain is another's loss when resources are limited."[46] Relatedness needs incorporate those needs which involve relationships with significant others. Significant others include family, co-workers, friends, enemies, and so forth. A basic characteristic of relatedness needs is that their satisfaction depends on a process of sharing or mutuality—mutually sharing thoughts and feelings. "This process markedly distinguishes relatedness needs from existence needs because the process of satisfaction for existence needs prohibits mutuality. The exchange of acceptance, confirmation, understanding, and influence are elements of the relatedness process."[47] Alderfer points out that formal power between two people need not be equal for relatedness need satisfaction to occur. "The essential conditions involve the willingness of both (or all) persons to share their thoughts and feelings as fully as possible while trying to enable the other(s) to do the same thing."[48] In addition, the outcome in satisfying relatedness needs may be positive as in an expression of warmth and closeness or negative in an exchange or expression of anger and hostility, an important part of meaningful interpersonal relationships. A sense of distance or lack of connectedness, not necessarily anger, is considered the opposite of relatedness need satisfaction.[49]

All needs which involve human beings making productive or creative efforts on self or environment are growth needs.[50] Satisfaction of these needs is dependent upon persons engaging in problems which require them to use their capabilities fully and may even require the development of additional capacities.[51] "A person experiences a greater sense of wholeness and fullness as a human being by satisfying growth needs."[52] Growth needs satisfaction depends on persons finding the opportunities to be what they are most fully and to become what they can. Alderfer stated that classification of human needs is not the same as explanation and prediction, "but some categorization (or variable definition) is necessary in order to formulate a theory."[53]

The propositions developed from ERG theory related to the format that the less a need is satisfied, the more it will be desired. For example, the less existence needs are satisfied, the more they will be desired. Then, the less relatedness are satisfied, the more existence needs will be desired. Then, the more existence needs are satisfied, the more relatedness needs will be desired, and so on.[54]

Alderfer concluded that a specific need in either category that is not being satisfied will result in that specific desire being heightened. Frustration of need fulfillment often increases motivation. No ordering of human needs among the separate and distinct categories were made by Alderfer. He did view the needs on a continuum in terms of their concreteness—existence needs most concrete, relatedness needs less concrete than existence needs, and growth needs the least concrete.[55] "The continuum from more to less concreteness is also a continuum from more to less verifiability and from less to more potential uncertainty for the person."[56] Alderfer used the term frustration regression to mean persons have a tendency to desire more concrete ends as a consequence of being unable to obtain more differentiated, less concrete ends. He uses the term satisfaction progression to explain when persons fulfill the more concrete aspects of their desires, more of their energy becomes available to deal with less concrete, more personal, and more uncertain aspects of living. "As he is able to fulfill existence needs, he needs to spend less of his energy in search of material things."[57] Alderfer applied classical aspiration level theory in formulating the propositions related to growth needs with the expectation that persons tend to raise their aspiration level when they reach self-determined goals and lower aspiration levels when they fail to attain their goals. Thus, growth needs, by their very nature, are intrinsically satisfying. The more a person grows, the more the person wants to grow. Conversely, the less a person grows, the less the person desires to grow. Research findings employed by Alderfer tended to favor ERG theory over the simple frustration hypothesis and Maslow's theory.[58]

Combs et al. propose a variation of the works of Maslow, Montagu, and Alderfer on human need theory. They have defined man's basic need, singularly, as a need for adequacy—a representation in the person of a universal tendency of all things. The expression of this tendency is comparable to the description of the need of self-actualization, self-fulfillment, or self-realization as expressed by others such as Maslow. It is believed by Combs et al. that this singular biologically determined fundamental need is a force within by which we continually seek to make ourselves more adequate to cope with life.[59] The need for adequacy stems from the characteristic of the universe, i.e., the maintenance and enhancement of organization. This basic need is expressed as the self of each person—that self of which he is aware and which he considers his personality.[60] A prime requirement for the satisfaction of the need for adequacy is a healthy body, which does the perceiving.[61]

Combs et al. state that the maintenance of the perceived self is each person's most crucial task. Each person seeks the development of an adequate self capable of dealing with life's circumstances effectively and efficiently now and in the future. The person constantly strives to meet a need for adequacy, i.e., the accomplishment of the adequate self, an adequate organization.[62] The core of the need for adequacy requires a view of motivation that is inherent in the person and not a problem of external manipulations or how one person influences another. Motivation is an internal force related to what a person is or has. It provides the direction, drive, and organization for functioning.[63]

Combs et al. view goals, values, and techniques as the ends and means to achieve need fulfillment. They consider the physiological, safety, security, and love and belonging needs specified by Maslow, Montagu, and others as goals, the achievement of which satisfy the fundamental need of the person for adequacy or self-actualization.[64] The most valuable techniques are those that maximize long-term need fulfillment for the person and society by contributing significantly to the enhancement of the persons and the groups represented.[65]

A person's perceptions contribute to his awareness. Thus, he does his best to fulfill his need for adequacy based on a perception of events at a given moment, be it a positive or negative perception. Thus, if the idea is accurate, blaming a person for a certain behavior is misdirected or even futile. The problem is not the need, per se, but the means to achieve its fulfillment. Negative acts or behaviors result when perceptions are incorrect. A negative response most likely seemed appropriate as a course of action at the time.[66] This point of view should be particularly helpful in facilitating interactional behaviors and outcomes for nurses whose practice involves encounters with numerous clients, colleagues, and co-workers and with the community of nurses-at-large.

Since the mid and late 1970s, interest in human need theory has taken on international significance. Scholars from varying nations have come together to develop a framework for action on meeting the human needs of the developed and developing nations of the world. The fruits of their intellectual efforts are summarized in the following paragraphs. They demonstrate the usefulness of human need theory to assure that individuals and collectives of individuals—the families, the states, and the nations of the world—have their human needs met. Using human needs as the framework for action, decisions that have international implications for the allocation of services and resources and for human need satisfaction would be more effective. These decisions would recognize and comply with the cultural heritage and diversity of the peoples of the world with the eventual goal of maximal satisfaction of the biosocial, psychocultural, and spiritual needs of human beings. In a report to the United Nations Environment Programme in 1977, Cleveland wrote that "basic human needs have 'arrived' " and ". . . the appearance of 'basic human needs' at center stage begins a new act in the continuing drama of world development."[67] He further indicated that during the years 1974 to 1977 a conceptual change occurred in national development strategies and in international and global negotiations: organizations realized, simply, that "the purpose of economic development and international cooperation is to meet the human requirements of people, and especially the minimum needs of the neediest."[68] McHale and McHale have invented a method of analysis that would operationalize the new imperative of meeting the basic human needs for the world community. This method attempts to set a minimum human need satisfaction by considering the diversity in climate, geography, access to resources, cultural and social tradition, stages of life, and time.[69] This method or framework recognizes that human needs may be individual (varying greatly in kind and quantity as the person moves through the life cycle); some relate to a family or a cluster of persons (termed a household unit) and some relate to the community and society-at-large. This global variation is not limited to human needs alone, but refers also to the resources to meet them. Resources vary greatly from place to place and country to country.[70]

The McHales, recognizing the interrelationships and dimensions of basic human needs for the world community, prescribed assessment approaches for the country/community, the family/unit household, and the life-style and have developed quantitative estimates of basic human needs of food, health, education, shelter, and clothing. Consideration included the extended services and support systems which incorporated energy fuels and materials supply, water and sanitation systems, transportation, communications, education and health facilities, construction, social institutions, and other dimensions which constitute the environment for working and living.[71] The McHales emphasize that personal and collective values have a powerful impact on the way human needs are defined and satisfied. They point out that in any interpretation of numerical calculations using data related to human needs, we can err on the side of misplaced concreteness if we do not take into account individual, social, and cultural diversity. The framework for action developed by the McHales includes (1) biophysical needs of food, health, shelter, and clothing; and (2) psychosocial needs encompassing education, employment, communication, mobility, recreation, security, self-realization, growth and development, and participation in social and cultural life.[72] These two categories of human needs are further subcategorized as (a) deficiency needs (mainly biophysical)—those threshold needs that must be maintained for survival; (b) sufficiency needs—those which should be met to maintain a standard of living at a desirable level, i.e., above marginal survival; and (c) growth needs—those above the minimum standard, the satisfaction of which allows the individual to develop above material sufficiency and to enjoy nonmaterial ends and aspirations.[73] Strategies for basic human needs must take into account the interdependency and comprehensiveness of the human needs rather than focus on one need at a time.[74]

Society emerges from the obligation to meet basic human needs on a larger scale, as nations determine the indicators for need fulfullment and need priorities. The family or unit household focuses more closely on individual human needs. The unit household may extend to the unit community and to extended kinship and other groups or settings more applicable in different cultural and social settings. The family more closely focuses on the human needs of the individual because these vary widely and are usually satisfied within a social context. The life cycle, which deals with the individual life span and with shifts in population cohorts, deals with the changing pattern of needs over time.[75] Consideration should be given to the influence of and demand for services based on the numbers of persons at different ages in the population.[76] These data would be particularly significant for the nurse who, in the course of professional practice, will make family and community diagnoses within the systems and human needs frame of reference.

Galtung, another international scholar who views the basic human needs approach as an indispensable ingredient for human, national, and international development, sees development as a process of satisfaction of more and more human needs dimensions and at progressively higher levels. He speaks of classes of human needs as security needs, welfare needs, identity needs, and freedom needs.[77] He, too, supports the belief that individual human beings develop their need consciousness in a social context and that most human needs are met there. ". . . Groups, cities, and countries do not have minds in which needs can be reflected or articulated." While human needs (material and nonmaterial) are located in and perceived by human beings, and the need-subject is a person, the term need can be used to refer to nonsubjects as national or community or social need. When basic human needs are not satisfied, some kind of disintegration takes place. As distinguished from the need-subject, a satisfier is produced in and by a social context and is dependent upon that context.[78] Galtung lists basic human needs as a working hypothesis using the four categories of security or survival needs (to avoid violence), welfare or sufficiency needs (to avoid misery), identity or closeness needs (to avoid alienation) and freedom needs or freedom to choose (to avoid repression) with their satisfiers. Readers will note the close relationship of these categories to the existence, relatedness, and growth categories of Alderfer. For example, identity or closeness needs include those for self-expression, creativity, praxis, work; for self-actualization, realizing potentials; for well-being, happiness, joy; for being active; for challenge and new experiences; for affection, love, sex; for roots, belongingness; for understanding social forces; for partnership with nature; for sense of purpose, meaning in life, closeness to the transcendental, transpersonal. Examples of the satisfiers for these closeness needs include jobs, leisure, recreation, the family primary group, secondary groups, political activity, natural parks, religion, ideology.[79] Galtung believes that a theory of needs should serve as a rich image of human beings and should demand that this richness be respected by social constructions. Further, human need theory can serve as a guide for warning of possible problems that result if priorities for need fulfillment are such that important classes of human needs are relegated to low or no priority for large sections of society and for a considerable period of time.[80]

Mallmann proposed a systematic approach to society, human needs, and rights. He defines need as the generic requirement for all human beings in order not to be ill, by the mere fact of being members of the human species.[81] He expands the definition by relating to vital needs as a group of independent needs whose satisfaction guarantees human beings the indispensable physiological and psychological vigor needed to live and to start to co-live, grow, and perfect. A satisfier is defined as an element whose use or consumption human beings require in order not to become ill.[82] Mallmann has developed a simplified, holistic, and systematic view of the dynamic interaction between human beings in a society and themselves and their political, social, and ecological environments.

Mallmann's human needs system includes a classification of needs according to the 24 following categories of needs: maintenance, protection, subsistence, love, security, existence, understanding, belongingness, autonomous participation, dignity, coexistence, recreation, development, creation, renewal, growth, meaning, transcendence, synergy, maturity, perfection, living, actualizing, and health. Mallmann then developed the classification of needs satisfiers according to personal (psychosomatic or intrahuman) and extrapersonal (psychosocial or interhuman, and psychoecological or extrahuman) categories. For example, for the need for maintenance, the personal satisfiers of nutrition, rest, and exercise are designated, the interhuman satisfiers of earning, work, reproduction, and social habitability are specified, and for the extrahuman, shelter, clothing, and physical habitability are included. Satisfiers, as such, were specified for all categories of human needs. The given and acquired structures of human beings were considered, as well as nature's innate structures. Mallmann believed that the study of motivational states and inherent structures of human beings and the dynamic interaction between these states and structures with the political, social, and ecological environments of society may be useful to analyze human needs and goals.[83] The measures of these objective conditions and their diffusion are a prerequisite to need satisfaction and are an important measure of the quality of life.[84]

Nudler views human needs as a dimension of the person as an open system and refers to this as sophisticated holism. The person is able to maintain identity throughout a process of exchange with the environment.[85] The maintenance of an identity—the most fundamental need of the person as a system—constitutes an achievement of the open system, in contrast to the alternatives of disorganization and death. The need to grow is the second most fundamental need. This need involves an increase in size, energy, and skills (physical and intellectual); however, it also implies differentiation, i.e., dividing into subsystems, and integration, i.e., connecting the subsystems and relating them to the environment. He states that the needs for identity and growth are characteristic of all living systems, but it is the third fundamental need, the need to transcend, that is a specifically human need. To transcend means to overcome the imbalance of man with nature. Nudler derives additional needs from these fundamental needs. From identity can be derived those of physical and psychological survival (food, shelter, affection, security, self-esteem, enjoyment, and meaningfulness); from growth stems the need to explore, to know, to be stimulated, and to have new and deep experiences; from the need to transcend arises the need to create, participate, love, mediate, and unite with nature.[86] The derived needs reflect the system to which a person belongs—the culture and natural environment as the larger systems; to the family and other primary groups as smaller systems. Nudler concluded that a satisfactory theory of human needs can only be constructed by studying the transformation that needs undergo in the subsystems of the person's system.[87]

Klineberg adds emphasis and specificity to the works of the previously cited international scholars. He states that social and cultural factors play an important part in the expression of biophysical needs. For example, relating to the need for food, social and cultural factors determine the kind of food eaten, the number and times of eating, with whom we eat and where, and the food taboos and restrictions imposed, particularly from a religious standpoint. These preferences are further complicated by dictates of subgroup and subcultures. He points out that need satisfaction must account for differences related to age, sex, socioeconomic status, occupation, and educational level.[88] Klineberg reminds us that a person is like all other persons as determined by a common human biological heritage or by universal features of social life; the person is like some other persons if that person belongs to the same cultural group or performs a similar role in society. Yet, the person is unique because no other person experiences the same sequence of human experiences.[89] What is regarded as lacking by a person should be accepted as a human need. What is needed is a criterion to identify those human needs that are more widely experienced. Regarding mental health, Klineberg points out a relationship of positive mental health with a satisfaction of human needs. The outcome is that if human needs are unsatisfied, strong feelings of deprivation or frustration may lead to aggression or resentment, to regression to a more primitive childlike level of behavior, to depression, or to various states of unhappiness.[90]

NURSING'S HUMAN NEED THEORETIC FRAMEWORK

Nursing's human need theory has its origin in the works of the international need scholars. Using deductive reasoning, 35 human needs were identified for use with the person, the family,* and the community—the clients of nursing. To facilitate use with the nursing process, the human needs were grouped as survival, closeness, and freedom needs. This grouping was adapted from the work of Johan Galtung and is particularly useful when applied to the family and community. No priority is used with the groupings.

The arrangement of human needs according to survival, closeness, and freedom needs groups is the following:

Survival needs (N = 15)	Closeness needs (N = 10)	Freedom needs (N = 10)
Activity	Acceptance of self and others	Autonomy, choice
Adaptation, to manage stress	Appreciation, attention	Beauty and aesthetic experiences
Air	Belonging	Challenge
Elimination	Confidence	Conceptualization, rationality, problem solving
Fluids (intake) and electrolytes	Humor	Freedom from pain
Interchange of gases	To love and be loved	Self-control, self-determination, responsibility
Nutrition	Personal recognition, esteem, respect	Self-fulfillment, to be, to become
Protection from excessive fear, anxiety, and chaos	Sexual integrity	Spiritual experience
Effective perception of reality.	Tenderness	Territoriality
Rest and leisure	Wholesome body image	Value system
Safety		
Sensory integrity		
Skin integrity		
Sleep		
Structure, law, and limits		

Nursing's human need theory was developed in the context of the four major concepts that comprise professional nursing, namely: *human beings, society/environment, health,* and *nursing.*[91] Definitions have been developed for the human needs and models have been constructed to explicate the theory. This modeling accounts for nursing's four major concepts and incorporates the schema for human needs. Propositions are stated, again reflecting the four major concepts, and the substance about human needs is explained. The goal of this theoretical effort is to enhance the professional nurse's ability to describe, explain, predict, and control nursing practice. The schema for nursing's human need theory is presented in Figure 2–2.

---

*The term family incorporates the prevailing forms of nurturing human beings bound by ties of blood and/or marriage as well as significant other persons.

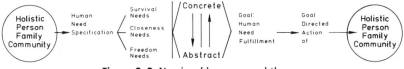

Figure 2–2. Nursings' human need theory.

This human need theory framework can be utilized with or within other broad theoretical frameworks, such as systems theory, and as a complement to other developing nursing theories.

While human needs may be defined and dealt with as discrete entities, the person is viewed holistically with the goal of nursing to foster the integrity of the person (Fig. 2–3). This analysis is academic in character and helps the nurse to view, care for, and care about the client from the appropriate perspective. There is less chance of overvaluing some human needs while ignoring others or erring in setting priorities for nursing interventions when human needs may be excessively or partially or fully unmet.

Human Being ⟶ Human Needs ⟶ Human Need Fulfillment ⟶ Wholeness

Figure 2–3. Holistic human being model.

Human Need Fulfillment. The state in which the person experiences satisfaction of human needs with the appropriate or target satisfier in a sufficiency to create a wellness state for the person as individual, family member, or community member.

Human Need Fulfillment Deprivation. A state in which the person experiences a partial or full lack of fulfillment with the appropriate or target satisfier for one or more human needs so that the deficiency creates a compromised wellness state or an illness state for the person as individual, family member, or community member.

DEFINITIONS AND DESCRIPTORS OF HUMAN NEEDS[92–98]

Definitions and descriptors for each human need were developed to be general yet specific enough to maximize their use in nursing practice. The descriptors provide additional detail stemming from the definition that portrays the variety of elements that could be considered. The combination of definition and descriptors presents a *word picture* for the nurse and the client. Selected data that describe fulfilled human needs appear in Appendix D at the end of the book.

Human Need for Acceptance of Self and Others, by Others

Definition: A receptive attitude toward self and others, and by others, which recognizes the value or worth of the person without implying approval of particular human behaviors and without implying affection.

Descriptors: Recognition of abilities and limitations; recognition of virtues and faults; feeling of contentment and satisfaction with one's self; experiences positive regard from others.

Human Need for Activity

Definition: A behavior or action requiring an expenditure of energy by the person with volition and intent.

Descriptors: Muscular action/organic functioning; a changed relationship between person and environment; organized response toward a specific result; purposeful use of memory.

Human Need for Adaptation, to Manage Stress

Definition: The harmonious accommodation of the person with changed demands in his or her internal and/or external environment resulting in a balanced relationship with these environments.

Descriptors: Adjustment poised for survival; response toward avoidance of undue tensions in one's life; coping with physical, psychological, social, economic, cultural strains; reconciliation; composure.

Human Need for Air

Definition: The intake of the mixture of gases, particularly oxygen, from the atmosphere through the nose and mouth to the alveoli and the transport of carbon dioxide and other excretory gases from the alveoli to the atmosphere.

Descriptors: Moisture; humidity; inspiration; expiration; condition and composition of air in the person's breathing environment; adequate air flow to communicate—talk, cry; structural integrity; pulmonary ventilation.

Human Need for Appreciation, Attention

Definition: The act of taking critical notice of and giving a determination of the quality, the value of the person.

Descriptors: Understanding and enjoyment; consideration; courtesy; thoughtfulness; response to another person's behavior; caring; cognizant of importance and uniqueness of person.

Human Need for Autonomy, Choice

Definition: Maintenance of ego-identity when making decisions and selections with independence from external control.

Descriptors: Relative lack of dependence on others; the right and the power to rule oneself; emotional independence; purposeful selection; conscious deliberation; knowledge of alternatives.

Human Need for Beauty and Aesthetic Experiences

Definition: The experience of pleasure or satisfaction arising from sensory manifestations or the mind.

Descriptors: Satisfying as to color, shape, sound, attitude, texture, design, pattern, tone, behavior, arrangement; lovely; concerned with pure emotion/sensation in contrast to the purely intellectual; artistic.

Human Need for Belonging

Definition: Being a part of, having a secure position in a group, as a family, of significant others, a community, a social/cultural group and having possessions, goods, or personal effects that are one's own.

Descriptors: One's place within the family, an occupation, an organization; a bonding with; membership; affinity; connectedness; close caring relationship; interrelatedness.

Human Need for Challenge

Definition: An act of striving to accomplish a goal through the expenditure of special effort or dedication.

Descriptors: Response to a call for a cause; action-oriented; make demands upon the imagination; take issue with; focused energy; thought provoking; stimulate.

Human Need for Conceptualization, Rationality, Problem Solving

Definition: The ability to grasp ideas and abstractions, to reason, to make sound judgments about one's life and circumstances, to resolve situational uncertainties, answer perplexing questions requiring solutions and resolution.

Descriptors: Acquisition and use of knowledge; decision making; induction; deduction; generalization; ordering of data; intellectual discrimination of facts and opinions; hypothesizing; critical thinking; understanding cues and responding.

Human Need for Confidence

Definition: The belief in the sureness, reliability of self and one's ability, other persons, and things.

Descriptors: Trust; certitude; assured expectation of experiences based on past similar or comparable experiences; having faith in oneself; self-reliance; consistency.

Human Need for Elimination

Definition: The removal, expulsion of the end products of metabolism from the urinary bladder and colon.

Descriptors: Food residues; gases and by-products; nitrogenous wastes; chemicals; drugs and toxic substances; urine; stool; flatus; fiber.

Human Need for Fluids (Intake) and Electrolytes

Definition: Taking in and utilizing water, liquids, and electrolytes to accommodate body function.

Descriptors: Intra-, inter-, extracellular fluid; diffusion and active transport; blood volume regulation; temperature regulation.

Human Need for Freedom from Pain

Definition: Exemption from superficial (skin, mucosa), deep (muscle tendons, joints, fascia, bone), and visceral and emotional discomforts which may be interrelated and interdependent.

Descriptors: Intact triggering and modulating systems; multiple receptors in body tissues—free nerve endings; pattern theory; gate control theory; protective stimulus signaling tissue damage; stimulus and response; individual differences in perception; comfort; absence of restraint in life work due to discomfort.

Human Need for Humor

Definition: The perception, the frame of mind to enjoy and express a sense of the clever, the funny, the comical.

Descriptors: Amusement; light heartedness and wit; recognition of the incongruencies and peculiarities in a situation; looking on the "bright side"; laughter; comedy; mood elevating.

Human Need for Interchange of Gases

Definition: The diffusion of oxygen and carbon dioxide at the alveolar level and the transport of oxygen in the blood to the tissues with the interchange and removal of CO_2 from the tissues through the blood circulation through to the alveoli.

Descriptors: Alveolar ventilation; arterial circulation; intact neurological respiratory-circulatory centers.

Human Need to Love and Be Loved

Definition: The experience of human energy given and/or received freely and honestly in the form of warm personal attachment and strong affection directly to self, God, parents and kin, spouse, children, significant others, friends and neighbors, the community of human beings; and reciprocated in kind.

Descriptors: Devotion; passion; charity; compatibility; adoration; affinity; erotic love; attraction; to hold dear; affectionate concern; friendship.

Human Need for Nutrition

Definition: The ingestion and assimilation of sufficient amounts of carbohydrates, proteins, fats, vitamins, minerals, trace elements, and fiber required for growth, repair, and maintenance of body function via structurally competent bodily parts.

Descriptors: Physical, psychological, religious, social determinants; eating habits; customs and beliefs; calories; food; actual body weight; skin fold thickness; age and gender requirements; energy input/output; hunger/satiation; feeding.

Human Need for Effective Perception of Reality

Definition: The act of comprehending by means of the senses or the mind, an experience or event as an actual, rather than imaginary occurrence of the self and the world around the self.

Descriptors: Deep and vivid impressions; understanding; excitation of sensory receptors; influence of person's life history; perceptual field; sensation; meaning of experience; visual, auditory, olfactory, tactile, gustatory, kinesthetic, visceral sensory modalities; intact sensory-perceptual system; awareness.

Human Need for Personal Recognition, Esteem, Respect

Definition: The experience of acknowledgment of achievement, worth, service, or merit, to be regarded favorably, with admiration and approval by others.

Descriptors: Reward; public honor; homage; reverence; high regard, approbation; to be looked up to; privileged position; favorable impression; experience of success.

Human Need for Protection from Excessive Fear, Anxiety, and Chaos

Definition: The act of shielding from danger or pain, from distress or uneasiness of mind caused by apprehension, by threat of danger or by misfortune, and from confusion and disorder.

Descriptors: Relief from foreboding or dread; order; organization; reduction of fright; lessened threat; secure; comfortable with self, surroundings/environment; at ease.

Human Need for Rest and Leisure

Definition: The experience of a period of restoration evidenced by limited activity or inactivity, repose, tranquility, mental and spiritual calm, freedom from the demands of role and responsibility.

Descriptors: Opportunity to enjoy nature, creative experiences, diversion, replenishment; self-determined inactivity; quiet; recreation; distraction; digression in focus of attention; relaxation.

Human Need for Safety

Definition: The experience of freedom from harm, danger or undue risk, injury, hazards involving the integrity of the body's structure, the environment around the person and its interpretation by the person.

Descriptors: Sense of an orderly, predictable future; lessened vulnerability; protection from susceptibility to alterations related to kinetic force, thermal energy, electricity, radiation, chemicals, microbes; integrity of defense mechanism; control of environmental factors of space, ventilation, light, cleanliness, sanitation, noise, weather; protection of the self.

Human Need for Self-Control, Self-Determination, Responsibility

Definition: The exercise of personal restraint, firmness of purpose and accountability for one's behavior and actions as a result of interaction between the person's internal powers of thought and emotions and the external forces in the physical and social environment.

Descriptors: Regulation of one's self; doing what one ought to do; deciding for oneself; accountability.

Human Need for Self-Fulfillment, to Be, to Become

Definition: The act of realizing one's ambition, desires, purpose in life through one's own efforts as knowing and understanding oneself and the environment in which the person finds oneself, then achieving one's potential and culminating in the fullest state of being for the person.

Descriptors: Self-understanding; goal-fulfillment; time-honored self-achievement; futuristic striving; personhood; striving for meaning; Creator's purpose for human beings; satisfaction; self-actualization.

Human Need for Sensory Integrity

Definition: The act of receiving and interpreting bodily and environmental stimuli through efficient sense organs for seeing, hearing, tasting, smelling, and touching and a complete and competent brain and nervous system.

Descriptors: Reception; acuity; intensity of stimuli; satisfaction of curiosity regarding self and the changing world around; self-protection; discriminate among sense data of differing intensity, extent, duration, position, temporal order and/or quality; impressions.

Human Need for Sexual Integrity

Definition: The state of integrated wholeness of one's maleness or femaleness with the physical, psychological, social, cultural, and spiritual self within a framework of dependence upon and interdependence with other persons.

Descriptors: Holistic being; self-expression; fulfillment of gender role and responsibility; sexual being; sexual attitudes, values, and beliefs; satisfying relationship; control of sexual self; procreation; family; intimacy.

Human Need for Skin Integrity

Definition: An intact and functioning covering of the person's body including the mucous membranes, which defends against harmful microbes; prevents water loss; regulates body temperature; provides sensory information; resists injurious substances, trauma, selected rays and waves and heat and cold.

Descriptors: Identity; dermis and epidermis; sweat and sebaceous glands; protection; touch/pressure; communication.

Human Need for Sleep

Definition: An organized behavior performed daily for a specified time in which a person experiences a suspension of voluntary exercise of bodily function, natural suspension of consciousness and in which one ceases to be awake.

Descriptors: Biological rhythmicity; dreams; REM sleep; NREM sleep; self-preservation; movement.

Human Need for Spiritual Integrity

Definition: An essential, nonmaterial element which inspires one to transcend the realm of the material toward one's ultimate end.

Descriptors: Belief in a Supreme Being; religion; experience of the holy; body-spirit interaction; inspirational influence; life or vital principle; faith development; religious belief system; determinant of the meaning of life; hope.

Human Need for Structure, Law, and Limits

Definition: A state of conduct in accordance with stated and learned principles which are sanctioned by one's conscience, natural law, God, and are within the boundaries of the rules, customs and practices of one's family, community, and culture providing a stable organized environment in which to live.

Descriptors: Protection; stability; authority; obedience; preservation of self and others.

Human Need for Tenderness

Definition: The state of being treated with consideration, gentleness, concern by others and reciprocation of this to others.

Descriptors: A gentle word; protective of vulnerable others; sensitivity to feelings of others; compassionate; caring; cherishing.

Human Need for Territoriality

Definition: The possession of a prescribed area of space or knowledge that a person denotes as one's own, over which the person maintains control, defends it if necessary, and receives acknowledgment from others of the identification of this space as owned.

Descriptors: Possession; defense against loss, violation, and devaluing of self; privacy; public and social distance; boundary/space; pattern of spacing.

Human Need for Wholesome Body Image

Definiton: The state of a positive mental representation of one's own body boundary and how it looks to others.

Descriptors: Body interior and exterior; body awareness; mirror image; physical and mental representation of self.

Human Need for Value System

Definition: An internalized designation of the importance of or worth of people, institutions, things, activities, and experiences in one's life.

Descriptors: Intrinsic desirability; judgment; set of beliefs, norms, and goals; intrinsic worth.

MODELS

A model is a representation of the structure of an idea or concept. Diagrammatically, the model demonstrates the relationship between and among concepts and facilitates logical consideration of the concepts. The concepts of human beings, society/environment, health, and nursing are diagrammed in Figures 2–4 through 2–7. These models visualize the core of nursing's human need theory.

PROPOSITIONS

The propositions developed about human need theory show how they impact human beings, society/environment, health, and nursing. Through these propositions, assumptions are made and relationships are stated that will serve to explain the practice of nursing. More specifically, the propositions direct the application of the triad of processes that comprise professional nursing—the nursing process, the leadership process, the research process. The end result is the validation of nursing's human need theory and the fulfillment of the purposes of theory, namely: to describe, explain, predict, and control professional nursing practice. The propositions are given in the following list.

Human Beings

1. Human beings are holistically integrated beings endowed with worth and dignity.
2. Human beings respond as total beings to life situations.
3. Human beings have human needs that must be met to achieve optimal wellness.
4. Human beings as adults are responsible for fulfillment of human needs for themselves.
5. Human beings determine the priority of their human needs for fulfillment.
6. Human beings' effort toward human need fulfillment is continuous throughout the lifespan.
7. Human beings' effort toward human need fulfillment requires modification to accommodate variables as growth and development, age, role responsibilities, gender, life-style, and knowledge acquisition.
8. A singular action by the human being toward human need fulfillment may meet multiple human needs simultaneously.
9. Human needs of human beings consist of 35 human needs which can be grouped as those relating to survival, to

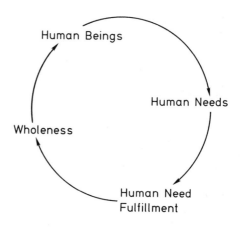

Figure 2–4. Model for human needs and concept of human beings.

closeness, and to freedom. Human needs may be concrete or abstract or have elements of concreteness and abstractness.
10. A human need of a human being can be studied from a physical, psychological, sociocultural, or spiritual focus or from any combination of these at a given point in time.

Society/Environment

1. The family,† the community, the state, the nation, and the community of nations exist to facilitate meeting the human needs of their membership.
2. The family is the primary unit for human need fulfillment of the person.
3. Human needs which cannot be met by the primary unit are assumed by other societal units as the neighborhood, the community, the organization, the state, and the nation.
4. The family takes responsibility for human need fulfillment for themselves as well as persons dependent upon them, e.g., infants, children, elders.
5. Societal/environmental dimensions as climate, geography, politics, economics, education, and socioethnocultural factors influence the manner, the mode, and the level of human need fulfillment for the person, the family, and the community.

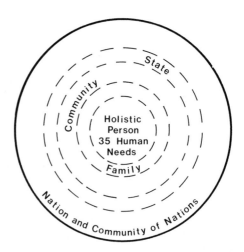

Figure 2–5. Model for human needs and concept of society/environment.

---

†The term family incorporates significant others.

Health

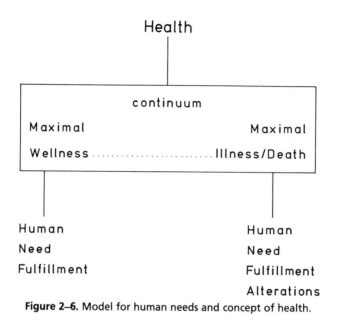

Figure 2–6. Model for human needs and concept of health.

Health

1. Wellness and illness are dimensions of the state of health viewed on a continuum.
2. The end points of the health continuum are maximal wellness to maximum illness or death.
3. The higher the level of human need fulfillment, the more *optimal* the state of wellness for the client.†
4. Clients may achieve their optimal wellness even though ill.
5. Human need fulfillment alterations contribute to a health status ranging from diminished wellness to maximal illness or death.
6. Human need fulfillment alterations occur when human needs are met excessively, when partially or fully unmet, or when there is a disturbance in the pattern of human need fulfillment.
7. The causes of human need fulfillment alterations can be categorized as personal/situational occurrences; environmental affronts; health-related therapies (commissions and omissions); pathophysiological states; psychopathological states; physiological miscalculation and/or nonacceptance; congeni-

---

†The term client incorporates the person, the family/significant other(s), and the community.

tal alterations (reparable, irreparable): philosophical, ethical, cultural, and religious impositions; social, economical affronts; educational/informational/knowledge deficits; growth and developmental alterations.

8. Subjective and objective data validate human need fulfillment and human need fulfillment alterations of the client.

9. The more concrete the human need, the more likely is the validation of human need fulfillment or its alteration by *objective* as well as subjective data in verifying the state of health.

10. The more abstract the human need, the more likely is the validation of human need fulfillment or its alteration by *subjective* as well as objective data in verifying the state of health.

11. The time interval for the human being's tolerance of human need fulfillment alterations may range from minutes for some and days, weeks, months and years for others.

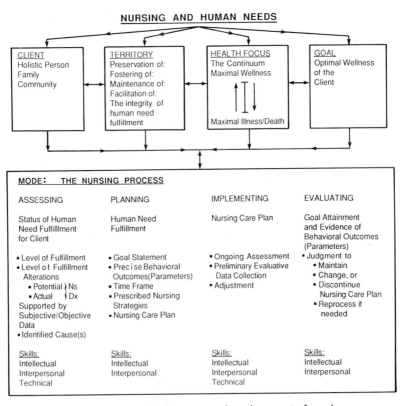

Figure 2–7. Model for human needs and concept of nursing.

Nursing

1. The nurse participates with clients§ in the wellness and illness dimensions of the health continuum.
2. The goal of nursing is the achievement of optimal wellness for the client.
3. Optimal wellness is achieved through fulfillment of 35 human needs of the client.
4. The preservation of, the fostering of, the maintenance of, and the facilitation of the integrity of human need fulfillment of the client is the territory of nursing.
5. The goal of nursing is achieved through the utilization of the nursing process.
6. The nurse and the client are partners in the application of the nursing process.
7. The nurse accommodates that the client responds as a total being to life situations through utilization of the nursing process.
8. The nurse uses the 35 human needs as the framework for assessing, planning, implementing, and evaluating nursing care for the client.
9. The nurse verifies the human needs that are met for the client during application of the nursing process.
10. The nurse verifies the human needs that are excessively met, or partially or fully unmet, or have a disturbance in the pattern of fulfillment for the client during application of the nursing process.
11. Human needs that are excessively met, partially or fully unmet, or have a disturbance in pattern of fulfillment for the client are termed nursing diagnoses.
12. Nursing diagnoses are verified on completion of the assessment phase of the nursing process and may be termed actual or potential.

    - subjective and objective data constitute the bases in designating human needs as met and/or with fulfillment aterations.
    - cause(s) of human need fulfillment alterations is determined and the nature of the cause(s) impacts the outcomes for the client.

13. The goal expectation resulting from nursing intervention is the client's human need(s) in the fulfilled or met state.

---

§The term client incorporates the person, family/significant other(s), and the community.

14. The client goal with behavioral/outcome criteria or parameters constitute the focal point for the prescription of nursing strategies and the evaluation of their effectiveness.
15. Prescribed nursing strategies incorporate support for and maintenance of human needs that are fulfilled and offset existing fulfillment alterations.
16. A singular action by the nurse toward human need fulfillment for the client may result in meeting multiple human needs simultaneously.
17. The nurse's effort toward the client's human need fulfillment reflects accommodation of the variables as level of growth, stage of development, age, gender, role, life-style, and level of knowledge acquisition.
18. Evaluation of outcomes resulting from the application of the nursing process is always in client terms.
19. The nurse validates that a particular human need of the client may be viewed as having a physical, a psychological, a sociocultural, or a spiritual focus or any combination at a given point in time.

Propositions will be validated by the research and practice of professional nurses and thereby verify the theory.

CONCLUSION

Designated human needs form the substance of nursing's human need theory and the arena for the practice of nursing. They are the tangible components for the use of the nursing process and for efforts toward a coordinated holistic approach to the client. These needs and their maintenance and integrity relate to physical, emotional, intellectual, social, cultural, and spiritual dimensions of the client. They are vital to the development of the person, to the family, and to society-at-large. Human needs range from those that are life sustaining to those that enhance the way we live with ourselves and others. They can be grouped as survival needs, closeness needs, and freedom needs.

Framed by the four major concepts (presently considered nursing's metaparadigm), definitions, models, and propositions were specified for nursing's human need theory. The theory is operationalized by the nursing process. Through the nursing process, the nurse supports, fosters, facilitates, and intervenes with well or ill clients to fulfill their human needs, achieving an optimal level of wellness. The ease, utility, and vitality of nursing's human need theory will be seen when incorporated within each of the components of the nursing process developed in Chapter 3.

REFERENCES

1. Maslow, A. *Motivation and personality*. New York: Harper & Row, 1970.
2. Montagu, A. *The direction of human development*. New York: Hawthorn, 1970.
3. Combs, A., Richards, A.C., & Richards, F. *Perceptual psychology: A humanistic approach to the study of persons*. New York: Harper & Row, 1976, p. 52.
4. Murray, H.A. (Ed.). *Explorations in personality*. New York: Oxford University Press, 1938.
5. Malinowski, B.A. *Scientific theory of culture*. Chapel Hill, N.C.: University of North Carolina Press, 1944.
6. Kubie, L. Instincts and homeostasis. *Psychosomatic Medicine*. 1948, *10*, 15–30.
7. Freeman, G.L. *The energetics of human behavior*. Ithaca, N.Y.: Cornell University Press, 1948.
8. Linton, R. *The cultural background of the personality*. New York: Appleton-Century, 1945.
9. Montagu, *op cit*, p. 113.
10. Montagu, A. *On being human*. New York: Hawthorn, 1966, p. 49.
11. Maslow, *op cit*, p. xxv.
12. *Ibid*, p. 2.
13. Montagu, *op cit*, p. 117.
14. Maslow, *op cit*, p. 20.
15. *Ibid*, p. 22.
16. *Ibid*, pp. 26, 28.
17. *Ibid*, p. 29.
18. McHale, J., & McHale, M. *Basic human needs: A framework for action*. New Brunswick, N.J.: Transaction Books, 1978.
19. Lederer, K. (Ed.). *Human needs*. Cambridge, Mass.: Oelgeschlager Gunn & Horn, 1980.
20. Maslow, *op cit*, pp. 36–38.
21. Montagu, *On being human*, p. 50.
22. Maslow, *op cit*, pp. 36–37.
23. Montagu, *On being human*, pp. 50–51.
24. Maslow, *op cit*, p. 38.
25. *Ibid*, p. 39.
26. Montagu, *The direction of human development*, p. 117.
27. Maslow, *op cit*, pp. 40–41.
28. *Ibid*, p. 41.
29. *Ibid*, p. 43.
30. Montagu, *op cit*, p. 51.
31. Maslow, *op cit*, pp. 44–45.
32. *Ibid*, pp. 45–46.
33. *Ibid*, p. 46.
34. Montagu, *op cit*, p. 52.
35. Maslow, *op cit*, pp. 137, 153–154, 159, 160–165, 168–171.
36. *Ibid*, pp. 51–57.

37. Montagu, *op cit*, p. 133.
38. *Ibid*, p. 134.
39. Maslow, *op cit*, pp. 57–58.
40. *Ibid*, p. 72.
41. *Ibid*, pp. 97–100.
42. *Ibid*, p. 135.
43. Alderfer, C. An empirical test of a new theory of human needs. *Organizational Behavior and Human Performance*, 1969, *4*, 142–175.
44. *Ibid*, p. 143.
45. *Ibid*, p. 145.
46. *Ibid*.
47. *Ibid*, p. 146.
48. *Ibid*.
49. *Ibid*.
50. *Ibid*.
51. *Ibid*, p. 147.
52. *Ibid*.
53. *Ibid*.
54. *Ibid*, p. 148.
55. *Ibid*, p. 150–151.
56. *Ibid*, p. 151.
57. *Ibid*, pp. 151–152.
58. *Ibid*, p. 173.
59. Combs, *op cit*, p. 57.
60. *Ibid*, p. 54.
61. *Ibid*, p. 80.
62. *Ibid*, pp. 56–57.
63. *Ibid*, p. 64.
64. *Ibid*, p. 133.
65. *Ibid*, p. 151.
66. *Ibid*, p. 68.
67. McHale, *op cit*, p. 3.
68. *Ibid*.
69. *Ibid*, p. 15.
70. *Ibid*, pp. 16, 18, 19.
71. *Ibid*, p. 22.
72. *Ibid*, p. 30.
73. *Ibid*, pp. 30–31.
74. *Ibid*, p. 31.
75. *Ibid*, pp. 39–40.
76. *Ibid*, p. 52.
77. Lederer, *op cit*, pp. 58, 59.
78. *Ibid*, pp. 60. 62.
79. *Ibid*, p. 66.
80. *Ibid*, pp. 69–70.
81. *Ibid*, p. 37.
82. *Ibid*, p. 38.
83. *Ibid*, pp. 45–46.

84. *Ibid*, p. 53.

85. *Ibid*, p. 143,

86. *Ibid*, p. 146.

87. *Ibid*, p. 148.

88. *Ibid*, p. 27.

89. *Ibid*, p. 28.

90. *Ibid*, p. 33.

91. Torres, G., & Yura, H. *Today's conceptual framework: Its relationship to the curriculum development process*. New York: National League for Nursing, 1974.

92. English, H., & English, A.C. *A comprehensive dictionary of psychological and psychoanalytical terms*. New York: D. McKay Co., Inc., 1958.

93. Guralnik, D. (Ed.). *Webster's New World Dictionary of the American Language*. 2nd college edition. New York: William Collins and World Publishing Co., Inc., 1978.

94. Mitchell. G.D. *A new dictionary of sociology*. London: Routledge and Kegan, Paul, 1968.

95. Stein, J. (Ed.). *The Random House Dictionary of the English Language*. Unabridged Edition. New York: Random House, 1973.

96. Yura, H., & Walsh, M.B. *Human needs and the nursing process*. New York: Appleton-Century-Crofts, 1978.

97. Yura, H., & Walsh, M.B. *Human needs 2 and the nursing process*. E. Norwalk, Conn.: Appleton-Century-Crofts, 1982.

98. Yura, H., & Walsh, M.B. *Human needs 3 and the nursing process*. E. Norwalk, Conn.: Appleton-Century-Crofts, 1983.

3

Components of the Nursing Process

The maintenance of the integrity and fulfillment of human needs to assure optimal wellness comprises the territory for nursing practice. Nursing is concerned with all of the human needs of the client viewed as the person, the family, and the community and fosters the meeting of these needs. When one or more needs are not met owing to psychopathophysiology, immaturity, or lack of knowledge or resources, the nurse intervenes to offset the lack of need fulfillment as well as to assure the maintenance of the integrity of all other human needs of the client. Health care colleagues may focus on selected unmet or partially met needs, designating the pathological basis for the unmet status and prescribing medical or related therapies to eliminate or diminish the source of the problem. The nurse may refer selected unmet needs to appropriate health care colleagues such as the physician, the clergyman, the social worker, or the dentist, and will collaborate with this person(s) as long as is needed. The nurse views clients in their wholeness, as part of a family and a neighborhood, to assure that all needs continue to be met despite the lack of fulfillment of one or more needs. Thus, the nurse is involved in preserving both the wellness of the person and the healthy aspects of the ill person, continually seeking optimal enhancement of wellness and diminution of illness. He or she is involved with the health and welfare of the family and the community as clients.

The nursing process is the designated series of actions intended to fulfill the purposes of nursing, i.e., to maintain the client's optimal wellness, and, if this state changes, to provide the amount and quality of nursing care the situation demands to direct the client back to wellness. If wellness cannot be achieved, then the nursing process should contribute to the client's quality of life, maximizing the client's resources to achieve the highest quality of living possible for as long as possible. The nursing process applies to the family and the community as well. The four components of the nursing process are: *assessing, planning, implementing,* and *evaluating.*

PREPROCESS

To conduct the nursing process, a minimum of two persons (the client and the nurse) is necessary. Usually more than two persons are significant to the client or nurse, or both, in a given situation. The number of interacting persons increases significantly when the client is the family or the community. As the number of persons increases in a situation, the complexity of the situation increases. Each person in the situation brings unique experiences and attributes to the encounter that is nursing, and it is these variables that alter, modify, simplify, or complicate each event experienced in an encounter.

As the nurse prepares to initiate the process of nursing, he or she considers the health status of the client (well or ill) by asking him or herself such questions as: What experiences does the client bring to this situation? What knowledge does the client possess and lack? Which strengths will help the client cope? In what situations will the client be dependent on others, independent, interdependent?

Initiating the process of nursing requires a consideration of the status of the nurse as well as that of the client; for example, the nurse asks him or herself, What approach will be the best to use for this client? How can I most efficiently and effectively set the stage for the provision of nursing? What assistance will I need, and from whom, to best care for this client? When will use of intuition be useful as an adjunct to the nursing process?

Within this framework the nurse anticipates the initiation of the nursing process and prepares for a productive client–nurse encounter. The tone of the meeting will be established by the degree of interest and trust that can be communicated to the client at the outset of the process. Greeting the client and introducing the nurse are amenities that are expected but sometimes overlooked. Through a deliberate approach to the nursing process the following preprocess expectations are achieved:

1. Establishment of a degree of trust between client and nurse.
2. Definition of the roles the nurse and client will play in the client's care.
3. An opportunity for the client to voice initial fears, raise pressing questions, begin to feel a degree of comfort in the client role.

4. A positive environment in which to permit successful pursuit of the nursing process.

Whether or not the nurse accomplishes these identified expectations prior to the initiation of or within the nursing process, is not so important as the nurse's awareness that their accomplishment is necessary to pursue the nursing process effectively. In some instances pursuit of the preprocess goals enables the process to be initiated with increased ease; in other situations, it is easier to incorporate these preprocess goals within the assessment phase of the nursing process.

Based on its framework, drawn from nursing's human need theory, each component or phase of the nursing process will be developed and analyzed, according to the persons, both nurses and clients, involved in the process. The goal of analysis will be to suggest nursing actions appropriate to the components of the process, considering such human factors as cultural background, age, level of wellness, degree of illness, as well as socioeconomic and educational levels. The unique aspect of each component as well as the interrelationships among components are considered. The components of the nursing process follow a logical progression, but two or more may be operational at the same time. The time span for using the process will vary with the client's situation and may portray immediate and long-term results.

The nurse and the client are viewed as partners in nursing, a subsystem of the health care system. Each person is viewed as a unique member of the family and the community—units of a social system. The family as a unit can be the client as can the community—an aggregate of persons, families, and groups unified with the goal of meeting human needs for the constituents. In addition to human need theory, the nurse draws heavily on perception, communication, and decision-making theories in his or her use of the nursing process. The clients utilize these skills in their roles by participating in their care.

The Four Components of the Nursing Process

The four phases or components of the nursing process (*assessing, planning, implementing,* and *evaluating*) used in this text are useful and inclusive and are utilized by the majority of practitioners of nursing. The nursing process is systematized, appropriate for the well person or the family or for the acutely or chronically ill according to the situation. It can be used by nurse practitioners in whatever setting the client as the person, the family, the community is found. It is important for the nurse to designate the client's wellness state as well as the client's actual and potential problems. There is a cyclic nature to the nursing process, and the movement is continuous between and among its components (Fig. 3–1).

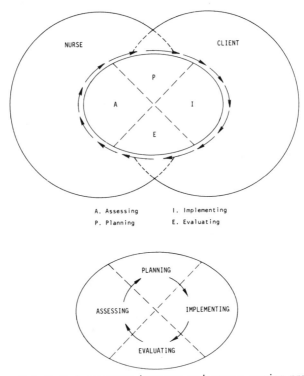

A. Assessing   I. Implementing
P. Planning   E. Evaluating

Figure 3–1. Cyclical movement between and among nursing process components.

The skills the nurse must have to use the nursing process are intellectual, interpersonal, and technical. Intellectual skills entail problem solving, critical thinking, and making nursing judgments. Interpersonal skills are related to the ability to communicate, listen, and convey interest, compassion, knowledge, and information, and to obtain needed data in a manner that enhances the individuality of the client as a person, the integrity of the family, and contributes to the viability of the community. These skills foster relationships with the client and the client's family, co-workers, and community members. Technical skills relate to methods, procedures, and the use of equipment to collect data and to bring about specific results or the desired behavioral responses of the client. Decisions and decision making are a part of every component.

Involvement in the nursing process assumes concern for persons, families, groups, and communities. To engage successfully in this process, the nurse and client must be aware of the following pertinent premises that apply to both.

statements / assumptions

The Client

1. Limitations in physical, emotional, spiritual, social, and economic capability and in the availability of resources impact human need fulfillment for the client and may cause problems when human needs are excessively met, partially or fully unmet, or there is a disturbance in pattern of fulfillment.
2. Inability to fulfill one's human needs may entail the intervention of another individual who can help a person fill those needs or fill the needs directly until such a time as the person can resume that responsibility unassisted.
3. Persons or families presenting themselves for health care desire a client-centered approach that enhances their value.
4. The person or family demonstrate a willingness to share information, feelings, and concerns so that their efforts to achieve optimal wellness will be realized and any problems can be identified and solutions sought.
5. When the human need framework is applied to the family and the community as clients in contrast to its use for the person as client, the reason for the fulfillment or alteration in need fulfillment differs as do the satisfiers for the human need. Data about the community are drawn from demography; census outcomes; morbidity and mortality rates; agriculture, business and industry; and educational, cultural, religious, social, legal, political, and social institutions and services.
6. Every citizen has the right to quality health and nursing care rendered with interest, competence, and compassion.

The Nurse

1. The nurse is interested in rendering high quality service to persons and families, no matter what their life-style, economic status, or cultural or religious beliefs might be.
2. To utilize the nursing process and develop goal-directed nursing care plans the nurse must have up-to-date knowledge of theories from the physical, biologic, social, behavioral, and nursing sciences.
3. The practice of nursing involves the ability to focus on another person(s) and requires the full attention and energy of the nurse when engaged in the practice of nursing.
4. Communication with the client is a necessary and continuous activity which permeates every aspect of the nursing process.
5. The heart of the nurse–client interaction is the development of a helping relationship in which the nurse fosters the client's personal development and growth by means of empathetic under-

standing, faith in the client's growth potential, respect and care for and about the client in an unconditional manner, willingly being available, and freely being one's genuine self.

6. Successful nursing practice results from continued study, both formal and informal, and from an ongoing self-evaluation of one's development and nursing practice, with plans to maximize strengths and minimize limitations.

7. The nurse strives to realize his or her own self-development through the practice of nursing.

8. Nurse practitioners focus on *preventing disease, maintaining wellness,* and *rendering care* to the sick and disabled, for persons, families, and groups of persons and families.

ASSESSING

Assessing is the act of reviewing a human situation from a data base in order to affirm the wellness state and diagnose potential client problems; to affirm an illness state, diagnosing the client's prevailing problems; determining the potential for problems; and identifying the wellness aspects of the ill client. The purpose of this phase is to identify and obtain the data about the client utilizing the framework of the 35 human needs specified in Chapter 2.

The assessment phase begins with the taking of the nursing history and the performance of a health assessment and ends with the verification of the wellness or illness state and the designation of the potential or actual nursing diagnoses. Both the nurse and the client or the client's family designate problems relating to wellness and illness. If potential or actual problems, or both, exist, then the first step toward a solution is to identify them.

The nurse's function is to assess the extent of human need fulfillment for the client as the basis for designating the client's place on the wellness–illness continuum. Human needs refer to those that all people must satisfy to enhance their image of themselves as persons. When these needs are considered as a totality, they provide a holistic, unified approach to the study of human beings and care of clients for the nurse. In contrast to goals of other members of the health profession, the nurse is involved with human needs that affect the *total* person rather than one aspect, one problem, or a limited segment of need fulfillment. The objective is to enable the meeting of *all* human needs. The nurse will try to foster satisfaction of the human needs for each person individually. In viewing the person holistically, consideration is given to the person's uniqueness, and the variation that characterizes the person's patterns of action, self-awareness, and view of others. The person is part of a family or group of significant others. The family, in turn, is a unit of the larger society—a neighborhood, a community, a state, a nation.

Inherent in the idea that each person is unique is the acceptance of one's own individuality. Nurses must first understand their own strengths, limitations, patterns of response, views, and values, before they can be receptive to and accept those of clients. A nurse's ability to assess and deal with his or her own behavior and that of the client presupposes a knowledge of human behavior. The nurse, as the helping person, must be willing to understand clients from their own frames of reference. The nurse senses and seeks to understand what is real and meaningful to clients at any point in time and must know how clients see things or feel about themselves. The nurse is sensitive to clients' conscious feelings and the meanings underlying outward communication. The nurse maintains a clear distinction between meaning that originates in him or herself and that which originates in the client. The nurse attempts to understand these meanings at a particular moment with the idea that this understanding is subject to correction and change as new data become available. Caring for and about the client is unqualified; that is, no conditions are attached to it. The client does not need to earn approval or liking by expressing some desires and suppressing others, by portraying certain attitudes or beliefs and denying others, or by being one type of person and not another. These beliefs are conveyed to clients during all phases of the nursing process. Efforts to establish a helping relationship begin with the first nurse–client interaction, at the time the client enters the health care system, and it continues as long as this interaction is needed.

At times of stress, crisis, or illness, problems may arise in meeting some or all of these needs. Illness does not mean that these human needs do not have to be satisfied; in fact, it may create heavier demands for fulfilling particular needs; the way in which they would be met; or even by whom they would be met and when. Physiologically oriented (survival) needs must be met in preference to others only when their deprivation is life threatening. As soon as the threat diminishes, attention must be paid to other human needs. Factors that influence human needs and their satisfiers include age and gender; intellectual, emotional, educational, social, and financial capability; level of wellness or illness; type, location, and extent of pathophysiology or psychopathology, or both; and the type, availability, and effectiveness of the therapeutic regimen.

It is not possible to separate a person into his or her physical, psychological, emotional, spiritual, educational, social, and cultural aspects. This is attempted academically, but in reality, a person is a unified entity. Rarely does a client have a physical problem that does not give rise to a psychological component, a social and economic impact; likewise, a psychological problem does not exist without a physical response to the situation experienced. This was the basis for the support of categories of survival needs, closeness needs, and freedom needs for the 35 human needs (Chapter 2). This categorization accommodates the level of concreteness and/or abstractness of the specific human need. Human need fulfillment is a motivating force. The choice of satisfier depends on whether the client is a person, a family, or a community. Needs motivate behavior directed toward achieving satisfaction or fulfillment; each person's particular needs are met in an individual manner.

By becoming aware of and by gaining knowledge about one's own inner experiences, a person develops a reliable basis from which the inner experience of others can be assessed. Within everyone, there is a basic drive for growth and development in the direction of optimal realization of his or her potential. Motivation and perception are trustworthy bases for constructive action. The nurse can facilitate and nourish the client's own basic drive for widening development; however, any attempt to force this motivation into being or into activity will usually defeat its own purpose. The client is responsible for him or herself. The nurse really cannot be responsible for the client, although he or she is accountable and responsible for his or her own behavior toward the client.

Human Needs and General Assessment Factors

The nurse adapts the human need framework to incorporate the unique aspects of a particular person or family, or both, and to suit the settings in which the client is found and in which the nurse is functioning. For example, factors for assessment of human needs of clients may have dimensions different for the school nurse, the office nurse, the nurse in the community health center, the nurse in a health maintenance organization, the nurse in a nursing home, the nurse in a rural setting, an urban setting, in an acute care or chronic care setting, or the nurse working with persons of a particular age group, such as infants, adolescents, or elders, with men or women, or with those who are physically or mentally handicapped. Initially the nurse starts with a prescribed list of general factors related to human needs.

Among these general factors are age, gender, education, growth and development, socioeconomic, cultural and religious elements, biological and physical status, emotional status, coping patterns, interactional patterns, life-styles, employment, and clients' views of wellness and illness as it relates to themselves, their families, and the community in which they live. In addition, consideration must be given to clients' expectations of health care and their awareness of the roles of health care practitioners, particularly the role of the nurse; the physical, social, emotional, and ecological environment in which they live and work; and the human and material resources available and accessible to them.

When assessing *human needs* and factors related to *age* the nurse should know the roles, expectations, and behaviors relative to infancy, childhood, adolescence, adulthood, and maturity for both men and women. Age and gender are extremely important factors when considering a person, whether client or nurse. These factors are combined with all others and influence each other significantly. A genogram may serve as a useful tool to portray these data for a person and a family.[1] Genogram symbols are presented in Figure 3–2. (Their utilization is demonstrated in Chapter 4.) Similar data may be plotted for the community viewed as a collective of persons, families, and groups of persons and families.

When assessing factors relating to the *human needs* of persons from different *racial groups*, the nurse should know their customs, rites, rituals, traditions, expectations, and views, including their implications for wellness, for the sick role, for suffering, illness, dying, and death.

When assessing the *human needs* of persons from different *nationalities* and *geographic* and *climatic areas*, the nurse should know their customs, rites, rituals, traditions, roles, and expectations as they relate to wellness and illness. The nurse needs to consider these clients' adaptability to their present environment when assessing their human needs.

When assessing *human needs* and *religious factors*, the nurse must know the various religions of this era as well as the beliefs, rites, and rituals of each. A knowledge of the rules (with implications) freeing individuals from participating in religious rites and rituals because of illness or handicap, of the rites and rituals of the different religions, as they apply or are available to the sick, disabled, the suffering, the dying, and to the person who has died, is necessary.

A person's *human needs* and *formal* or *informal education*, acquired through experience, must be considered. Included would be an investigation into any specialized language used by the client acquired during education or employment. Specialized interpretations or uses of words and phrases or of foreign words or phrases are important to know. For example, the nurse should know how the 2-year-old shows the need to urinate or defecate. Failure to understand this may create a problem for the child where none existed before. This is particularly significant when the child is away from the home setting—as in a child

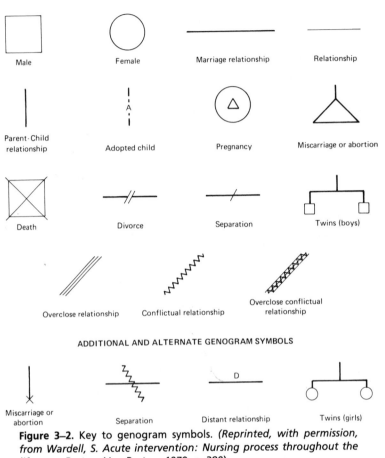

Figure 3–2. Key to genogram symbols. *(Reprinted, with permission, from Wardell, S. Acute intervention: Nursing process throughout the life span. Reston, Va.: Reston. 1979, p. 380)*

health clinic, a day care center, or a pediatric unit of a general hospital. Another important facet of the educational factor is to assess the client's problem-solving ability.

As to *socioeconomic status* and *human needs* it is important to assess clients' perceptions of their status. The perception and expectation of clients with varied socioeconomic backgrounds—from the deprived to the wealthy—must be considered. The impact of the client's job as well as the needs fulfilled by it must be determined.

The assessment of *human needs* and *growth and development* should be broadened to include physical, social, intellectual, and psychological elements in establishing growth and development patterns. Age, gender, and culture are inextricably bound to growth and development and may be assessed simultaneously.

To assess *biologic, physical,* and *emotional status*, the nurse utilizes the human need model of wellness to serve as a base. Models of wellness may differ for different age groups, for men and women, and for persons from varied socioeconomic and cultural backgrounds. Knowing what is expected or normal for bodily and psychic functions provides the framework within which the status of each can be assessed for a person or a family. The nurse must know what constitutes normal nutrition, fluid and electrolyte balance, oxygen demand, elimination of wastes, rest and sleep activity, skin integrity, perception of reality, comfort (freedom from pain and discomfort), recreation and diversion, and sensory integrity, to mention a few.

This knowledge gives the nurse a broad framework within which to work and from which he or she will determine the normal variation for a specific client for each specific human need. When additional data are forthcoming about this person, judgments are made from these initial data. For example, if a person's blood pressure is 110/80 mm Hg, it may be considered normal. However, it may also be a sign of organic disorder in an aged person who normally has a blood pressure of 150/90 mm Hg. A clear picture of what is normal for each particular person is of primary importance.

The nurse must have a knowledge of major pathological and psychopathological insults to the person at various age levels, for each gender, for the major racial and cultural groups, and of those prevalent in specific geographic areas or in certain environments. For example, structural abnormalities, malnutrition, infections, cancer, and accidents are major problems among infants and young children; for the preschooler, communicable diseases, dental caries, schizophrenia, retardation, speech defects, leukemia, and kidney infections must be considered. The older child, the adolescent, and the young adult are prone to accidents, respiratory conditions, allergies, cancer, obesity, suicide, schizophrenia, communicable diseases, behavioral problems (such as faulty eating and sleep patterns), interpersonal maladjustment, speech disorders, learning difficulties, and acne. As a person advances in age, conditions causing illness and death become more numerous. Major disabilities are related to cardiovascular-renal disease, cancer, diabetes, pneumonia and respiratory impairments, suicide, and accidents.

The nurse assesses a person's *human needs* and *interactional patterns* with family, significant others, nursing and health care personnel, and the person's ability to cope with problems. The nurse determines ways and means available to the person should a crisis or stressful situation arise. Coping patterns vary greatly among individuals and within family groups. The number of variables that constitute a stress situation may determine a person's ability to cope successfully with a problem. This ability may differ from time to time and is influenced by the person's view as to what constitutes a stressful situation. In family settings, the abililty to cope with a problem or problems may be pooled and some of the detrimental effects of a stressful situation may be offset by the strengths of individuals in the family. Interactional ability may bear on how, when, and in what manner particular human needs are met.

Considering persons' life-styles, expectations of health care, views of their own health or illness, or both, and expectations of health practitioners, as well as the availability and accessibility of human, health, and material resources may help to determine whether they will present themselves for a health status evaluation or for the diagnosis and correction of a health problem, or if the therapy that is instituted will be successful. Life-style and environment cannot be separated from the person if that person is to be viewed in his or her entirety.

Human Needs and Specific Assessment Factors

Nursing History and Health Assessment
A nursing history is taken to obtain needed data systematically, through a planned interview with a client. The collection of this information, the analysis of data, and the designation of problems for nursing intervention are the responsibility of the professional nurse. A time is specified to obtain the history, and the place where it is to be taken—an inner city clinic, the client's home, a hospital room, a physician's office, an industrial camp, or community mental health center—should be private. The history should be taken as soon as the nurse and the client encounter each other. As much information as possible should be obtained in an unhurried manner. The data may be subjective in nature in that it is experienced solely by the person and shared with another (e.g., nausea, dizziness) or objective in that it can be seen and/or measured by another. It is possible that objective data may or may not be known by the client. A low hemoglobin or a diffuse mass on a mammogram are examples of objective data that may not have the awareness of the client. Time should be given to impart information to the client. The Human Need Nursing History Starter Question Samples (Fig. 3–3) patterned after the 35 human needs described in Chapter 2 may be used during the nursing history and the health assessment. The content may be modified to fit the client situation. The format of the interview may also vary according to the setting and services rendered and to the role functions of the nurse. Although core data about the client as a person will always be needed, specific areas of information will differ if the nurse is admitting a woman in labor, if the client is being admitted into the health

Figure 3–3. Samples of human need nursing history starter questions. Starter questions invite answers from which additional questions can be developed.

Starter questions formulated within nursing's human need theory framework are those which the nurse initiates with the client and from which additional questions may be developed. The following starter questions are suggested. The nurse may retain, omit, substitute, refine, or reword the starter questions to accommodate the client's situation and level of understanding.

Acceptance of self and others, by others

- Describe your personal strengths or qualities. How do you feel about them?
- Describe what personal limitations you have. How do you feel about them?
- Describe your acceptance of family members, friends, significant others. How do you feel about their acceptance of you?

Activity

- How do you use your energy in a given day?
- What do you do to keep your muscles, bones, joints, etc., in shape?
- What intellectual activity do you pursue to keep abreast of happenings in your environment?

Adaptation, to manage stress

- Describe your ability to handle the stresses and strains you have in life.
- What stresses and strains are you experiencing about health? Your illness?
- What have you found to work best for you in managing stress or strain?

Air

- How would you judge the air quality where you live? work? play?
- Are you able to take air in through your nose, throat, and windpipe into your lungs comfortably?
- Are you able to breathe air out from your lungs through your windpipe, throat, and nose comfortably?

Appreciation, attention

- Which of your qualities and accomplishments have been positively noticed by your family, friends, significant others?
- What type(s) of response that you get from others is most meaningful to you in terms of appreciation, attention?
- Have you received attention for your efforts to achieve the highest level of wellness possible for you?

Autonomy, choice

- How do you handle the important decisions in your life? in matters of health?
- Would you describe yourself as an independent person? Explain.
- When you are confronted with choices for yourself, your work, your play, how do you handle these?

(continued)

Figure 3–3. (continued)

Beauty and aesthetic experiences

- What do you do that adds beauty to your life? your environment?
- What beauty do you find in yourself? your family? friends? significant others?
- Do you view beauty as a dimension of a healthy self? Explain.

Belonging

- Describe your relationship with your family; significant others; your friends.
- With what person(s) and group(s) do you have the closest relationship?
- Have you sought or been involved in membership in any community, church, work, social group in the past year?

Challenge

- If you had to describe a challenging situation in your life, what would it be?
- Do you derive satisfaction from taking on a challenge and dedicating your time and energy to it? Explain.
- What challenges are you experiencing in maintaining the highest level of wellness for you?

Conceptualization, rationality, problem solving

- Describe your ability to make judgments for and about yourself; your health; your work; your family.
- When you identify a problem that must be solved, how do you go about finding the best solution?
- What do you do to keep informed, especially in matters of health?

Confidence

- In what circumstances, activities, places or with whom do you feel most sure of yourself?
- How would you describe your confidence in your ability to be well and stay well?
- What do you know and/or do that makes you feel most confident in yourself? Least confident?

Elimination

- Describe your usual pattern of elimination from your colon.
- Describe your usual pattern of elimination from your urinary bladder.
- Have you noticed anything different from your usual pattern of elimination from your colon and/or urinary bladder?

Fluids

- What is your usual pattern of taking in fluids in a 24-hour period of time? In a week's time?
- Describe the kind, amount, and timing of your fluid intake.
- How does your body respond to fluids?
- Have you experienced any recent change(s) in fluid intake and your body's response to these fluids?

Freedom from pain

- Are you able to conduct your daily life free from physical pain or discomfort? Explain. From emotional pain or discomfort? Explain.
- How do you handle brief, periodic experiences of physical and/or emotional pain or discomfort that comes from overdoing or inattention?
- Describe pain or discomfort you are experiencing.

Humor

- What place does humor play in getting you through the day?
- Can you describe any experience in which humor or amusement had a healing effect on you?
- What type of humor is most likely to lift your spirit and help you look at your bright side?

Interchange of gases

- Describe the state of health of your heart and lungs. In this state usual to you?
- Describe the state of health of your blood circulation. Is this state usual for you?
- Are your body tissues free of swelling, coldness, unusual color (as grey or blue tones)? Explain.

To love and be loved

- Who are the persons significant to you and for whom you have a personal attachment and strong affection exists?
- Who are the persons who have a personal attachment and strong affection for you?
- Which of these attachments are reciprocal and enhance your state of wellness?

Nutrition

- Describe your food and nutrient intake in a 24-hour period.
- What additions, changes, omissions in food and nutrient intake have you initiated in the past month? For what purpose?
- Describe your pattern of weight in the past year. Does it differ from previous years? How? Explain.

Effective perception of reality

- How would you describe your impressions about what happens within you and around you?
- Are these impressions similar and/or different from the impressions of people significant to you? Explain.
- What is your impression of your state of wellness? Of illness and its cause?

Personal recognition, esteem, respect

- What is it that you know or do that brings recognition and esteem to you? Or should bring recognition and esteem to you?
- Who are the persons/groups that give you recognition? Why?

(continued)

Figure 3–3. (continued)

- What form(s) does this recognition, esteem, respect take?

Protection from excessive fear, anxiety, and chaos

- In what areas or what circumstances, including health, do you feel vulnerable to excessive fear? excessive anxiety? confusion and disorder?
- What is it within yourself and/or your environment that protects you from excessive fear? excessive anxiety? from confusion and disorder?
- What techniques and/or resources have you developed and found effective in maintaining this protection?

Rest and leisure

- Describe what you do for rest and leisure. When? How often?
- What experiences are most likely to be restorative for you?
- How do rest and leisure figure in your efforts to achieve the highest level of wellness for you?

Safety

- Explain your efforts to protect yourself from harm, infection, communicable diseases, injury, and hazards within your self and environment.
- What is the area(s) of greatest vulnerability for your safety?
- In what practices do you engage that would impact negatively on your health? That impact positively?

Self-control, self-determination, responsibility

- How would you describe your ability to control and be responsible for yourself?
- What is it within you and the environment around you that facilitates your ability to control and determine for yourself? What detracts?
- How do you account for your state of wellness? State of illness?

Self-fulfillment, to be, to become

- Describe your efforts toward realizing your life's purpose. Goal. Do you believe your life has meaning?
- What future do you see for yourself, particularly in matters of health?
- What gives meaning to your striving to achieve wellness? To confront illness?

Sensory integrity

- How would you describe your ability to see? to hear? to taste? to smell? to touch?
- Are the data from your sense organs such that you can make accurate impressions of what is happening to you or to your environment? Example.
- Have you noted any differences in the function of your sense organs or in your ability to interpret stimuli? Example.

Sexual integrity

- How does your gender impact your physical self? psychosocial self? cultural self? spiritual self?

- What role, responsibilities, and relationships in your life are affected by your gender? How? Your patterns of sexual expression? How?
- How does your gender affect your efforts to achieve optimal wellness? Your sexuality?
- Are you satisfied (or comfortable) with your personal pattern of sexual expression?

Skin integrity

- Describe how your skin and mucous membranes look and feel when in a usual state of wellness.
- What do you do to maintain your skin and mucous membranes in a state of wellness?
- Have you noticed anything different about your skin and mucous membranes from the usual experience—temperature, lesions, texture, moisture, trauma, sensation, pressure, infection, inflammation, for example?

Sleep

- Describe the pattern of sleep that is normal or usual for you: Pre-sleep rituals? Length of sleep time? Time of retiring and waking? Awakenings during sleep? Naps?
- What do you do to enhance sleep?
- Are you experiencing any differences from your normal or usual sleep pattern? Describe.

Spiritual integrity

- Do you subscribe to a spiritual, nonmaterial being or focus that brings meaning to your life? Describe.
- How does your spiritual element interact with your self as a person, your body, your state of health?
- Are you experiencing any differences or concerns with the spiritual element that is impacting your state of wellness? Your state of illness? Describe.

Structure, law, limits

- Describe the personal rules, customs, and practices you follow which impact positively on your health. Which impact negatively?
- Describe the rules, customs, and practices within your family or group of significant others in matters of health which you follow. Which are helpful? Which are not?
- What rules, customs, and practices within your community impact positively on your health? Which impact negatively? Within your work place? Within your socio-cultural group?

Tenderness

- What practices do you experience which convey gentleness and being treated with consideration for you? From whom?
- How do you convey caring and sensitivity to the feelings of others—to your family, friends, significant others?
- Are there ways and circumstances that you wish you could experience to convey concern, tenderness to you? Explain.

(continued)

Figure 3–3. (continued)

Territoriality

- Do you have a space to call your own—that you control and one that others recognize as yours? Describe.
- What actions or techniques offer you privacy of body, feelings, communications as these relate to health?
- Are there any affronts to your control of your space, your privacy? Explain.

Wholesome body image

- Describe the way you and your body look to you. The way your body functions.
- How would you describe how others view you and the image of your body?
- Does your body's image reflect wholeness? Wellness? Illness? Explain.

Value system

- What beliefs do you hold that designate the worth of people, things, activities, and experiences in your life?
- How are these beliefs incorporated into your experience of living on a day to day basis?
- Do these beliefs impact on your health positively? negatively? Explain.

care system for the first time, or if the client is being interviewed in a self-care unit, a long-term care facility, in an emergency unit, or at home.

In some instances, checklists and questionnaires have been devised for the convenience of the nurse and to save time. These may contribute a negative factor if only items on the form are addressed, or if they are merely filled out and filed away with no use made of obtained data. At times, it may be appropriate for the client to fill out information sheets. This, of course, is only appropriate if the client can read, write, and is oriented and aware, having the strength and will to do so. In any case, an interview with the nurse should verify, clarify, and yield any additional information deemed necessary. The interview gives the nurse the opportunity to see the person and the family, and to use perceptual abilities not only to obtain information but to communicate concern, interest, and willingness to understand. It gives the nurse the opportunity to reinforce those behaviors conducive to wellness.

The nurse should strive to develop his or her own format for the nursing history and health assessment, which should allow for flexibility and adaptability with persons having a variety of problems and accommodate the nurse's knowledge base and expertise. Eventually a specific guide may no longer be necessary. The nurse focuses on general specific topics, making adjustments as they are needed, to obtain the data needed to assess the client's status of human need fulfillment and delineate any problems accurately. While the data are being collected, the nurse validates inferences to assure accuracy in interpretation and acknowledges his or her intuitive feelings or responses. When the nurse infers the existence of a problem, or assumes a condition from known facts or evidences, he or she should confirm or validate the problem, condition, or situation with the client. Making inferences about information and validating them with the client emphasizes the nurse's desire to get an accurate picture of the client's experience and minimizes the possibility of imposing a judgment based on inadequate information, a few symptoms, or a limited social history. This will also protect the client from becoming the recipient of stereotypes, prejudices, or generalizations held by the nurse.

The time involved in obtaining a nursing history is well spent; it may be a significant factor in saving time in any service or care rendered to the client. Failure to obtain and validate data about the client before problems are assumed or solutions imposed may be more time consuming, may drain the physical and emotional energy of the nurse as well as the client, and create a climate of mistrust and insecurity. It could also add considerably to the cost of client care.

During the interview, the nurse should seek to clarify points that are not understood. The nurse should allow the client to express him or herself completely and obtain a clear picture of his or her expectations. Should the client be unable to express his or her problems, concerns, and perceptions of these directly because of age, sickness, unconsciousness, or a life-threatening situation, a person who knows the client well should supply the necessary information. All efforts should be made to involve the client as soon and as much as possible. This holds true for all clients who are unable to participate temporarily, can participate partially, or only on a nonverbal level. The nurse will use his or her own senses to collect information as well as to consult with family members, neighbors, co-workers, and other health team members during the interim in which the client cannot participate. As soon as possible, the nurse will continue the nursing history with the client.

Up to this point, verbal interaction between nurse and client has been emphasized. The nurse uses various communication techniques, such as open-end questions and reflection to aid communication. The selection of techniques is based on how they are used and if they facilitate exchange of data. A technique is not good or bad within itself. How appropriately it has been used and the outcome will designate its value. The nurse and client may have picked up nonverbal cues that must be clarified and verified.

In conjunction with the nursing history, the nurse performs a health assessment. A health assessment includes the systematic collection of data relating to physical, psychological, emotional, social, and spiritual dimensions of the person, family, and neighborhood, with the nurse fully utilizing the five senses as well as his or her intellect and any data-gathering tools available to provide needed information.

Inspection, palpation, percussion, and auscultation as formal methods of physical and psychosocial examination require the use of hands (touch), eyes (sight), ears (hearing), and nose (smelling), as well as keen perception, astute judgment, and sound decision making. The use of all these skills is crucial to the nurse as he or she collects data about the client's status of human need fulfillment. Subjective and objective data are compiled within the human need framework. A selection of observations and data obtained through the senses of sight, hearing, touch, and smell may be found in Appendix C. Limiting the health assessment to the physical dimension alone would fail to provide data that reflect the wholeness of the person. The challenge faced by the nurse is the development and efficient use of the appropriate intellectual, interpersonal, and technical skills as dictated by the client's health state and the presenting problems—viewed as alterations in human need fulfillment.

To further enhance the organized and systematic process of health assessment, it is wise to use some plan for data collection. For example, a physical examination can proceed from head to toe to ensure a consideration of every part of the body. A body system plan is another framework that can be used. Either of these can be incorporated into or utilized with the human needs framework. For example, inspection and palpation of the skin will provide data about the level of fulfillment for the human need for skin integrity. Many authors have contributed via texts and audiovisual media to the technique of physical examination, and no attempt will be made to duplicate this information here.

The nurse exercises perceptual and judgmental skills to note the client's posture; facial expression; manner of dress; physical limitations, such as the loss of use of a hand, arm, or leg; deformities; absence of parts, such as teeth or extremities; presence of scars, discolorations, cuts; and the use of eyeglasses, contact lenses, hearing appliances, crutches, and canes. The nurse uses sight, hearing, touch, and smell to collect these and related data. Critical judgments are made about the relationship and interrelationship of selected data, as well as the absence of data relative to human needs.

In addition to the nurse's sight and hearing, which are used extensively throughout the interaction, touch can elicit data about skin temperature, muscle tension, skin moisture, variation in strength of extremities, swellings and masses, palpable distortions in configuration, areas of pain and tenderness, and tremors. Moreover, the nurse's sense of smell can supply data relative to usual and unusual odors: (a) pinpoint specific breath odors, such as tobacco, alcohol, mustiness, sweetness, use of commercial mouthwashes, and agents that are unknown or not easily recognizable; (b) determine smells that denote a pattern of living or job; and (c) identify smells of wounds, particularly those infected or with decomposed or dead tissue; odors of bodily excretory products—urine, feces, vomitus, sweat; and such odors as perfumes, medicines, liniments, and salves.

The nurse can measure bodily function, using palpation, percussion, auscultation, observation, and can use tools, such as the thermometer, stethoscope, or sphygmomanometer, to obtain readings of body temperature, heart rate (and its quality and characteristics), respiratory rate, and blood pressure. Other data gathering tools as attitude tests, rating scales, and self-administered questionnaires may be used in conjunction with or separately to obtain data about specific human needs or categories of human needs. These tools are particularly helpful in obtaining data for human needs designated as more abstract as well as for those considered concrete. Such specimens as urine, stool, vomitus, sputum, and secretions from other bodily parts or draining wounds may be collected. Some tests can be done immediately, using chemical tapes and kits. Others must be sent to the laboratory for analysis. The nurse could assign supportive health and nursing personnel, qualified to collect specimens and proceed with analyses, to assemble these laboratory data.

After the client has been given the opportunity to express feelings, concerns, goals, desires, expectations, and the nurse has affirmed and validated any inferences and determined that there are no gaps in the information, the interview can be terminated. At this point the client can be told how these data will be used, what conclusions will be drawn, and the plan for continuing the interaction into the planning, implementing, and evaluating phases. Clients should have felt that the nurse was interested in them and that this was conveyed, both verbally and nonverbally, with respect and dignity. Using the client's name, listening with full attention, anticipating questions, and speaking *with* rather than *to* the client, all convey respect. The nurse should refrain from using language unfamiliar to the client, and guard against responding to questions in a condescending manner. If the client's condition is critical, with life-threatening problems, there should be intervention to relieve the crisis and a focus immediately on joint participation. The nurse should be attentive to the desires and concerns of the persons important to the client.

During this interview and performance of the health assessment, the nurse and client begin a relationship based on trust, respect, concern, and interest. Clients should feel that the nurse is truly interested in them as persons, that he or she is concerned about their welfare, and that he or she recognizes and respects each as a co-partner, designating and meeting their expectations for health and nursing care. Clients know that they not only are viewed as valued persons, but as members of a family or group of significant others, and members of a neighborhood and a community.

When this nursing history interview is terminated, clients should know who the nurse is; who will be responsible for their care; that some one person knows their views, fears, concerns, and expectations; that someone knows the human needs that they can fulfill and those they cannot. They know how to summon the nurse, where the nurse will be, when and how they can communicate with this nurse, and when this nurse will see them again. If the client is an inpatient in a health care facility, orientation to the environment and available services may be included in the interview. The nurse may consider it prudent to delegate this orientation to another member of the nursing team.

Analysis of Assessment Data

After the data are collected, the nurse seeks additional relevant data from family members, from persons accompanying the client, or from persons in the household. Other members of the health and nursing teams, significant members of the community, and available records and reports are also used to obtain data.

The nurse sorts, organizes, groups, categorizes, compares, analyzes, and synthesizes the data about the client obtained up to this point. Decision making and judgment are inherent in every phase of the nursing process and are particularly significant during assessment. The nurse decides what to ask, when to ask it, and how to ask it; decides when to listen, how to listen, and how long to listen; uses judgment throughout the interview and health assessment by focusing on some areas in depth and by passing more briefly over others (see Appendix D for selected data that describe fulfilled human needs); judges when there may be more to the meaning of a topic than that which the client has stated; summarizes all available data, then makes judgments as follows:

1. The client's human needs are met to a reasonable extent.
   a. No problem(s) exists and the client's state of wellness is affirmed. A plan to maintain wellness is developed with the client that the client then implements. Periodic reassessment of wellness will be made, and the client will be present for these at

given intervals. The client will seek reassessment sooner if a problem is suspected.

b. No problem exists, but there is a potential problem that may be offset by giving the client information on prevention and planning for a future interview. It may be necessary to refer the client to another health care member.

2. Some of the client's human needs are met to a reasonable extent and some show alterations by being met excessively, or a disturbance in the pattern of fulfillment, or in a deficient manner.

a. A problem(s) exists but is being handled successfully by the client, the family, or both. Plans for periodic reassessment will be formulated, but the client will return for these at nonscheduled times if the client thinks it necessary. The problem may be new or it may be a long-standing one. Pharmacological and mechanical aids may be used to resolve the problem, for example, medications, crutches, hearing aids, colostomy or ileostomy appliances, or prostheses.

b. A problem(s) exists that the client needs help in handling. Providing this assistance—whether it is informational, caring, socioeconomic, pharmacological, or mechanical, will either resolve the problem or make it easier for the client, family, neighbors, or some combination to handle it. Appropriate provision, including referrals to health team members and social agencies, will be planned with the client. The client, nurse, and other health team members share in implementing the plans. Implementation continues until evaluation indicates that the problem has been resolved or has decreased or reassessment deems a change in plans is necessary.

c. A problem(s) exists that the client cannot handle at this time and its nature prevents family and neighbors from helping to resolve it. Health care intervention is needed. Specific members of the health care team, such as the nurse, physician, dentist, psychiatrist, physiotherapist, or nutritionist, may be assigned to help the client. With health care intervention, the problem can be specifically diagnosed, treated, and resolved. An example of such a situation is dental caries.

d. A problem(s) exists that must be studied further and diagnosed to resolve or to keep it within manageable proportions. Ambulatory or inpatient health and nursing services may be needed. The problem(s) may be solved completely; for example, a foreign body or obstruction of some kind is removed. In other situations, an elevated blood sugar may be diagnosed, treated, and provisions then made for continued management on an ambulatory service.

e. A problem(s) exists that is not incapacitating to the client at present, but its resolution requires intervention that would render the client dependent for a specific period or indefinitely. Surgical interventions and certain medical regimens are examples. Inpatient care is generally necessary. A specific medical diagnosis may have been made before the initial nurse–client interaction. Acute care followed by extended care or ambulatory care may be part of the planning.

f. A problem(s) exists that places heavy demands on the client's ability to cope with it and that the family cannot resolve; they could, however, contribute emotional and financial support for intervention by members of the health care and nursing teams. These problems may be due to life-threatening medical conditions, e.g., myocardial infarction, cerebrovascular accident, diabetic acidosis, cirrhosis of the liver, bleeding peptic ulcer, drug addiction, or depression. Immediate and continued intervention by members of the health care team, on an inpatient basis, is required.

g. A problem(s) is imposed unexpectedly on the client or the family because of an accident, injury, or natural disaster, or is self-imposed (attempted suicide). The problem may or may not be a threat to life. If it is life threatening, health team members must attend to it immediately to reduce the crisis situation, if possible. If not, the crisis imposes problems on family members. If the crisis is resolved or the situation is more incapacitating than life threatening, situations discussed in judgments 1 through 2.f. may prevail. An example would be the child who is found to have an obstruction in the respiratory tract. Removing the obstruction, e.g., a bottle top or balloon, quickly and effectively relieves the problem, with no residual disability. If the problem cannot be resolved, immediate surgical intervention may be required. When the crisis is due to a natural disaster, such as a flood, food, water, and shelter become unavailable. Although the lack of these can be tolerated for some time, illness is a direct result of such deprivation, with survival threatened as the time without these necessities lengthens.

h. Problems exist that are long-term and permanent. The client is able to cope with some but not all problems, and other persons, such as family, nursing and health team members, clergy, lawyers, or social workers, may have to intervene to cope with the problem and provide care on a continuing basis. Long-term health and nursing care must be provided within the home, community health center, community mental health center, an extended care facility, or a combination of these. An example would be the person with a congenital anomaly such as spina bifida.

The judgment made by the nurse designates the place of the client on the wellness–illness continuum at a particular point in time. The nurse then, designates specific potential and actual nursing diagnoses. If the client is the family or the community, the nurse makes comparable judgments based on assessment data that relate to human need fulfillment and alterations in fulfillment. One proposed grouping of human needs labeled as survival needs, closeness needs, and freedom needs plus the subgroup of human needs serve as the focal point from which judgments about the family and the community can be made—family and community nursing diagnoses.

Nursing Diagnosis

The nurse concludes the assessment phase with the verification of the status of human need fulfillment for the client including the specification of potential and actual nursing diagnoses. *A nursing diagnosis is the judgment or conclusion reached by the nurse based on assessment data that indicates the potential for or actual human need fulfillment alteration viewed as an excess, disturbed pattern of expression, or a deficit, lack, or limitation for the client as person, family, or community.* This diagnosis specifically (a) indicates that no obvious problems exist that demand the intervention of the nurse, though the potential for alteration in human need fulfillment exists, or (b) identifies those human need fulfillment alterations to be resolved so that the client can experience optimal wellness.

Making a nursing diagnosis requires a high level of intellectual skills. This most strategic aspect of the nursing process concludes the assessment component. Without a nursing diagnosis for potential or actual human need alteration there is no reason to continue to other components of the process in an effort to solve a client's problem(s). There will be no basis for planning or intervention, or for evaluative judgments about this client's problems.

A nursing diagnosis may be further qualified by prefixing the diagnosis with such adjectives as acute, chronic, full, complete, partial, minimal, intermittent, internally induced or externally induced. In addition, the statement of the nursing diagnosis is followed by the identified supporting evidence (subjective and objective data) and the selected reason(s), causes(s), or "due to" that may be categorized as follows:

1. Personal and situational occurrences
2. Environmental affronts

3. Medical, dental, pharmacologic, and nursing therapies (commissions and omissions)
4. Pathophysiologic states
5. Psychopathologic states
6. Legal states and occurrences
7. Physiologic miscalculation and/or nonacceptance
8. Congenital alterations (reparable and irreparable)
9. Philosophic, ethical, and religious impositions
10. Social and economic affronts
11. Education, information, or knowledge deficits
12. Growth and developmental alterations
13. Heredity and genetic impacts
14. Cultural imposition
15. Geographic and climate affronts
16. Functional role structure and impact
17. Political impacts and impositions
18. Communication alterations

This format will clearly, logically, and succinctly provide the information needed to determine the appropriate goal achievement for the client. This facilitates the selection of nursing strategies to improve the client's health state.

For example, sleep is a human need. Sleep patterns have been described quantitatively and qualitatively in the literature. Thus, the pattern for a specific person can be designated. To follow the pattern and then awake refreshed to accomplish the tasks of the day would be the expectation. Lack of fulfillment or failure to meet this need would be designated as sleep deprivation, excessive sleep, or disturbed sleep. Sleep deprivation may be acute, chronic, occasional, or sporadic. It can be due to a noisy environment, excessive use of caffeine, failure to allow time for sleep, fear of the dark, brain neoplasm, continued disturbance resulting from medical therapy (as in an intensive care unit), or to the onset of disease yet undiagnosed.

Proposed nursing diagnoses for the person, family, and community have been developed and are outlined in Tables 3–1 and 3–2. The pattern for designating nursing diagnoses based on human need theory is *too much, too little*, or a *disturbed pattern* of human need fulfillment. This level of specificity is required to facilitate problem solving. The term alteration should be used *only* to designate a deviation from human need fulfillment. The vagueness of the term defies solution. A nursing diagnosis may be singular or numerous depending on the client's health status and the amount of human need fulfillment alterations evident. Nursing diagnoses may cluster according to the reason for the diagnoses, e.g., pathophysiologic or psychopathological states

TABLE 3–1. PROPOSED NURSING DIAGNOSES BASED ON THE FRAMEWORK OF HUMAN NEEDS FOR THE PERSON[a,b,c]

Human Need	Nursing Diagnosis
Acceptance of self and others, by others	Overacceptance of self and others, by others
	Disturbance in patterns of expression and/or fulfillment of acceptance
	Rejection of self and others
	Rejection by others
Activity	Excessive activity (hyperactivity)
	Disturbance in patterns of expression and/or fulfillment of activity
	Insufficient activity
Adaptation, to manage stress	Excessive adaptation
	Disturbance in patterns of expression and/or fulfillment of adaptation, management of stress
	Insufficient adaptation
Air	Excessive aeration, hyperaeration
	Disturbance in patterns of expression and/or fulfillment for aeration
	Insufficient aeration
Appreciation, attention	Excessive appreciation and attention
	Disturbance in patterns of expression and/or fulfillment of appreciation, attention
	Lack of appreciation, attention
Autonomy, choice	Excessive autonomy, choice
	Disturbance in patterns of expression and/or fulfillment of autonomy, choice
	Lack of autonomy, choice
Beauty and aesthetic experiences	Preoccupation with beauty and aesthetic experiences
	Disturbance in patterns of expression and/or fulfillment of beauty and aesthetic experiences
	Lack of beauty and aesthetic experiences
Belonging	Excessive belonging
	Disturbance in patterns of expression and/or fulfillment of belonging
	Lack of belonging
Challenge	Excessive challenge
	Disturbance in patterns of expression

(continued)

TABLE 3–1   *(continued)*

Human Need	Nursing Diagnosis
	and/or fulfillment of challenge
	Lack of challenge
Conceptualization, rationality, problem solving	Preoccupation with conceptualization, rationality, problem solving
	Disturbance in patterns of expression and/or fulfillment of conceptualization, rationality, problem solving
	Inability to conceptualize, rationalize, problem solve
Confidence	Overconfidence
	Disturbance in patterns of expression and/or fulfillment of confidence
	Lack of confidence
Elimination (end products of metabolism, toxins, poisons, chemicals, drugs)	Excessive elimination of metabolic end products, nutrients, fluids, chemicals, electrolytes, drugs
	Disturbance in patterns of expression and/or fulfillment of elimination, nutrients, fluids, chemicals, electrolytes, toxins, drugs
	Lack of or diminished elimination of metabolic end products, nutrients, electrolytes, chemicals, toxins, drugs
Fluids (intake)	Excessive hydration and electrolytes
	Disturbance in patterns of expression and/or fulfillment of fluid hydration, and electrolyte intake
	Depletion of fluids and electrolytes
Freedom from pain	Excessive freedom from pain, lack of appropriate pain signals
	Disturbance in patterns of expression of pain sensation and/or patterns of relief of pain
	Inability to experience pain relief
Humor	Excessive or continuous use of humor, hilarity
	Disturbance in patterns of expression and/or use of humor
	Inability to experience humor
Interchange of gases	Excessive gaseous exchange
	Disturbance in patterns of expression and/or fulfillment of gaseous exchange
	Insufficient gaseous exchange
To love and be loved	Excessive expression of love and requirement to be loved

(continued)

TABLE 3–1 *(continued)*

Human Need	Nursing Diagnosis
	Disturbance in patterns of expression and/or fulfillment of love
	Diminished or lack of ability to love and be loved
Nutrition	Excessive nutritional intake
	Disturbance in patterns of intake of nutrients
	Insufficient or lack of nutritional intake
Effective perception of reality	Hypersensitive perception of reality
	Disturbance in patterns of expression and/or fulfillment of perception of reality
	Ineffective, inaccurate perception of reality
Personal recognition, esteem, respect	Overrecognition, respect, excessive esteem
	Disturbance in patterns of expression and/or fulfillment of recognition, esteem, respect
	Lack of recognition, esteem, and respect
Protection from excessive fear, anxiety, and chaos	Excessive fear, anxiety, chaos
	Disturbance in patterns of expression and/or fulfillment of protection from excessive fear, anxiety, chaos
	Lack of expression of fear and anxiety, lack of protection
Rest and leisure	Excessive rest, over-use of leisure
	Disturbance in patterns of expression and/or fulfillment of rest, and leisure
	Restlessness, lack of rest, and/or leisure
Safety	Excessive thwarting of safety
	Disturbance in patterns of expression and/or fulfillment of safety
	Diminished or lack of safety
Self-control, self-determination, responsibility	Excessive self-control, self-determination, responsibility
	Disturbance in patterns of expression and/or fulfillment of self-control, self-determination, responsibility
	Diminished or lack of self-control, self-determination, responsibility
Self-fulfillment, to be, to become	Independency, preoccupation with becoming

(continued)

TABLE 3–1 *(continued)*

Human Need	Nursing Diagnosis
	Disturbance in patterns of expression and/or fulfillment of self-fulfillment, becoming
	Lack of fulfillment of self, of feeling of becoming, prolonged dependency
Sensory integrity	Sensory overload
	Disturbance in patterns of expression and/or fulfillment of sensory integrity
	Sensory deprivation
Sexual integrity	Preoccupation with sexual dimension
	Disturbance in patterns of expression and/or fulfillment of sexual integrity
	Lack of attention to sexual integrity
Skin integrity	Preoccupation with maintenance of skin integrity
	Disturbance in patterns of expression and/or fulfillment of skin integrity
	Diminished or lack of skin integrity
Sleep	Excessive sleep
	Disturbance in patterns of expression and/or fulfillment of sleep
	Insufficient or lack of sleep
Spiritual integrity	Preoccupation with spiritual dimension
	Disturbance in patterns of expression and/or fulfillment of spiritual integrity
	Diminished or lack of spiritual integrity
Structure, law, and limits	Excessive structure, law, and limits
	Disturbance in patterns of expression and/or fulfillment of structure, law, and limits
	Diminished or lack of structure, law, and limits
Tenderness	Excessive, smothering tenderness
	Disturbance in patterns of expression and/or fulfillment of tenderness
	Diminished or lack of tenderness
Territoriality	Excessive territorial requirement
	Disturbance in patterns of expression and/or fulfillment of territoriality
	Diminished or lack of territorial space
Wholesome body image	Excessive valuation of overall image and/or selected body parts
	Disturbance in patterns of expression

(continued)

TABLE 3–1 *(continued)*

Human Need	Nursing Diagnosis
	and/or fulfillment of wholesome body image
	Diminished or poor body image, un-wholesome body image
Value system	Excessive or rigid application of value system
	Disturbance in patterns of expression and/or fulfillment of value system
	Diminished or lack of value system

[a]*Prefixes:* Acute, chronic, intermittent, internally induced, externally induced, potential for.
[b]Categories of reasons (specificity to be added):*Reasons:* Personal and situational occurrences; environmental affronts; medical, pharmacologic, and nursing therapies (commissions and omissions); pathophysiologic states; psychopathological states; physiologic miscalculation and/or nonacceptance; congenital alterations (reparable, irreparable); philosophic, ethical, and religious impositions; social, economic affronts; educational deficits; growth and developmental alterations.
[c]*Nursing strategies:* The goal to be achieved is specified. The human need is satisfactorily met or excesses, disturbances, limitations are diminished or compensated for.
Specifically prescribed nursing strategies related to each human need and/or its nursing diagnoses based on the reason(s) for (1) excessive fulfillment, (2) disturbance in pattern of expression and/or fulfillment, or (3) diminished, lack of fulfillment are stated.
Where excesses, disturbances, and limitations are due to irreversible pathophysiologic, psychopathological, developmental or congenital states, nursing strategies reflect those that maximize available ability of the person in relation to specific human needs.
The timing for evaluative purposes is specified.

TABLE 3–2. PROPOSED NURSING DIAGNOSES BASED ON THE FRAMEWORK OF HUMAN NEEDS FOR THE FAMILY (OR COMMUNITY)[a,b,c]

Human Need Categories and Needs	Family (or Community) Nursing Diagnosis
Survival needs	Excess in survival need fulfillment
Air	Disturbed pattern in provision for survival need fulfillment
Nutrition	
Sleep	Deprivation in survival need fulfillment
Activity	
Structure, law, and limits	
Protection from excessive fear, anxiety, and chaos	
Interchange of gases	
Adaptation, to manage stress	
Safety	
Fluids	
Elimination	
Rest and leisure	
Sensory integrity	
Effective perception of reality	
Skin integrity	

(continued)

TABLE 3–2 *(continued)*

Human Need Categories and Needs	Family (or Community) Nursing Diagnosis
Closeness needs	Excess in closeness need fulfillment
To love and be loved	Disturbed pattern in provision for close-
Tenderness	ness need fulfillment
Confidence	
Sexual integrity	Deprivation of closeness need fulfill-
Acceptance of self and others	ment
Belonging	
Personal recognition, esteem, respect	
Appreciation, attention	
Humor	
Wholesome body image	
Freedom needs	Excess in freedom need fulfillment
Territoriality	Disturbed pattern in provision for free-
Spiritual experience	dom need fulfillment
Autonomy, choice	
Conceptualization, rationality, prob-	Deprivation of freedom need fulfill-
lem solving	ment
Challenge	
Self-fulfillment, to be, to become	
Value system	
Self-control, self-determination, re-	
sponsibility	
Beauty and aesthetic experiences	
Freedom from pain	

[a]*Prefixes:* Acute, chronic, intermittent, internally induced, externally induced, potential for.
[b]Categories of reasons (specificity to be added): *Reasons:* Personal and situational occurrences; environmental affronts; medical, dental, pharmacological, and nursing therapies; legal states and occurrences; political impacts and impositions; functional role structure and impact; pathophysiologic and psychopathological states; physiologic miscalculation and/or nonacceptance; hereditary and genetic impacts; philosophic, ethical, and religious impacts; social, economic affronts; educational and informational deficits; growth and developmental alterations; communication alterations; cultural imposition; geographic, climatic affronts.
[c]*Nursing strategies:* The goal to be achieved is specified. The human needs of the members of the family are met by the collective action of the family (or community).
Specifically prescribed nursing strategies related to the human need categories and the specific related human needs based on the reason(s) for (1) excessive fulfillment, (2) disturbed pattern of provision for fulfillment, or (3) deprived, diminished, lack of fulfillment are stated.
Where excesses, disturbances, and limitations are due to irreversible pathophysiologic, psychopathological, developmental or congenital states, for example, nursing strategies reflect those that maximize available ability of the family (or community members—persons, families, groups) in relation to specific human need categories and needs.
The timing for evaluative purposes is specified.

such as diabetes mellitus, myocardial infarction, depression, cancer of the breast.

Some common errors[1a] in stating nursing diagnoses include:

1. The use of the word "need" in the statement of nursing diagnosis. Misuse of the word *need* may connote a nurse prescription for the client, e.g., the client needs to sleep. This statement by-

passes the precise statement of the client's problem, in this case, sleep deficit. Or "the need for sleep" may connote the human need for sleep applicable to all human beings. This error does not give the diagnosis but jumps to what the client requires to offset the problem. It completely bypasses the problem which is to answer the question "why?" when confronted with "need for sleep."

> Incorrect nursing diagnosis: "Need for sleep."
> Correct nursing diagnosis: "Sleep deficit."

2. The use of medical diagnosis (e.g., diabetes mellitus, cancer of the lung) with the label of nursing diagnosis.
3. The use of the vague statement of *alteration* in the diagnostic statement. This lacks the precision needed for resolution of the problem. It is necessary to determine if the "alteration in sleep" is too much sleep, too little sleep, or a disturbed pattern in the fulfillment of the human need for sleep.
4. The combination of two unrelated problems in one statement, e.g., sleep deficit and increased fear and anxiety related to spouse's Alzheimer's disease and behavior of nighttime wandering. Even though both problems may have the same cause, the evidence, the goal statements with behavioral outcomes, and nursing strategies operationalized to assure goal achievement differ.

> Correct nursing diagnoses: "Sleep deficit related to spouse's Alzheimer's disease and nighttime wandering behavior." "Increased fear and anxiety related to spouse's Alzheimer's disease and nighttime wandering behavior."

5. The use of a legally inadvisable statement.

> Incorrect nursing diagnosis: "Potential for physical injury related to lack of safety precautions."
> Correct nursing diagnosis: "Potential for physical injury related to pathological state of Alzheimer's disease."

6. When both the nursing diagnosis statement and the cause statement connote the same problem, e.g., "sleep deficit due to inability to sleep."

> Incorrect nursing diagnosis: "Sleep deficit due to inability to sleep."
> Correct nursing diagnosis: "Sleep deficit due to deterioration of the brain's sleep center (Alzheimer's disease)."

Thus, the realistic fulfillment of human needs of the client is the goal of nursing intervention. The planning to enhance human need fulfillment and offset fulfillment alterations (client problems), with evaluation of the achievement of this goal will follow a nursing diagnosis. The determination that the human need is fulfilled is the objective for the evaluation phase of the nursing process.

PLANNING

Planning is the determination of a plan of action to assist the client toward the goal of optimal wellness based on the highest level of fulfillment of human needs and to resolve the nursing diagnosis (diagnoses). The planning phase begins with the utilization of judgments made about human need fulfillment, i.e., human needs that are met and those with fulfillment alterations, nursing diagnosis (diagnoses), the outcome of the assessment phase. Plans are made with the client and family to support the maintenance of human needs that are met and to deal with alterations in need fulfillment. It is expected that the goal with behavioral outcomes desired will be the resolution of the problem diagnosed, i.e., human need fulfillment. For example, if sensory deprivation because of isolation from stimuli is the problem, then sensory integrity will be the goal. All efforts will be exerted to achieve this goal and the specified behavioral outcomes stemming from the goal. Precise problem identification with specific actions planned to achieve the outcome will provide the framework and data for the evaluation phase of the nursing process. If sensory deprivation, however, is due to permanent blindness, then the goal of sensory integrity is still realistic, but goal expectation with behavioral outcomes and specific nurse actions will be directed toward maximizing hearing, touch, smell, and taste, while acknowledging the absence of sight.

The purposes of the planning phase are to (a) assign priority to all potential and/or actual nursing diagnoses; (b) specify the goal expectation with behavioral outcomes for the client including the expected time of achievement; (c) differentiate client problems that could be resolved by nursing intervention, those that could be handled by the client or members of the family, and those that would have to be referred to other members of the health team or handled in conjunction with health team members; (d) designate specific actions and the frequency of these actions in accordance with the specified goal and behavioral outcomes/expectations and to accommodate the reason or cause; and (e) write out the human need, the client problems (nursing diagnoses), the cause(s) or reason(s), the subjective/objective data base, the goal with behavioral outcomes and time frame, prescription of nursing strategies and their frequency on the nursing care plan. The planning phase terminates with the development of the nursing care plan, which is the *blueprint for action*, providing direction for implementing the plan and providing the framework for evaluation.

If no obvious problem exists and the nurse verifies the client's state of wellness with human needs reasonably well met, a plan for periodic reevaluation of the client's state of wellness is formulated jointly. Plans to continue wholesome living patterns will be reinforced, and specific information the client requests or requires will be given, such as immunization, accident prevention, poison control information, or disease prevention. Brochures may support and reinforce or expand the information. The client is requested to return immediately if symptoms appear in relation to or if the client feels there is a problem. Thus, in an interaction with the well client, the nurse and the client participate together in the assessing and planning phases; in the implementation and evaluation phases, the client is responsible for performing those actions that will maintain human need fulfillment—optimal wellness.

Goal Designation

The goal with expected behavioral outcomes for the client is specified in relation to *each* actual or potential nursing diagnosis. The goal is stated as the human need satisfactorily met. Fulfillment excesses, limitations, and disturbances in pattern are diminished or compensated for. The goal would be specified for a family or community nursing diagnosis. For example, if the nursing diagnosis is sleep deprivation, the expected result of intervention for the client would be attainment of a normal sleep pattern, and the human need would be fulfilled. The goal with behavioral expectations is always stated in *client* terms. For example:

Goal Description
Client will resume normal sleep pattern within 3 days.

Expected Behavioral Outcomes Stemming from Stated Goal

- Able to fall asleep within 20 minutes and stay asleep for at least 6 hours.
- Awake only once during sleep and able to resume sleep with no difficulty.
- Accept available social support to keep the vigil for ill spouse during the night (1 day).
- Yawning behavior diminished (2 days).
- Eyes clear and alert (2 days).
- Able to stay awake during the day and care for spouse.
- Decreased stumbling (2 days).

- Longer attention span; states that mind can be kept on a task.
- Irritability and depression diminished.

The level of human need fulfillment that can be achieved by the client should be stated realistically by considering the reason for the alteration initially and accommodating the subjective and objective data base. For example:

- Related to: Situational occurrence—caring responsibility for spouse with Alzheimer's disease.
- Related to: Socioeconomic affront—insufficient finances to purchase home care services.
- Related to: Personal occurrence—feels personally responsible to provide care for spouse. Spouses made pact with each other to keep disabled one at home.

Evidenced by subjective data	Evidenced by objective data
Short tempered.	Yawning.
States, "I get 2 to 3 hours of sleep at night."	Red, itchy eyes.
"I'm afraid to go to sleep for fear I won't hear my husband if he starts to wander."	Had great difficulty concentrating during interview; short attention span.
Dozes when sitting quietly at home.	Ecchymosis on both knees and ankles.
States she sleeps in a lounge chair outside her spouse's room.	
Exhaustion.	
States she feels "depressed all the time."	
States she stumbles, bumps into furniture.	

As noted earlier, if a client has a nursing diagnosis of sensory deprivation and the client is blind, having a congenital absence of the optic nerve, it would be unrealistic to expect the client to see. The nurse would focus on strategies that would maximize the intact senses—touch, hearing, smell, and taste. The stated goal would be sensory integrity for the client's remaining four senses. Further goal and behavioral outcome statements reflect the highest level of human need fulfillment available or possible to the client whether the cause for the alteration was reversible or irreversible. If a nursing diagnosis is malnutrition due to cancer of the stomach, a state of normal nutrition is the expected goal. The consistency of the food may be liquid; the food may be introduced directly into the stomach by tube; food may be given continuously rather than following the client's prepathology state. Medical, surgical, and chemical interventions may accompany nursing interventions.

When the goal has been stated for each actual or potential nursing diagnosis, the nurse indicates the date when the goal with behavioral result is expected. The specification of the date will reflect the best judgment of the nurse considering the time needed to reverse the alteration, the condition of the client, the availability of support systems (family, friends, neighbors, etc.), the impact of the alteration for the client, and the type and duration of interventions required. For example, 24 to 48 hours would be a realistic time to offset sleep deprivation if the deprivation was self-imposed. If the deprivation was due to injury of the brain's sleep center, it may take weeks or months for a normal sleep pattern to be restored. A significant level of logical thinking and critical judgment by the nurse is needed to realistically designate the expected goal and the date for realization of the goal.

If the client is the family or community, the expected goal(s) for the alteration in survival, closeness, and freedom need categories are specified and the date for achievement of the goal(s) is targeted. For example, if malnutrition of family members is the family nursing diagnosis and the alteration is due to lack of money, an improved nutritional state may be evidenced within days or a week if a consistent money source and nutritious food become available. However, if malnutrition of family members is due to rejection and irresponsibility rather than money, a much longer time (weeks, even months) may be needed before the family members are well-nourished. If survival of a community is threatened because of food shortages, the time until the shortage is over will be dependent on the cause. Food shortages can be offset in a few days if caused by a heavy snowfall which temporarily disrupted shipments of food stuffs. This is in contrast to a long-term problem in food production because of geographic and climatic affronts, such as an extended drought in an isolated rural community.

The description and specification of each goal with date and time of expected achievement and the time interval for measurement of achievement of human need fulfillment not only serves to give direction to the planning and implementation phases, but is the core for the evaluation phase as will be noted later in this chapter.

Priority Setting

If specific client problems in relation to human need fulfillment are diagnosed, effort is exerted to assign priority to each. The nurse uses his or her own judgment and considers the client's views in assigning priorities. During priority setting, problems can be conveniently classified as high, medium, or low priority. As high priority problems are resolved fully or in part, the order in which remaining problems are resolved may have to be reevaluated. Problems in the medium or low priority categories may be given a higher rating at a later time. The more life threatening the problem is, the higher the priority assigned. A number of problems may be considered high priority simultaneously, such as severe deprivation of oxygen caused by an obstructed airway and evidenced by ineffective breathing and severe loss of fluids and electrolytes, caused by impaired circulation or gross hemorrhage.

Each client problem should be classified so that the integrity and unity of the person are maintained. Although physically oriented survival needs for air, nutrition, fluids, and safety may take precedence when life is threatened, as soon as problems that stem from an inability to meet these human needs are diminished, high priority must be transferred to problems that arise because other human needs have not yet been satisfied effectively. In some nursing situations, there may be no problems with survival needs initially, and high priority is given to needs for closeness and self-esteem. For example, the client who has a poor self-image may disregard safety measures and refuse to eat. Resolving the problem with self-esteem may also solve problems regarding other needs that stem from the original problem area.

In all situations, the client should be closely involved in decisions that set levels of priority. In instances in which the nurse and client assign different priorities to the same problem, the difference can be resolved by mutual communication of the reasons for setting a particular priority. Priorities set by the client should be considered whenever possible. Other factors that influence the priorities set for clients include the availability of personnel and resources, the cost of needed services, and the approximate time needed to resolve their problems, particularly from each one's point of view.

Once priorities have been identified by the client and the nurse, an ordering of these priorities is established. The nurse specifies the goal with behavioral outcomes for the client in relation to human need fulfillment. Specific outcome measures should be established for each goal and specific measurement intervals should be specified. A determination should be made regarding the point in time goal achievement is expected and what outcome data will be required to determine goal achievement. The nurse designates possible solutions for each client problem diagnosed, but solutions offered by the client should be included. The possible success of each solution to a problem is estimated, based on scientific principles and sound research. A highly developed intuitive sense of the nurse may come into play in making the final judgment about the best solution for the clients' problem. Client variables such as age, gender, life-style, education, socioeconomic and cultural background, ability to cope with problems, and physiologic and emotional status, as they relate to and effect suggested solutions, should be considered. The nurse predicts, as accurately as possible, the consequences of each solution. Then, in cooperation with the client, the nurse selects the solution most likely to be successful in resolving or diminishing the problem. If the client endorses the solution, efforts and cooperation by the client in implementing that solution will ensure its success. If the client is the family, family members participate in the selection of the solution(s). Similarly, significant community members participate in the specification of solutions for community problems or diagnoses.

The solution may be multifaceted, with immediate, intermediate, and long-range implications. A solution with an immediate result is one that can be accomplished in a short span of time. One with an intermediate result can be attained over a period of time—teaching, supporting, preventing acute problems; whereas a solution with a long-range result is oriented toward the future. Solutions and results for the client include preventive and rehabilitative aspects as well as crisis or immediate aspects relative to the present wellness–illness status. For example, if the client's problem is constipation and this difficulty has been a long-standing one aggravated by the frequent use of laxatives and self-administered enemas, to relieve the condition temporarily would neither resolve the problem (nursing diagnosis) nor provide long-term benefits. The client may experience immediate relief, but requires sustained relief if an impact is to be made on the problem and if discomfort, inconvenience, and the cost of relief measures are to decrease. For example, one solution may be specified to provide immediate relief by using pharmacological or mechanical agents. Additional solutions may have intermediate and long-range effects, such as developing a regimen to increase fluid intake, increase fruits and vegetables in the diet, plan specific time for defecation, and provide privacy and an unhurried atmosphere, as enemas and laxatives are gradually withdrawn. This regimen would be instituted after pathological conditions that cause constipation, such as strictures, tumors, and congenital anomalies, have been ruled out. To relieve constipation only for the present would not have a lasting impact on the problem and thus could cause the client to return repeatedly to obtain relief.

Intermediate and long-range results that stem from solutions to the problems will be concerned with preventing complications, with rehabilitation, and with health instruction. Continuity of care is enhanced by this farsightedness, and the cost of health care, both in time and money, to the client and health personnel will be considerably less. Immediate, intermediate, and long-range results of the solutions are appropriate if the problem can be resolved. Long-range results may focus on preventing additional problems or on preventing intensification of the present problem. This would be true, for example, when the problem is permanent blindness. Failure to designate long-term expectations may mean the difference between a client who can become maximally independent or one who remains dependent and therefore derives only limited joy from living because of multiple complications and problems.

When a problem that can be resolved by nursing intervention has been identified and the best solution has been selected based on the strengths and resources of the client or family, or community, the availability and competency of nursing and health personnel, and the resources available for health and nursing care, specific nursing actions or strategies (and their frequency) are prescribed to bring about the expected outcomes for the client's problems.

Problems of the person, the family, and the community that can be resolved by nursing intervention must be differentiated from those that require not only the attention of a nurse but also that of one or more members of the health care team, such as a physician, physical therapist, or clinical pharmacist, and from those problems that can best be resolved by other members of the health care team or by specific members of the community, such as a lawyer, employer, or legislator. A well-designated and developed referral system should be established so that appropriate persons can be involved with a minimal loss in time and so that maximum use can be made of persons and agencies qualified to solve various client problems. Methods and forms are generally available for use by agency health care personnel.

Nursing Strategies

The solution to any one client problem or nursing diagnosis may be an adaptation of a known solution or it may be designed specifically for that problem. When the solution most likely to be successful is selected, specific nurse actions designed to achieve the short-term, intermediate, and long-range results of that solution must be delineated. These prescribed actions directed toward human need fulfillment for the client are called *nursing strategies*. For example, a sample of nursing strategies that might be developed for the client with sleep deprivation to achieve the goal of resumption of normal sleep pattern within 3 days follows.

Nursing Strategies with Frequencies

1. Complete the assessment of client's normal sleep pattern within the next 24 hours.

2. Investigate the support services available to client for assistance with nightly vigil with spouse. Consult with social worker (within 24 hours).
   - Plan the strategy with the person(s) hired to keep vigil with spouse to handle spouse's behavior.
   - Assist the client to orient hired person(s) to household and expectations so client will not require nighttime awakening.
   - Assure that client will be awakened for emergency and only then.
   - Check outcome of above strategy in 2 days.
3. Workout the strategy with the client to reestablish normal sleep pattern.
   - Assist the client to: arrange for conducive sleep environment (away from spouse's bedroom and person hired to care for spouse during the night);
     - arrange for appropriate security of household;
     - provide level of darkness, humidity, temperature, controlled tolerable noise level, and freedom from other disturbances, e.g., noxious odors.
   - Encourage the client:
     - to wear comfortable bedtime clothes;
     - to resume pre-sleep rituals that promote sleep.
4. Teach the client relaxation exercises to bring about sleep. Begin by alternate tensing/relaxing of muscles while lying in bed—starting either with the toes and proceeding upward to head or from head and proceeding downward. Have client pay particular attention to relaxation of jaw.
5. Use suggestion as a mechanism to bring about sleep.
6. Encourage the client to keep a diary or log of activities related to sleep (length and quality of sleep; time, length, and number of awakenings) for 1 week. Review the diary with the client.
7. Plan a dietary regime with client to assure that foods (i.e., milk, cheese, peanut butter) containing the protein tryptophan are included, especially with the evening meal or bedtime snack.
8. Encourage client to avoid foods and beverages containing caffeine throughout the day, but particularly with the evening meal and at bedtime.

Nursing actions should be clear, purposeful, moral, capable of being accomplished, and adapted to the particular life situation, beliefs, and expectations of the client. Because nursing action is designed to solve the problem, the goal and behavioral outcomes expected as a result of that action should be stated in terms of the *client's behavior*, reflecting a human need that is fulfilled or met. The nurse can judge the impact of actions only by specifying and recording the client's behaviors. Statements of nurse behaviors can be a basis for evaluating the nurse's competency, but if the effectiveness of the care rendered is to be evaluated, expected outcomes must be stated in client terms.

In some health care settings, established policy may dictate the kind of action to be implemented and the person who will implement that action. Policies pertaining to nursing care should be formulated by nursing personnel. Health team members may develop policies and procedures for handling particular problems or governing some particular area in a health care facility. Policies bypass thinking; the person involved in implementing a policy must know the specific circumstances under which it applies. When the situation is recognized, the policy is applied. Policies may vary from designating the number of visitors per hospitalized client to the established policies and procedures formulated in the event of cardiac arrest. They appear to be more numerous in settings where personnel tend to be less prepared. Thus, there are policies to safeguard clients. For example, a policy stating that every hospitalized client 65 years of age or over must have bed side rails probably resulted from evidence that older clients often fall from their beds during their periods of hospitalization. This policy does not protect the 50-year-old with an orientation or behavior pattern that might result in a fall. Nursing judgment is needed to interpret policies and make appropriate adaptations in the best interest of the client. Policies and procedures need to be reviewed from time to time. Circumstances under which they were formulated may no longer exist and other policies may be needed. The nurse should be informed of prevailing policies, for and by whom they were instituted, of the allowable latitude in their interpretation, and what procedures must be followed to change the policy. The nurse is obligated to bring to the attention of the appropriate persons those policies potentially detrimental to clients or those which are misinterpreted or overly implemented by personnel. Clear, precise policies and procedures developed for such units as coronary care, kidney dialysis, or intensive care help these facilities function quickly and smoothly. These policies should also be reviewed periodically, particularly if clients demonstrate high levels of anxiety, signs of sensory overload, or sensory or sleep deprivation. Precise data to support any request for a policy change that would improve care and enhance the individuality of the client would be helpful. All policies should be expressed in writing and dated to safeguard the nurse against pressures that perpetuate patterns of action that are custom rather than policy.

The quality and quantity of nursing actions delineated to solve a client problem and effect a specific behavioral change will be determined by the nurse's knowledge and experience. The nurse's knowledge of biological, physical, and behavioral sciences, as well as nursing knowledge, clinical experience, research orientation, and knowledge of resources—nurse consultants, researchers, interdisciplinary health team members, nursing and health literature—broadens the options, variations in actions, and the application and expectations from the actions. The nurse designates actions that will most likely effect a behavioral change and that have been approved by the client. Documenting these nurse actions—what should be done, when, and how—constitutes nursing strategies.

When actions are designated to offset human need fulfillment alterations or nursing diagnoses, according to priority, a decision is made as to who will carry out these actions, when, and how. The nurse may select those he or she will do for and with the client, those the client can perform unassisted, those that can be performed by the family with or without supervision, and those actions that can be accomplished by certain members of the nursing team. To assign the nurse who is best able to perform the nursing actions—making adaptations and modifications to suit the client's strengths, limitations, level of wellness, illness, and personal preferences—a team conference may be appropriate for planning. It not only serves to orient nursing team members involved in the care of the client but may also be useful to ensure that the client's interests and preferences will be considered, the human needs met, and the problem solved.

It must be obvious to the reader that both the assessment and the planning phases draw heavily on intellectual skills—critical thinking, decision making, judgment, observation—and interpersonal skills. The latter are used to establish rapport through verbal and nonverbal communication, including active attentive listening. Technical skills are used mainly in the assessment phase to obtain data but to a lesser extent than are intellectual and interpersonal skills. Intellectual and interpersonal skills are paramount in the planning phase.

During the entire planning phase, activity is directed toward the quality and quantity of nurse actions that will be needed to resolve or minimize client's problems within the human need framework. This activity effects specified behavioral change within the context of immediate, intermediate, and long-term results of nursing actions, and culminates in the formulation of the nursing care plan for the person, the family, or the community as clients.

Nursing Care Plan

The nursing care plan includes precise data about a specific client. These data are organized in a systematic, concise manner that facilitates overall nursing and health goals. It clearly communicates the nature of the client's problems. It contains all information about the client, the actual and potential nursing diagnoses and the priorities assigned to each, problems and complications to be prevented, and expected outcomes with prescribed nursing actions.

The format for the nursing care plan should flow from the goals set. Space should be provided to designate client problems, solutions, nurse actions, and expected outcomes. A suggested human need framework for a nursing care plan for the person, the family, and the community is presented in Figure 3–4. The health care agency may have an operational nursing care plan form. This form can be adjusted to accommodate human needs and be appropriate to clients and to problems that are most likely to be seen in the health care facility. Or, the plan may be developed and included as part of the problem-oriented system that may be utilized by multidisciplinary health personnel whose focus is the resolving of client problems relating to wellness–illness (nursing as well as medical, dental, dietary, etc.).

A well-written nursing care plan provides a central source of information about the client, with a description of the client's specific problems (nursing diagnoses) based on human need fulfillment alterations (too much, too little, or disturbed pattern) and a plan of action to solve them. A nursing care plan has become increasingly important with the increased number of professional and nonprofessional personnel involved in the nursing and health-related services rendered to the client.

The plan is developed by the professional nurse who obtained the data for the nursing history and the health examination; this nurse is most knowledgeable about the client and has the data needed for planning effective nursing care. The plan developed incorporates elements in the medical care plan so that designated regimens complement rather than conflict with each other. When the most knowledgeable nurse creates the nursing care plan, recognition of the client's individuality is most likely to be enhanced. This nurse is the one who is most likely to know the client's ability to cope with situations; thus, intervention will not be planned where none is needed and at those times when the client is coping with problems satisfactorily. The right to appropriate independence, as well as to interdependence and dependence in the management of wellness and illness is fostered in the client.

Once the nursing care plan is developed, it can be utilized as a separate entity or be included as a component part of the prevailing system utilized in the health care agency, provided this system is truly client-focused and problem-oriented.

The development of the nursing care plan is, therefore, a knowledgeable, creative, and intellectual activity and should be so designed as to mark its identity explicitly, even if the client's name is omitted. When one nurse is responsible for developing and keeping the plan

Client Data: _____

Human Need	Nursing Diagnosis	Due to or Related to	As Evidenced by	Goal Description and Expected Behavorial Outcomes

Nursing Strategies with Frequencies

Figure 3–4. Human need framework for nursing care plan (person, family, community).

viable, additional data about the client obtained by other nursing and health care personnel can be directed to this nurse. Often, important data are lost or given low priority when they are submitted to the wrong person, or the receiver places little value on the information because he or she has no knowledge of the client's problems or goal or does not view the data in relation to other available client data.

A clearly stated nursing care plan is the most effective means of assuring the client that problems will be solved and human needs fulfilled. The drain on the time and energy of nursing personnel and the frustration and anxiety experienced by clients when the staff is not interested in or unaware of their human needs and preferences can be eliminated. If clients know the nurse is interested in them, if they know what to expect and whom to summon, they are likely to be more relaxed and less anxious. They also are less likely to make frequent requests for errands or small favors—often only as an assurance that someone cares and knows that they exist. If the clients' problems, preferences, and life-styles are known, the actions of the nursing staff will be more useful and purposeful. Time wasted through ineffective or multiple actions by many nursing personnel because goals are lacking, communication is poor, and facts about the client are not being used properly can be reduced substantially.

The time used in preparing a nursing history and health assessment, a nursing diagnosis, and a nursing care plan is time well spent. Failure to take the time to assess and plan before intervening contributes to the misuse of time and to wasted efforts and talents of nursing and health care personnel. The cost in economic, physical, and emotional terms can hardly be estimated. Economically and morally, the profession of nursing cannot permit this misuse of human and material resources.

An additional dimension of planning which fosters the logical progression of nurse actions has its greatest impact when the nurse and client interact on a continuing basis throughout a 24-hour period. This planning includes timing specific actions, paying special attention not only to human needs but also to the client's circadian rhythms. For example, if the nurse is required to perform numerous actions and there are accompanying actions by other members of the health team, such as a physical therapist, occupational therapist, medical technologist, or physician, actions should be planned to permit undisturbed periods of sleep and undisturbed meals. Not to include these considerations during the planning phase may cause problems for clients and divert some of the energy required to heal and improve their state of health. Thus, time is a major consideration in planning. It considers not only when nursing actions will take place, but the biological timing of the client, which must be known and preserved. Considerable research literature is available concerning biological rhythms. It has direct bearing on the nurse's understanding of self and the meeting of human needs for the nurse and the client.

Once developed, the nursing care plan is ready to be implemented. At this point, the plan should not be considered a finished product. It is merely a guide to actions and must be kept viable by additions and changes based on the status of the client's problems, on evidence of resolution of these problems, and on continuous collection of data as nurse and client get to know and trust each other.

The format of the nursing care plan should be such that it is easy to use and contains enough space to record everything that should be written. Although brevity and clarity are characteristics of a useful nursing care plan, its use will be diminished considerably if brevity becomes the exclusive goal. The development of the nursing care plan is the nurse's privilege and expression of his or her knowledge, ability, and focus in regard to the client. It will also serve as the model for all actions initiated by other members of the nursing team. Thus, the nurse contributes to the effectiveness and goal direction of others, all of which benefit the client. If the nurse's clientele have similar human variables and/or types of pathophysiology or psychopathology, for example, it is recommended that a *model* nursing care plan be developed utilizing all 35 human needs and incorporating the variables. The model nursing care plan will serve as a ready reference when formulating an individualized nursing care plan. A sample nursing care plan for the client with Alzheimer's disease is presented in the next chapter.

Every effort should be made to develop a method of displaying and storing the nursing care plan so that it is readily available to the nurse when it is needed. No one should have to wait to review the plan because someone else is using the folder that contains it. For study and research, the nursing care plan and information about how it evolved should be preserved, since it contains first-hand data about persons, families, communities, their human needs, solutions to these fulfillment problems, and evidence of the status of goal achievement that may be useful in further developing nursing's human need theory.

Bertha Harmer made similar statements in 1926 in her book entitled *Methods and Principles of Teaching the Principles and Practice of Nursing*. She suggested that nurses develop a written program of nursing care and that these programs be kept and filed under a classification of diseases. She believed that nurses would collect a mass of information about nursing specific persons and about nursing in general. Organized knowledge would be available in a form that permits the nurse to go back and check his or her work, to note progress in content and method, and ". . . to compare facts presented for the study of a great many cases of the same class, and of different classes, and to select facts common to all cases of the same class; in other words, to formulate principles, to organize knowledge—the process of making knowledge, which is science."[2]

Also, the plan can serve as the basis for a model for the care of other persons with similar problems, with a similar ability to cope with problems, or it can serve as a point of self-improvement for the nurse as well as for all members of the nursing team.

Sharing the nursing care plan with nursing and appropriate health team members fosters a better understanding of the client, and the efforts of all health and nursing personnel are more likely to complement each other. Team members will find that they can function in their roles more effectively and successfully when their associates' roles are clarified. Health team members should be encouraged to utilize the nursing care plan as a resource. In situations where a joint plan of care is formulated by the interdisciplinary health team, the nursing care plan will be incorporated into the joint plan. Nursing diagnoses, client goals and outcomes, and specifically determined nursing strategies should be clearly visible in the joint plan or problem-oriented system.

The planning phase ends when the nursing care plan has been designed and developed. This plan is an effective medium for transmitting information for planned care in that all team members can accurately perceive and implement the care intended. It should be designed so that it can be utilized quickly and can result in nurse actions that are meaningful and directed toward resolving the client's problems.

In some situations, client problems, particularly those that are critical in nature, may be preplanned for use within the framework of the nursing process. Preplanning involves the use of nursing or problem-solving processes to develop plans of action when time is important and life may depend on a predetermined plan of action. An example of such preplanning would be actions to be taken in case of fire. Available data about fires, how they start, various types of fires, combatting various types of fires (electrical, chemical, etc.), the combustibility of materials, level of vulnerability of a particular setting, fire regulations, materials available to extinguish fires, techniques for safety of personnel and clients, and methods of prevention should be sought. In addition to the literature and manuals, a specialist in fire fighting should be sought for consultation. A plan could be drawn up by nursing and health team members, clients, and other interested persons, then tested for accuracy and efficiency, including dissemination of the plan, instructing personnel about their roles, and testing equipment. A periodic review to reinforce the plan should be scheduled. Thus, as soon as the nurse assesses the fire, the plan indicated by the situation is implemented. The applicability and effectiveness of the plan can only be evaluated after it has been used. Preplanning may include all members of the nursing team, health team members, and citizens. Other situations in which preplanning is valuable include such crises as cardiac arrest, mass disasters, such as floods and earthquakes, drownings, explosions, and emergency treatment for accidents (poisonings, burns). The more intense the crisis and the greater the immediate threat to life, the less time there is for thinking and problem solving, the more important preplanning becomes. The plan is revised as new knowledge of how different crises should be handled becomes known. Thus, there is less time between the assessment and implementation phases. When the crisis has passed or diminished, the usual problem-solving methods prevail.

In addition to preplanning by health and nursing team members and citizens, the nurse may find it necessary to preplan a selected number of problems to enhance the safety, security, and life of the client, and which could be used until the problem is relieved or its intensity and immediacy diminishes. For example, if the nurse is working in a school setting and among the students there are a few with epilepsy, she may preplan the care they should receive for a seizure. This preplanning involves collecting a great deal of data about the clients' patterns and manifestations of convulsions; the presence or absence of an aura; the clients' methods of handling themselves before the onset; the characteristics and effects of the convulsion; data from the literature about convulsive seizures; identifying problems associated with convulsive seizures (falls); known methods of promoting safety and minimizing injury during or after a seizure; identifying persons likely to be involved, such as teachers and classmates; ramifications for each client when a seizure occurs, for example, during a swim class, in the science laboratory, or in the lecture hall; formulating a plan of action in the event of a seizure and communicating that plan among teachers, friends, the clients, or selected classmates who may become involved. Suggestions shared by these persons should be incorporated into the plan. Once the plan is implemented, it should be evaluated. Other plans might be devised by the nurse as they are needed; for example, what to do in the event of sudden death (in whatever setting this may occur), choking, obstructed airway, or hemorrhage.

Preplanning may be appropriate for anticipated crises and problems, where thinking and planning time is limited and where immediate action is necessary to enhance the client's safety. Preplanning focuses on an event and is often highly technical. Continued preplanning beyond the selected crisis, for more than "just in case," or outside the framework of the nursing care plan defeats its purpose. Preplanning should be used within the various phases of the nursing process, and incorporated into a client-centered, goal-directed human need framework. Excessive, exclusive, or inappropriate use may be dehumanizing and depersonalizing, focusing on an event or problem rather than on the client, or focusing on one problem to the exclusion of others. It can add a measure of confidence to the nurse and security for the client if the nurse knows what to do in an emergency. Preplanning may be strategic in that it may help the nurse to prevent a situation, and the plans should be shared with nursing and health team members, family members, and clients, if appropriate. When the design of the nursing care plan is completed, the planning phase is concluded. The viability of the nursing care plan is tested in the implementation phase of the nursing process.

IMPLEMENTING

Implementing is the initiation and completion of actions necessary to accomplish the defined goal of optimal wellness for the client through fulfillment of human needs. When the nursing care plan has been developed, the implementation phase begins. Depending on the nature of the client's problem and on the condition, ability, and resources of the client as well as the nature of the action planned, the nursing care plan may be implemented by the client, the nurse and client, the nurse alone, or with nursing team members who act and function under the nurse's supervision. Implementation may also be accomplished by the nurse assisted by nursing team members, in cooperation with health team members or in conjunction with family or community members. Any combination or all of these situations may prevail. In other words, in any one situation, some planned actions may be accomplished by the client, some by the nurse, and others by nursing team members. In other instances, only the client may be involved. This is particularly true if the client is well and prevention or maintenance of human need fulfillment is the goal. The client may be able to continue wholesome health practices or new health practices in place of faulty ones. Some or many care measures may also be performed by the client's family, not only for clients who are homebound, but also for inpatients in health care facilities.

The implementation phase of the nursing process draws heavily on the intellectual, interpersonal, and technical skills of the nurse. Decision making, observation, and communication are significant skills, enhancing the success of action. These skills are utilized with the client, the nurse, nursing team members, and health team members. Although the focus is action, this *action* is *intellectual, interpersonal,* and *technical* in nature.

With the nursing care plan as the blueprint and client goals with behavioral expectations and time frame firmly in focus, actions are put into practice. The plan is not carried out blindly as though all thinking and decision making had been completed during the two previous phases.

The nurse continues to collect data about the client as a person, about the client's condition, problems, reactions, and feelings. Additional information continues to be gleaned from other nursing and health care personnel, and from family, neighbors, teachers, and records. The same holds true if the client is the family or the community.

The success or failure of the nursing care plan depends on the nurse's intellectual, interpersonal, and technical abilities. This includes the ability to judge the value of new data that become available to the nurse during implementation, and the nurse's innovative and creative ability in making adaptations to compensate for unique characteristics—physical, emotional, cultural, and spiritual—that become known during interaction with the client. The nurse must have the ability to react to verbal and nonverbal cues, validating inferences based on observation. Paramount during the interaction is the nurse's acceptance of him or herself as a person and the confidence in his or her ability to perform the independent nursing functions inherent in the planned action, recognizing those that are interdependent and which contribute to fulfilling the medical care plan. The nurse must have a realistic understanding of self, recognizing and accepting strengths and limitations; be convinced of his or her own personal worth and find meaning in his or her life; meet his or her own human needs reasonably well, so that he or she can, with willingness and joy, give of him or herself to another—strength, courage, faith in the competency of the client, value for life, knowledge, skill, and time during the interim when these might be needed by another. The nurse must feel comfortable being him or herself, authentically him or herself. The nurse should feel secure and adequate in his or her relations with others. If the nurse's human needs are satisfied and his or her own thoughts, feelings, and actions can be controlled, then he or she will be able to focus on the thoughts, feelings, and human needs of another in a wholesome comfortable manner. Although the nurse meets many of his or her needs outside the nurse–client interaction, the nurse's needs for recognition, creative expression, conceptualization, problem solving, challenge, and self-fulfillment are satisfied in his or her function as a nurse through the interactions with clients, their families, co-workers, and colleagues. The more wholesome the nurse's view of him or herself as a person and the stronger the philosophy of life, the less likely the client will experience depersonalizing encounters with the nurse.

The nurse should feel confident, comfortable, and satisfied in relating to clients. The assessment and planning phases require these same qualities in the nurse; in addition, the implementation phase tests the nurse's endurance, love, intellectual ability, and interpersonal and technical skills.

The amount of time spent with the client, whether in the home or in the health care facility, varies significantly, ranging from a short to a prolonged interaction. This encounter could range from minutes and hours per day to a daily, weekly, monthly, or yearly continuation of the relationship; the interaction may be continuing or intermittent. Interaction should be planned precisely by the nurse and client, with allowances made for the unexpected.

It is strategic that each interaction be goal directed and purposeful. An atmosphere of intellectual and interpersonal "thereness" should prevail. In other words, the interaction demands alert, observant, and attentive behavior by the nurse. In this atmosphere, the nurse conveys his or her concern for the client, and an interest in helping the client achieve optimal wellness. The nurse imparts personal views of this person's dignity and value by manner of speech, tone of voice, gestures, and mannerisms. This means conveying dignity and value even though the client may not feel, look, or smell good, or act, look, or think differently.

In the client's presence, the nurse uses his or her perceptual skills to their fullest. The nurse looks at the client, maintaining eye contact as much as is comfortable, and observes posture, appearance, actions, the immediate environment, and the presence of other persons. The nurse may initiate conversation or allow the client to do so. The client is given the opportunity to direct the conversation and initiate topics of interest. The nurse actively listens to what is said, indicating by nods or short statements that what the client is saying is understood. The nurse asks for clarification if he or she does not understand and helps the client focus on a topic when it is difficult to do so. He or she adjusts and adapts his or her manner and the content of communication with the client when the situation is such that verbal expression is difficult, temporarily not possible (client has a tracheostomy), or permanently impossible. The nurse must be able to judge when it is necessary to listen more patiently, when an interpreter is needed, when technical or mechanical devices such as paper and pencil are needed, and when hand signals should be used. The nurse and the client will also need to know when verbal communication is not necessary, silence is appropriate, touch is useful and appropriate, as well as when and where it should not be used, or when words are conveying a message different from the nonverbal message coming through. The nurse judges how to word his or her statements and questions in a manner that will elicit responses within the client's capabilities (physical, emotional, social, educational), and uses repetition, as needed, without demeaning or demoralizing the client. If the nurse cannot understand the client's message, he or she freely admits this and seeks ways or persons who could enhance his or her understanding.

The nurse is fully aware of the requirement to communicate with the client who does not respond in the usual and expected manner. Talking to the infant or to the comatose or unconscious client is important, not only from the standpoint of conveying a message, but to maintain as much sensory integrity and contact as possible. The verbal as well as the accompanying nonverbal message may be received, even though the receiver is unable to return verbal messages. The nurse can meet human needs for safety, acceptance, love, tenderness, and territoriality, by talking to the client, by his or her manner or voice, particularly by holding a client's hand, feeling the brow, or supporting a shoulder. Further, very young or very old clients who are isolated, or who become disoriented, may feel alone or abandoned if human contacts are limited or task centered. It is extremely important to prevent sensory deprivation for these clients.

The nurse may find that the client needs the nurse's full attention and in this case, the nurse will choose to sit in full view of the client, yet with the privacy of their interaction protected. At other times, the nurse may find that opportunity for conversation will be available while bathing or feeding the client. Since the nurse has considerable data about the person, he or she will be able to use it to explore or suggest topics. The nurse may plan a caring activity, using this activity as a vehicle to foster conversation. The nurse will judge when technical activity will enhance the client's safety and security more than verbal assurances. Thus, by viewing action in terms of expectation of nursing care, based on client problems, the nurse's focus on achieving a client goal is facilitated, often meeting several human needs simultaneously by a particular action. For example, relieving dyspnea has physical as well as emotional implications for the client. If the nurse does not perceive or respond to the client's dyspneic state, his or her anxiety may increase, adding additional stress to any respiratory reserve which may result in a disturbance in interchange of gases.

When the purpose of the nurse–client interaction is to perform a technical action, the success of the nurse's activity can be heightened if he or she focuses on the recipient's immediate situation as well as on the technical procedure itself. Clients are entitled to an explanation of the action; their role and expected behavior during the action; the expected results of the action; the type of equipment, solution, and so on; the discomforts to be anticipated; the position to be maintained; and how much privacy will be afforded. Clients are not only informed, but also receive the message unmistakenly that the nurse is sensitive to their human needs, particularly freedom from excessive fear and territoriality, knows the technical aspects and expectations of the procedures, and considers each as a person. The equipment should be assembled outside the immediate environment, if possible, particularly when discomfort is associated with the technical action, the requisite equipment is not prepackaged, considerable time is needed to prepare the equipment, or the nurse requires more time to organize and familiarize him or herself with the use of the equipment and the procedural method, or desires to consult someone about the technical aspects of its use or the procedural method involved. If the technical aspects are to be performed by or in cooperation with another member of the health team, a mutual understanding of the role of each person (nurse, health professional, client) and the requisites for the procedure should be established in advance. The client's preparation and participation should be clarified before the technical action is initiated.

The nurse continually uses decision-making skills, judging when the procedural method and the timing of the technical action must be modified, or when consultation with or assistance from other persons is necessary to assure a safe, effective action.

In each contact with the client, the nurse not only focuses on the purpose or goal of the interaction but also continually expands his or her perceptual ability to obtain data about the client indicating that the planned action is correct. The nurse seeks data that would indicate other problems arising from unmet, poorly, or excessively met human needs. The nurse continually reviews the client's reaction to his or her thoughts and actions, for discrepancies are quickly picked up between verbal expressions of interest and concern and actual practice. When the client is not called by name, or when the nurse fails to look at the client, uses a brusque manner, is impatient, rough, or focuses on a body part or piece of equipment rather than on the client, then the nurse's disinterest is clearly evident to the client.

If another member of the nursing team assists the nurse with planned actions, special attention must be paid to the client-centered focus. Conversation between or among nursing personnel in the presence of the client should focus on and include the client. Social conversation or conversation pertaining to other clients, or about nursing and health care personnel, has no place in the immediate client setting. Further, the client quickly picks up the nurse's and his or her assistant's lack of interest, attention, and concern. The impact may be quite serious if the client's ability to cope with the situation is strained, if the client's self-image is poor, and if the client is apt to misinterpret motives. While light conversation may be very appropriate and may serve as needed diversion, it should include the client and be of interest.

As the nurse proceeds to implement the nursing care plan, he or she learns more about the client's reactions, feelings, strengths, limitations, coping ability, preferences, satisfactions, and dissatisfactions. The nurse learns the client's response to planned nurse actions, the additional ways available to him or her and the client to perform actions, the requirement for additional actions, and any untoward response to the planned actions. These data are synthesized and utilized to further develop the nursing care plan and are the basis for recording data about the client on appropriate client records. Similarly, the nurse learns more about the family and the community as clients, and continues to expand the data base for the nursing care plan.

If the nurse finds that some or selected actions should and could be performed safely by other members of the nursing team, these actions should be delegated. The nurse knows the capabilities of nursing team members and should also know the responsibilities of persons with a particular title and legal ramifications as well as those who have a specific role. The nurse needs to know the strengths and limitations of the individuals in these roles and should focus on selecting the most appropriate person to perform a specific action for the client. The person so designated should have as much information about the client as is needed so that any action is truly effective and the nursing team member is able to perform in an informed manner. Thus, delegated activities are part of the whole focus of action and contribute purposefully to expectations or results of care. The persons performing the delegated tasks are responsible for their own acts and are expected to report the outcome in terms of the client. The nurse supervises the performance of supportive nursing personnel.[3] Data about clients obtained by team members should be communicated to the nurse responsible for their care and for implementing the nursing care plan. If more than one nurse is involved in a client's care, particularly in inpatient settings, written and verbal reports concerning the client as well as an up-to-date nursing care plan are needed to ensure continuity and goal direction. Each nurse responsible for the client's care should participate in the changes needed to keep the nursing care plan viable. If conflict arises relative to the interpretation of goal or outcome specific to the action to be taken by the nurse, or the priority of action to meet the desired goal, or client responses differ at different times of the day, a conference should be planned with the nurses involved and with the client to resolve it. This does not necessarily mean that two different strategies could not be used to achieve the same end because the views, knowledge, or experiences of the nurses involved differ. Resolution is needed only when conflict involves a goal or priority opposing that planned with the client.

In designating the *who* in terms of planned nurse action, the nurse may feel that he or she is best prepared to perform the action at a particular time from an intellectual, interpersonal, or technical standpoint. The nurse may find that a performance of a particular action will serve as a vehicle to meet human needs for safety, love, and respect. The nurse may wish to use his or her presence or thereness, to give the client an opportunity for self-expression and to share any doubts, fears, and anxieties. The nurse may require assistance and will decide on who, the amount, and type he or she needs. This pattern may vary at any time and is always dictated by behavioral changes in the client, the available nurse manpower, and the coping ability of the client and family.

Just as the nurse's philosophy, education, and experience influence the type and character of nursing actions the nurse designs to meet client problems, so will these significantly affect implementing the actions. The nurse's emphasis, focus, and creativity will be affected by his or her own strengths, limitations, prejudices, stereotypes, knowledge of human behavior, convictions, and ability to both handle human closeness and use him or herself therapeutically. The nurse's willingness to share knowledge of his or her intellectual, emotional, social, and spiritual boundaries, will influence what the nurse will do, can do, and knows enough not to do.

Gentleness, sureness, and strength can be conveyed by the nurse, not only to alleviate associated discomfort, embarrassment, or frustration accompanying the problem, but to actually meet the human needs of love, safety, and acceptance.

If other persons are involved in the client's care, the nursing care plan gives direction to the actions of nursing and health care personnel. But the actions and activities of these persons need to be coordinated to make them person-centered and family-centered whether the client is in a health care setting or at home. Coordination takes into account who is doing what and when. This assures that actions are taken and that the client's biological rhythms and situation are benefited rather than overwhelmed. It is possible that an action may be ineffective simply because it is poorly timed, or is done in conjunction with other actions that may conflict or interfere with each other. For example, a health professional enters the room to treat a client with a poor appetite just as the client begins to eat. Or the nurse plans a care activity just as a visitor enters the room of a lonely client. Persons involved in activities with a client may influence the performance of a specific action because of the variation in approach. For example, the manner in which a client is helped out of bed and supported, and which side of the bed is used for this, may influence the client's desire to get out of bed, the amount of time spent out of bed, and what is done when out of bed.

Depending on the client's response during implementation, priorities may have to be reassigned; reassessing and replanning will then be required. Nursing judgment is required to know what to do with data, the additional data needed, what the data mean, whether a new nursing diagnosis is evident, and what the plan of action should be.

Thus, the implementation phase, although it does have an action focus, also includes assessing, planning, and evaluating activities by the nurse. The actions of implementation performed with and for the client could include the following: inserting, withdrawing, turning, cleansing, rubbing, massaging, flexing, irrigating, manipulating, teaching, exercising, offering, awakening, cuddling, holding, drying, applying, communicating, administering, influencing, altering, relieving, supporting, cooling, warming, providing, accompanying, sitting with, listening, walking, moving, touching, soothing, pulling, pushing, facilitating, interacting with, straightening, twisting, wrapping, folding, and on and on. Strategic to these actions are those related to assessing, planning, and evaluating, which complement the action implemented. These actions are needed to resolve, diminish, or dissolve the client's problem and facilitate the fulfillment of human needs.

The actions may be independent or interdependent functions of the nurse. The latter relate to the nurse's participation in the medical care plan and collaborating with multidisciplinary health team members to effect a specific outcome. Interdependent functioning does not imply following prescriptions of other health team members blindly and without question. Critical thinking and sound judgment must be exercised to make decisions about what, when, how much, and in what manner. For example, specific nursing action planned to relieve pain should follow a careful assessment of physiologic manifestations of the pain, its location, quality, and character, severity, what the pain being experienced means to the client, and other factors. The nurse needs to know the pattern of the pain, verbal and nonverbal evidences, and gestures. The nurse may be able to utilize pharmacological measures and manipulate clients' experiences by changing their positions, removing wrinkles or restrictions, and by taking actions that influence their behavioral responses to pain. McCaffery summarized the physiologic and physical factors influencing clients' sensation of pain and the behavior associated with it as (a) neurophysiologic processes underlying the sensation of pain, duration and intensity of pain, alterations in the level of consciousness, cutaneous versus visceral sites of pain, environmental conditions, sensory restriction, physical strain and fatigue; (b) cultural aspects, including sociocultural group membership, age, sex, religion, body part involved in the pain, roles ascribed to members of the health team; and (c) psychological factors, including emotionally traumatic life experiences, secondary gains of the client's complaint of pain, personal past experience with pain, knowledge, understanding, and cognitive level, powerlessness, attitude and feeling of others, perceptual dominance of pain.[4] Thus, the client's pain involves more than automatically administering a prescribed analgesic.

The implementation phase concludes when the nurse's actions are completed and the results of actions and the client's reaction to them have been recorded. Recording these actions and reactions is an important function of the nurse. The quality of the recording about the client and what the nurse chooses to document give direct evidence of the status of goal achievement and individual client reactions. It designates the status of and the direction for continued problem solving. Placing a low value on recording, or insufficient or inappropriate recording, is an affront to the client and demonstrates the nurse's limitations. Deliberate well-thought-out notations and specific statements about the client convey respect for the client's individuality, problem, and reactions to the planned action. The recordings are related to the problem; they describe the nurse's actions and the results, and include additional data. The written report of the nursing care given serves to direct continuing action. Communication, both oral and written, associated with the nursing history and health assessment, nursing diagnosis, nursing strategies and actions, and client actions and reactions, should be given a high priority by the nurse. Recording should reflect the client's unique situation and should be identified easily by the quality of content. The recording should contain the information needed to give a profile of the client whether the client is a person, a family, or a community. Rules that set limits on what and how much should be recorded and that have only one basis—to save time—can be a waste of time. The nurse should decide what to write, how much to write, when to write, and where to write. These are professional judgments. Where to write has the least significance compared with what and how much to write. The place is generally designated by the prevailing record system in an agency. If the prevailing record system is inadequate, action should be taken to institute a system worthy to receive the written observations and actions of the nurse. Writing associated with the development of the nursing history (including health assessment), nursing care plans, and recordings about an action performed is a professional, not a clerical, activity. Nor should it be delegated to persons who are not prepared to assume this important professional responsibility. Specific recording of data certainly may be delegated, but not the nursing history, the health assessment, the designation of nursing diagnoses, the goal statement with expected behavioral outcomes, the nursing care plan, or the recording of significant data about the client that stems from implementing the plan. Recordings are more frequent when the client's behavior changes rapidly. If these changes occur slowly and are infrequent, there will be less to record, but the information will not lose its significance. When recordings become copious or their use is minimized because there is not the time to review them, the information should be summarized periodically in coordination and in conjunction with the nursing care plan. It would be helpful to index recordings of client progress toward goal achievement. The process of indexing would be based on significant experiences or stages in the resolution of a problem, and would also be useful for nursing care plans. If plans have been developed over long periods of time, a new or revised nursing care plan should be developed. All previous plans or additions to it should be retained as long as the client has human need fulfillment alterations that have not been resolved or that are being dealt with but cannot be resolved. Plans developed with persons who are well or for whom health prevention and maintenance are major goals will be reactivated, as needed, for reassessment. These plans and records should be retained for evaluative purposes and future planning. These plans also provide valuable data for the cost of nursing care.

Thus, the implementation phase of the nursing process includes nurse actions determined by the nursing care plan. The nurse continues to focus on the client, conveying, through his or her intellectual, interpersonal, and technical skills, that the client and family are worthy of the nurse's respect and are imbued with dignity. Nursing actions are based on scientific rationale, research results, and directed toward promoting a suitable internal and external environment in which wellness is enhanced and illness diminished. Factors in the external environment include influencing significant legislative actions, particularly those related to the maintenance of health and a safe and viable neighborhood. Available resources and their appropriate use are inherent in the implementation phase. The appropriateness and direction of the nurse's action(s) is determined by the client's behavioral change in the direction of goal achievement. The direction and amount of change is evaluated.

EVALUATING

Evaluating is the appraisal of the changes experienced by the client in relation to goal achievement and realization of expected behavioral outcomes as a result of the actions of the nurse. Evaluation, the fourth component of the nursing process, follows the implementation of actions designated in the nursing care plan. Evaluation is *always considered in terms of how the client responded to the planned action*. Since specific nurse actions were planned to solve client problems resulting from excessively met, unmet, or partially met human needs, any judgment about how these problems are being resolved should originate with the client. It was noted earlier that the human need, nursing diagnosis, and the goal of resolution with expected behavioral outcomes of the client problem would serve as the framework for the evaluation component. The nursing care plan contains the framework for evaluation. The impact of all intellectual, interpersonal, and technical actions on the client as the person, the family, or the community, and the changes these produced are the focus of evaluation.

Although elements of evaluation, like those of assessment and planning, are concurrent and recurrent with other components, evaluating the effect of actions during and after the implementation phase determines the client's response and the extent to which immediate, intermediate, and long-range results are achieved. The evaluation must continue in a purposeful, goal-directed manner until the human need is at the highest level of fulfillment considering the cause. For example, if relief of pain for a person is to be expected from implementing the nursing action, the results would be known within a short period of time. The client would tell the nurse that the pain was or was not relieved. The nurse could compare the client's behavior prior to nursing action, noting posture, facial expression, pulse and respiratory rates, color of a bodily part, and the client's ability to focus on other topics and other persons rather than on the pain. Behavioral evidence would indicate whether the client's pain was fully relieved or not. If the client was the family, and the family nursing diagnosis was an alteration in closeness needs (belonging) because of a rejection of an aged family member, data about the acceptance of the client within the family unit, about relationships between and among family members, mode of addressing the aged person, type of reference statements, level of participation of the aged person in family affairs could be utilized to make a judgment about the state of acceptance of the aged person and level of resolution of the alteration in meeting closeness needs within the family. If the client was the community and the community nursing diagnosis was a deficit in the survival need of gaseous exchange due to an abnormally high level of toxic industrial chemicals in the air, analysis of air quality with specific data about the quantity of the total chemical in the air could give evidence for the necessity to resolve the problem and for effectiveness of strategies.

Evaluation is the natural intellectual activity completing the process phases because it indicates the degree to which the nursing diagnosis, the goal statement with behavioral outcomes, and nursing strategies have been correct. By evaluating nursing strategies the nurse demonstrates the acceptance of responsibility for these actions and shows an interest and involvement in enhancing the effectiveness of actions directed toward solving the client's problems. This also demonstrates that the actions are person-family-community-centered and there is less likelihood a nursing action will be continued if it is not helpful.

Evaluation will also pinpoint omissions during the assessment, planning, and implementation phases. In any given client situation, it is possible that some problems may be resolved at different time intervals. Since evaluation will be in terms of immediate, intermediate, and long-range expectations, the evaluation process is continued until goals are realized. The outcome of the evaluation of human need fulfillment may indicate that the care planned must be reassessed, replanned, modified, and the revised plan implemented and evaluated. Thus, the nursing process is a continuing cycle.

The nurse and the client are the agents of evaluation. Other persons, such as the client's family, nursing and health team personnel, and significant neighborhood and community members may also be involved. Based on the behavioral response of the client relative to the mutually agreed on goals and immediate, intermediate, and long-range behavioral expectations, measurement data are collected so that value judgments can be made. A number of measuring devices and methods are available to obtain these data. For example, these data may include the following: temperature, pulse rate, blood pressure recording, apex rate, electrocardiogram and electroencephalogram, weight, physiologic analyses of urine, blood sugar, blood urea nitrogen, cholesterol, results of attitude surveys, rating scales, and behavioral checklists. The condition and situation of the client—posture, appearance, color, level of orientation—and statements made by the client, family, and significant others should be used by the nurse in the evaluation. The nurse uses the senses to collect data; utilizes communication techniques to elicit subjective data (questioning the client about dizziness and nausea, for example), makes inferences and validates them, makes a decision about the client's behavioral responses and compares the response to the specified expected outcome.

Evaluative Data Gathering

Some of the questions the nurse can ask during this evaluation phase to complete the evaluative data base follow. What was the expected client goal and behavioral outcome in relation to the satisfaction of human needs? Was the expected behavior realistic, accurate? What data supported the judgment that the behavior was realistic and accurate? What behavior was manifested? What tools or instruments were utilized to obtain the data? What observable data were collected? What judgments were made concerning these data? Were significant data overlooked, omitted, or devalued? What subjective data were collected and documented? Were data synthesized and compared before any value judgment was made? Does the client agree with the judgment? Do other members of the nursing team and health team concur with the value judgment?

What additional data are needed? How should they be obtained? From whom should they be obtained—the client, the client's family and associates, the nurse, physician, clinical pharmacist, teacher, or employer? Are data needed from one or all of these sources?

Were the nursing diagnoses, nursing strategies, and nursing care plan developed during the assessment and planning phases accurate and realistic? What data demonstrate appropriate and accurate human need fulfillment? Were the time intervals and measurement expectations for the achievement of human need fulfillment accurate and realistic? What data demonstrate incomplete need fulfillment? Were nursing strategies planned to offset actual or potential nursing diagnoses? Were nursing diagnoses stated as potential or actual alterations in human need fulfillment? Was the plan of action accurate, but the action ineffective because it was not carried out accurately, was inept, or did not consider the client as a person? or as a family? or as a community? Was there input from the client? If not, why not? Was the nursing action accomplished by the wrong member of the nursing team? Should it have been a nursing action at all or should it have been accomplished by the client or family members or a member of the health team?

Were goals stated in light of fulfillment of human needs? What goals have been or are being met? If goals have been met, what are the plans to periodically reassess and maintain a problem-free status?

What factors influenced goal attainment? What factors influenced a limited or lack of goal achievement? Were these factors internal, external, or both? What factors were related to the setting in which the nursing care took place—the home, the clinic, industry, a health care facility? Were environmental, socioeconomic, cultural, or religious factors involved?

Are some client problems partially resolved? How is this partial response determined? Could the problem have been resolved completely if additional data had been sought or an alternative solution tried? Was the assessment complete? Was the nursing diagnosis (diagnoses) correct? Did the problem resolve itself despite omissions in assessment, planning, and implementation? What contributed to this resolution?

If the client's behavioral manifestations indicate that the problem (nursing diagnosis) was not resolved, what were the reasons? What data support the lack of problem resolution? Were there physiological, psychological, intellectual, socioeconomic, cultural, or religious reasons for the lack of resolution? What external factors are influencing this failure to solve the problems? If there is a medical care plan for the client, do the nursing care and medical care plans conflict rather than complement each other? Is there a lack of resources (human, financial, technical)? Is there a permanent handicap, an incomplete understanding of the problem and its impact?

Has the situation been labeled a problem when it is not a problem? Do the client and the nurse want to relinquish the problem? If nursing action was deemed appropriate but the results of the action were ineffective, what was the reason? Was timing incorrect? Did the appropriate member of the nursing team implement the action? Was consideration given to the age, gender, developmental level, and role of the client? Is there a limitation in the nurse's intellectual, interpersonal, or technical skills or in those of a team member?

Was communication effective? Was the message received identical to that sent? Did feedback verify the accuracy of the message?

Did the client suffer an affront to any feelings as a person, e.g., failure to identify the client by name, focusing on a part rather than on the whole person, attending to equipment rather than the client, ignoring persons significant to the client and their participation? Was recognition given to the psychological, emotional, religious, cultural, and socioeconomic influences inherent in the client situation and accompanying implementation of nursing actions?

Was the intent of the goals clear? Are new problems or nursing diagnoses evident? Are they related to other unresolved nursing diagnoses? What data are available about the new problem? Is the problem known to the client? If so, what is the reaction? Is the new problem the result of new pathology or changed socioeconomic status? Is it the result of limited scope in anticipating problems? Is it the result of a change in the client's role, a diminished ability to cope with the situation, or an affront to the client's value system? Are there changes within the family system? Within the community system?

Are there previous problems that have not been dealt with? How have long-range plans influenced these problems? Have they been realistic? Have these plans and related actions made an impact? Were the immediate, intermediate, and long-range expectations of nursing strategies geared to preventing disease and maintaining health, as well as to sickness care, if needed?

Were the nursing actions based on principles from the physical, biological, behavioral, and nursing sciences? Was the nursing action stifled by a rigid policy interpretation or the failure to accept that there are independent functions of the nurse?

Evaluative Outcomes

When the data for evaluation are collected, analyzed, and synthesized a new picture emerges. Either the problem is resolved with human needs fulfilled to an optimal level for the client and no further nursing action is needed or the problem is not resolved and new priorities are set and goals determined. The nursing care plan may no longer be needed or it may continue as designed; it may need to be revised partially or completely. Additions may be made or alternative action selected.

The *outcome* of evaluation may be any one or a combination of the following:

1. The client's human needs are reasonably fulfilled.
   a. The client responded as expected and the problem is resolved.
   b. No further nursing action is needed. A plan to maintain the client's state of optimal wellness is formulated jointly by the nurse and the client.
   c. Potential nursing diagnoses have been identified and appropriate strategies designed to assure continued human need fulfillment. An appointment may be made for a future date to reaffirm the client's problem-free status.
2. Some or all of the client's target human needs remain excessively met, partially or fully unmet, or with disturbed patterns of fulfillment.
   a. Behavioral manifestations of the client's situation indicate that the problem has not been resolved; evidence demonstrates that immediate results, but not intermediate and long-range expectations have been achieved. The nature of the client's problem is such that complete resolution, if it is possible, will be slow. The nursing action is then geared to fulfillment of human needs in the intermediate and extended range. The expectation includes preventing possible problems. Reevaluation is to continue.
   b. Behavioral manifestations of the client are similar to those evidenced during the assessment phase. Little or no evidence is available that the problem has been resolved. Immediate results have not been realized; there may or may not be evidence that intermediate or long-range expectations may begin to be realized. Anticipated and possible problems may or may not have been avoided. Reassessment with replanning is needed.
   c. Behavioral manifestations indicate new problems resulting from excessively met, unmet or poorly met, or disturbance in pattern of fulfillment of human needs. Assessing, planning, and implementing a plan of action to resolve these problems (nursing diagnoses) are in order. Planning action to resolve the

new problem must be coordinated with the planning for the previously diagnosed problems. Evaluation will follow implementation.

If the nurse has used the logical, goal-directed, problem-solving approach of the nursing process, evaluation should indicate a high level of success. Involving the client, the family, and community members in the nursing process contributes to this success. The likelihood that any or all of the client's problems will be resolved is increased.

As the nursing profession directs its efforts toward developing standards for the practice of nursing, these standards are broadly stated and are applicable to all clients who enter the health care system, particularly the nursing subsystem. Standards of nursing practice are stated in terms of a systematic, goal-directed, problem-solving approach. The profession fulfills its obligations to provide and improve nursing practice by developing these standards, which are recognized by nurse practitioners, nurse educators, and nurse administrators nationally. The standards convey to the citizenry a model of nursing service that can be expected from members of the profession and their associates. The nursing actions directed toward resolving client problems are guided by these standards, and action is measured and compared with the standards. Legal decisions affecting nurses are made with the standards of nursing practice as the authority. Evaluation of nursing actions purposely directed toward the client's problem, as included in the nursing care plan, is applicable to a specific client, whether person, family, or community.

As in all other phases, the client is involved in evaluation. Specific nursing actions may be found to be highly effective, moderately or minimally effective, or ineffective; however, these conclusions can only be reached after the degree to which the client's problem has been resolved is evaluated, based on the goal statement and behavioral manifestations demonstrated. Judgment during other phases may have resulted in immediate reassessment and replanning. But only during the evaluation phase is a *comprehensive appraisal* of *goal achievement* made. After client behavior is evaluated, the quality of nursing care and its impact on the client's health status are determined.

Modification is incorporated in the evaluation phase and also follows it, resulting in reprocessing activity, giving feedback for reassessment, and continuing the cycle of each phase. The cyclic process is continued as long as it is needed, in other words, as long as there are goals to be achieved. If the goal to be achieved is the maintenance of the client's well-being, periodic reassessment may continue for an unlimited time span. The nurse–client relationship may be a periodic rather than a continuous interaction. In viewing the use of the nursing process with a client longitudinally, the time interval of nurse–client interactions may be periodic, continuous, or both as evidenced by the client's wellness–illness profile over a span of years.

A changed client situation may result in a transfer, for example, from home to a health care facility, from an acute care facility to a nursing home or vice versa, a transfer to another unit of the same health care facility (from intensive care to a surgical unit), or a discharge to the home. Changes in the client situation or location within the health care system may involve other health professionals. The balance of action geared toward maintaining wellness, preventing illness, giving care during sickness, or fostering rehabilitation may show a directional shift toward the client or toward the nurse.

In addition, a changed client situation may result in disorientation because of sensory deprivation (nursing diagnosis). Behavioral evidence within the client must be sought to demonstrate whether the deprivation was relieved and the goal of sensory integrity achieved. By comparing the client's behavioral profile before and after nursing action, data are obtained to make an evaluative judgment. The basis of sensory deprivation may be factors within the client, e.g., congenital sensory deficit and inability to see, hear, or speak. There may be pathophysiologic and psychopathological reasons. The client may be very young or very old; be isolated from the mainstream of activity due to disease or therapy (staphylococcal infection, AIDS, radiation treatment), or geographic location; be unappealing, not look good, smell good, or have unwholesome habits. The clients may have no relatives or friends; be unconscious, nonverbal, or withdrawn. If the problem was diagnosed and a series of nursing actions was planned to relieve the deprivation, then evidence of increased orientation, cerebration, and sociability would be some of the behaviors the nurse would expect to see in the client. Of course, behavioral expectations would be limited to those the client is capable of. Behavioral manifestations of lessened sensory deprivation for the unconscious client would need to be specified and observed.

If the client is capable of verbal expression, the nurse will have a series of behaviors that designate a decrease in sensory deprivation and an increase in sensory input. Expecting clients to demonstrate that they are oriented in a way in which they were not capable at any time previously would result in failure to achieve a goal. For example, expecting a disoriented child to tell time and know the date may be beyond that which is able to be accomplished, considering the child's age and level of growth and development.

Nurses have supplied calendars and clocks, particularly if the client is in a room that does not have a window. A radio is helpful since time checks, weather reports, news events, as well as a variety of voice tones or music may stimulate the client in whom sensory deprivation is a problem. These aids are especially useful for the unconscious or blind person, and serve as adjuncts to human interaction on the verbal and nonverbal level.

The nurse will seek evidence that the client can recognize familiar and significant persons and things. The nurse can observe the number of human contacts the client has and the quality of the interaction. Does anyone speak to or touch the client? Does the client experience variations in sensation, such as coolness, warmth, softness, roughness, smoothness? Are family members encouraged and assisted to participate in maintaining sensory contact? Do they know how? What are the sounds, smells, sights, colors, temperature of the environment? What are the furnishings of the environment? What sensory stimulation is there for the client? Is the client an active or passive recipient of this stimulation? Does the client attempt sensory stimulation without assistance or encouragement?

Is the client lethargic, unresponsive, irritable, despairing? Are there complaints about limited human contacts? Are family members or significant others contacted and aware of the client's requirement for tenderness and belonging as well as sensory stimulation? Are family members and significant others encouraged and supported in their effort to maintain contact? Is there a clock or a calendar in sight? Is there a radio or television set in the room and is one or the other turned on? If the client is unconscious, does the nurse talk to the client and explain what is being done when lifting the client's leg or arm or elevating the bed? Does the nurse tell the client that the water is cold, warm, or if compresses are being used? Does he or she tell the time of day, day of the week, month of the year to the client? Does the client hear various voice tones—masculine, feminine, loud, soft? These might be some of the questions that must be answered to evaluate changes in client responses, using the initial assessment as a baseline. The results may indicate continuing sensory deprivation, indicating that the nursing actions planned should be continued. Modification in terms of the kind of nursing action, the person(s) doing the action, the intensity and timing of the action, increasing the length of human contact, changing the quality of the contact, and increasing the number of persons involved may be necessary.

If the client is a toddler and excessive crying is evidenced as a lack of fulfillment of nutrition, safety, and love needs, then crying should decrease after the nurse actions planned to offset these human need fulfillment deficits have been implemented. The actual amount of time spent in crying, the character of the cry, the amount of playful activity, evidence of contentment, improved appetite, and increased weight would be observed, recorded, and used to judge that the child's target human needs were being fulfilled. Nursing actions would be considered appropriate, based on the behavioral change noted in the client.

It is expected that if the nursing process is the key to solving these problems created by alterations in human need fulfillment as excesses, deficits, and disturbances in pattern which affect the client's wellness or illness, its use should be highly effective. The client is considered the nurse's partner throughout the phases of the process. In instances where goals and behavioral expectations have not been fully achieved and when a judgment has been made that a particular nursing action or series of nursing actions had little or no effect on the problem for which it was planned, as demonstrated by client behavior, the nurse looks for the reason.

Sources for reasons why predicted outcomes were not realized include the client, the nurse, significant others (to the client), nursing staff members, and health team members. Concerning the client, possible causes include sharing inaccuracies, insufficient information, or withholding important data about self and situation. Causes for failures to realize goals can include an increase in pathophysiology or psychopathology, or both, allergic manifestations, a drain on the client's expected ability to cope with problems because of multiple influencing variables acting simultaneously. Unrealistic expectations of one's self and predicament, loss of self-esteem, loss of job, inadequate finances, untoward reaction to therapeutic agents (chemical, mechanical, pharmacological), a lack of or an insufficient opportunity to participate in diagnosing problems and planning strategies, failure to seek immediate attention for high priority problems, a lack of interest in and attention to goal determination and behavioral outcome specification and planned strategies that have not been accepted by the client are other reasons.

If the nurse is the source, the reasons why the client's problem has not been resolved may include overlooking data; assigning high or low priorities inappropriately; a failure to validate a hunch or inference; a lack of knowledge about the client's situation, particularly socioeconomic, cultural, and religious; failure to recognize intellectual, interpersonal, and technical limitations; failure to use intellectual, interpersonal, and technical strengths; inappropriate delegation of nursing actions to nursing team members; failure to consider elements of the medical plan when formulating the nursing care plan; limited sharing of important information about the client with health team members; failure to consider the value of input from family members, employers, neighbors, or teachers; inadequate fulfillment of independent and interdependent nursing functions; deficiencies in taking a nursing history and performing a health assessment; failure to involve the client in planning; inadequacies in the development of the nursing care plan; failure to specify expectations in relation to human need fulfillment; failure to specify goals and outcomes for human need fulfillment that are realistic in terms of the causes; failure to designate and follow through on data collection at specified intervals in relation to human need fulfillment; failure to recognize client strengths and the desire for independence within the limits of wellness or illness; ineffective or infrequent communication; failure to consider significant others; and failure to recognize the impact a nurse can make on others.

For nursing team members, possible reasons contributing to ineffective goal achievement may be insufficient information about the client and the nursing diagnosis (diagnoses); failure to convey important data about the client to the nurse who is responsible for the nursing care plan; interpersonal affronts to the client as a person, i.e., not calling the client by name, commenting negatively about the client's family, failure to ensure privacy, conversing in the client's presence without including the client; failure to record important data such as intake–output or changes in quality and rate of pulse; giving information about the client to a nurse not knowledgeable about the client; focusing on "things" rather than on the client; being noisy, loud, insensitive, and forceful or domineering.

Concerning the significant others of the client, some of the reasons goals are not achieved are the following: they are not available or are not interested in the client; the problem, its solution, and expected behavioral change are not understood; the client has a limited ability to cope with the problem; fears and anxieties exist about self and client; they fail to see that a problem exists or resources—financial, physical, emotional, intellectual—are limited; lack of transportation; and moral, cultural, and religious influences.

Health team members may be responsible for the failure to achieve the goals planned for the client. Reasons for failures in these cases might include conflicting goals for the client, excessive possessiveness of the client, failure to discern when the focus is on a part of the client rather than the whole, inability to function as a team member, failure to see value in a nursing care plan, limited experience in communicating with members of the nursing team and other health team members, focus on technical aspects of contribution to the exclusion of the interpersonal component, and acts of depersonalizing the client.

The evaluation phase of the nursing process has been the most neglected part of the process, probably because it has been perceived as the most difficult. Evaluation requires measurement. Measurement involves a system of feedback through the use of standards, or a base, that indicates the extent to which there is deviation from the standard or the extent to which the standard is met. Identification of the progress that has been made, or remains to be made to meet a specified standard is an important element in health care. To identify such progress, some valid, reliable instruments are necessary, and these have been in short supply. Over the past 20 years, health care professionals have become more willing to study and to develop the necessary instruments for evaluation; professional nurses have been very active in striving to achieve qualitative evaluation of client care.

Other Evaluative Sources

The importance of evaluation has long been recognized. It was not until the 1970s that quality assurance programs became integral parts of the nurse's functioning. Federal legislation became one impetus for the evaluation of care; there were cries for consumer protection, health care consumers were demanding their rights, and there were concerns for a reasonable return in services for the high price that was being paid for health care. These demands and pressures are in existence today, and there are added stimuli that impact on the evaluation of health care, namely, the presence of Diagnostic Related Groups (DRGs) in the acute care facilities, and the increasing number of older persons who are residents of long-term care facilities.

Professional Standards Review Organizations (PSROs) were established as a result of legislation in 1972; the purpose of these groups is to monitor the appropriateness of those health services that are financed by federally funded programs, such as Medicare, Medicaid, and maternal and child health programs. Professional Standards Review Organizations were among the first visible efforts to comply with the federal mandate. Multiple health care professionals participated in this review effort with nurses functioning as integral parts of this evaluation system.

In 1973, the enactment of the Health Maintenance Organization Act included a request by Congress for a study to identify mechanisms for health care quality assurance.[5] The multifaceted nature of the concept of quality made it impossible to accept one definition of quality. However, characteristics of an ideal quality assurance program were specified. The results are the following:

1. An organizational entity for assessing quality does exist.

2. Standards or criteria exist against which quality is measured.
3. There is a regular system for gathering data.
4. The data sample is representative of the total population.
5. There is a process for reporting results to appropriate consumers and providers of services.
6. There are means for correcting deficiencies.[6]

A total quality assurance program should provide for input from the client, family, nurse and peers, and other health care workers. Efforts have been exerted by nurses and other health personnel involved in rendering health services to clients to determine the level of quality of health and nursing services and to establish if these services make a difference in outcome for the client. The nurse peer review is one method whereby practicing nurses, as peers, appraise the quality of client care rendered by equally qualified practitioners of nursing. This review (focusing on the developed nursing process and client behavioral outcomes) is based on prestated criteria or standards, thereby determining the level of quality of care. This review may be geared to one peer or to a group of peers in a specific health care agency. Such a review should benefit all clients as well as specific clients and should provide a means for an evaluation of the nurse's ability to assess, plan, implement, and evaluate nursing care, by his or her superiors. The expected outcomes for the nurse peer review are: (a) the support of a high level of client care; (b) the diagnosis of low-level care with definitive plans developed for implementation to offset the deficiency; (c) the accumulation of precise data to justify employment of prepared nurses capable of expert utilization of the nursing process and in a number sufficient to meet the health and nursing goals for clients; (d) direct feedback to individual nurses about care rendered by them; (e) specification of monetary and status awards based on high level of competency in the utilization of the nursing process; and (f) data to support and designate areas of need for orientation programs, inservice education, and continuing education.

In addition to the collaborative efforts of the interdisciplinary teams, nurses have moved deliberately on various levels of functioning to develop constructive evaluation systems. The American Nurses' Association's Standards of Nursing Practice are hallmarks of nursing goals to be achieved with all clients. These standards are client-oriented and are developed within a nursing process framework to assure the client of a sound standard from which nurses function (see Appendix B).

Nursing audits are essential elements of care and are the responsibility of all nurses who provide client care. The primary thrust of the audit is to review nurses' recordings of care that was provided for the client or care that was provided in collaboration with the client and family. A basic premise is that unless the data are recorded, the care has not been given. This puts the onus on the care-giver to communicate, via records, the essential facts about the client care provided. An associated challenge within this practice is the requirement to develop records that are complete yet are reasonable and efficient both in the presence of decreased numbers of personnel and with the increased cost of all facets of health services.

A secondary thrust in the audit system is observation of the client to determine a health status. This aspect of the system is not mandated in the same way as is the record-keeping aspect of the audit, yet the results of care surely must be consistent with the data recorded on the audit sheet. Hence, the ultimate intent is to determine how well the clients' human needs have been met; *who* has met them (whether nurse, physician, or client) becomes secondary in importance.

Another aspect of an audit is to observe the nurse as care is provided. This is of less concern when client-care goals have been focused on and the interdisciplinary record-keeping system is operational. However, when concerned about nursing actions and behaviors, this aspect of an audit is beneficial.

A variety of approaches to quality assurance programs can be followed. One that has been successful is that proposed by Donabedian.[7] He suggests that three aspects of quality should be considered: structure, process, and outcome.

Structure is the setting in which care is given. This can be an ambulatory setting in which the client is healthy, located in a home in the community, with family, and concerned about maintaining health. The setting can also be an acute care facility where the client may be hospitalized for a minor health problem or a major, critical illness. In addition to the physical parameters of the situation, the aspect of structure would also be concerned with such items as the equipment available, expertise of personnel, and how the various disciplines relate with each other.

Process is the events that enter into the actual care and the sequence of those events in the eventual care. This sequence usually follows a period of data collection, data analysis, conclusions reached, plan devised and carried out, and evaluation performed. These are the elements of the nursing process and are the essence of client care. The systematic, orderly means of providing care enables an organized system for auditing client care.

Outcome is the end result of client care. Inherent within this facet of the audit system is the satisfaction of the client. Despite the complexities of measuring outcomes, it is essential to the audit system so that the strengths and pluses of the system can be replicated and the weaknesses and errors can be reduced or deleted.

The development of audit outcome criteria has become a significant effort for nurses although it "is the most time-consuming and yet the most interesting aspect of the audit cycle."[8] The critical nature of the criteria are illustrated in the following audit process:

1. Select area of topic to be audited.
2. Draft objective criteria.
3. Ratify criteria.
4. Review client record.
5. Analyze problems.
6. Develop solutions.
7. Implement solution.
8. Evaluate and re-audit.
9. Repeat cycle with drafting of new criteria.[9]

To be considered valid, the audit outcome criteria should be relevant, understandable, measurable, behavioral, and achievable.[10]

A *nursing audit* is a review, by a nurse, of the client's care or records to determine the extent to which that care or records meet established standards. Auditing care plans developed for a client assume that the client's status has been assessed, a nursing history and health assessment have been done, a nursing diagnosis (diagnoses) has been made, the goals with expected outcomes have been established, and nursing strategies have been written to assure realization of the desired outcome. The recorded nursing care plans can be audited periodically by nurses who are less familiar with the client. The advantage of this type of audit is that it is an objective means for determining gaps in the plan, raising questions about areas of care that should be pursued, or areas of the plan that can be approached in another way.

The client's care can be audited by observing the client when that care has been completed. A semicomatose person in a hospital can be observed for such aspects as body position, body cleanliness, status of the environment, apparent comfort. An ambulatory amputee in a clinic can be observed to detect the correct use of body mechanics, the care given to the body area near the prosthesis, and exercising techniques. A diabetic person can be observed in the home as this person self-administers insulin to determine how well the instructions given about insulin administration were understood.

Records tell the auditor that data have been documented; to be certain of the quality of care that has been given, the most economical, effective, and direct way to audit this information is to observe the client. This offsets the question of whether the nurse who keeps detailed, well-written records also provides good nursing care. Auditing the care given to the client is a certain and sure way to determine the extent to which that care has met established standards. The results of the audit can have direct and immediate implications for the client under care.

Following the care rendered to any client, some type of documentation is done on a legal record; the specific type of record depends on the setting in which the care is provided. A review of these legal records is the type of nursing audit performed most frequently. It is a client-centered activity and is a form of hindsight or retrospective evaluation. Phaneuf developed the nursing audit process which is applicable to a variety of settings, and which has as its theoretical framework the independent and interdependent functions of nursing. She developed this process to determine the extent to which nursing care has measured up to the specified objectives; it is not designed to evaluate care while it is being given and is not designed to be used to evaluate the nurse's performance.[11]

The persons responsible for the nursing audit are the professional nurses who can function as individual auditors or as a group of auditors. They may be associated closely with the client, be completely unfamiliar with the client, or the group may comprise some nurses who know and some who do not know the client. The first task of the auditors is to establish standards against which their observations will be measured. Although several nurses may be responsible for developing these standards, performing the audit or aspects of it can be delegated to various members of the group. It is important that peers review the final audit data and draw conclusions, determining the required follow-up on the data.

The frequency with which audits are taken can be determined by the group, according to the type of client whose care is to be audited. The records of a critically ill person in a hospital should be audited more frequently than those of a person in an ambulatory clinic. The care of chronically ill persons in a nursing home or in home care can be audited more regularly and as mandated than that of clients in a facility designed for the acutely ill. Important factors in the conduct of the audit are that nurses should be convinced of its value, should develop standards and auditing instruments appropriate to clients for whom they are responsible, and should be motivated to continue to improve the auditing techniques for their own satisfaction and especially for the continued improvements of the care given to the client.

The audit contributes to a systematic method for evaluating client care and assigning a qualitative judgment to the care and services received by a client. The nursing audit serves to pursue excellence and to contribute to the nurse's moral and legal accountability for the service rendered. The nursing audit cannot only contribute to an improved quality of nursing care, but can also influence the total health care system. It can contribute to better communication and collaboration among nursing and health team members. The result of the audit should be shared with all persons concerned with client care. This openness, coupled with a knowledge of the goals of the auditing process, is strategic if the nursing care rendered is to be enhanced continuously and the quality of person-centered, family-centered, and community-centered health care increased. It may provide data needed to effect required changes in the health care system.

Jelinek et al., in a pioneering effort, developed a methodology for monitoring the quality of nursing care based on the nursing process and client human needs, simultaneously considering the persons, activities, and environmental elements that impinge on direct care as well as the administrative and organizational structure for the delivery of care.[12] This validated and reliable methodology utilizes the computer-generated worksheets and data analysis which allows for comparative interpretation of quality indices across health care agencies. Intensive testing and analysis of the quality instrument has demonstrated it to be valid and reliable. The results of testing have demonstrated that the nursing process relates to client outcomes and that such identified variables as registered nurse hours per client per day, continuity of care, and coordination of parts of the client care system related positively to quality care, whereas size and client census per unit and nonprofessional staffing related negatively.[13]

Another instrument in use is the Quality Patient Care Scale (Qualpacs) developed by Wandelt and Ager to evaluate quality of nursing care received by clients while the care is in progress. In addition to measuring objectively the quality of nurse interactions and interventions, it can be used to measure effects of changes in care, compare quality of care when differing staffing patterns are used, appraise the effects of in-service education, and provide data for research purposes as well as point out researchable problems.[14]

For many years the Joint Commission on Accreditation of Hospitals (JCAH) has had in existence a voluntary program for the accreditation of hospitals. Since 1966, this commission has also provided a voluntary program for Nursing Home accreditation. This accreditation agency, the JCAH, is recognized for its long-standing record of encouraging independent peer review and professional responsibility; both of these are significant factors in ensuring quality of care for the client.

With the advent of the Medicare Prospective Payment System (PPS) many changes are taking place in the three arenas for client care: the hospital, the nursing home, and home health care. Recently reported data are revealing major changes in hospitalization patterns and are acknowledging a significant impact on the nursing home industry. With a 4.5 percent drop in hospital length of stay for persons over age 65 between 1984 and 1985, and a 40 percent increase in hospital discharges to skilled nursing facilities and to home health care since October 1983, there is concern that fewer resources may be available for clients who need care and that quality of care may be compromised.[15] To determine the impact on these changes, extensive evaluation of care is being initiated in all these arenas, and "quality care" is linked in an integral way with "evaluation of care." It is assumed that there is a base, a standard, from which evaluators proceed to judge the extent to which personnel in each arena measure up to the standards to provide quality care for the clients.

Quality has been a difficult term for policymakers to define; however, to evaluate effectiveness of care, quality is being addressed by health policymakers and researchers as well as health care providers. Donabedian insists that quality health care must be evaluated according to two populations: the providers and the clients.

Despite the difficulty in defining the term "quality," there is more ready agreement that client satisfaction is a critical indicator of quality care. Structure and process criteria continue to be important in quality evaluation, but recent emphasis on outcome criteria as a component of evaluation has redirected research and accreditation activities. A major deficit in this evaluation process that health policy researchers readily acknowledge, is the lack of a unified national data base, hence limiting the scope of quality evaluations.

As the client populations swell in nursing homes, and in home health care, and as the PPS in the form of DRGs precipitate the movement of clients out of the acute care setting (some say they are moved out "sicker and quicker"), the resources of nursing homes and home health are strained immensely. The nursing home industry recognized the implications for evaluating client care in the early 1980s and leaders in the field have responded with the development of two instruments—one to evaluate quality care and one to regularize the recordings about care that is being (and was) delivered. The instrument for evaluating quality care was developed by and is available from the American Health Care Association.[16] Known as the Quest for Quality, specific tools are included in a comprehensive package that enables health care providers in a nursing home setting to collect data from all levels of staff, residents, and families. The process for data collection and analysis is clearly presented to the providers and the longitudinal focus of the evaluation activity suggests a positive direction for evaluating the quality of care that is provided for the nursing home residents.

A second instrument that has been developed is a patient care management system. The State of Maryland took the initiative in this endeavor and in 1982 published the Maryland Appraisal of Patient Progress (MAPP).[17] This system was the result of $2\frac{1}{2}$ years of development and testing. Those who follow the MAPP recording system realize the benefit of accomplishing an interdisciplinary coordinated plan of care for the resident; they are better able to identify the resident's needs, both met and unmet, and the system provides a base from which evaluation of care can be done. Some states now mandate the use of the MAPP system in all licensed and certified nursing homes.

Two major publications address the issue of quality care in nursing homes, namely: a report of the National Citizens Coalition for Nursing Home Reform (1985)[18] and a report by the Institute of Medicine on Improving the Quality of Care in Nursing Homes (1986).[19] In practice, the state survey process of inspecting nursing homes to determine the extent to which they are in compliance with state regulations has been changed from a paper-oriented process to one of people orientation. Emphasis is being placed on surveys measuring the quality of care that residents actually receive rather than the capability of the facility to provide care. Surveyors now (since June 1986), interview residents and families about the care received, they observe nursing home staff as they minister to the resident (medications, treatments), they accompany residents to their meals, observe the food that is served, and identify the support systems that are available for feeding those who need assistance. Through this person-to-person activity, the expectation is that more precise evaluation of quality care can be achieved.

The home health care industry has not recovered sufficiently from the increased demand for services to have in place all the necessary tools for evaluation of client care. In the mid-1980s (1986–1987), accreditation programs have been developed to provide added consumer protection in addition to Medicare certification and state licensing of agencies. Consumer groups are collaborating with professional nursing groups to provide leadership in this area of ensuring quality care in the home health setting. Evaluation of this care will be a critical factor in the immediate future.

CONCLUSION

The fourth component of the nursing process, evaluation, for which the framework has been prescribed, stems from the goal expectations and behavioral outcomes established during the planning phase and incorporated into the nursing care plan. Evaluation is always expressed in terms of achieving the goal and expected behavioral manifestations within the client related to the fulfillment of human needs. The entire focus of the nursing process is goal directed. It is systematically geared to foster optimal wellness for the well and the ill client, to solve diagnosed client problems by prescribing those specific nursing actions which would denote the client's problem had been resolved. Evaluation aids the nurse and client to determine those human needs that are reasonably well met and those that require reprocessing (which includes reassessment and replanning), as well as the diagnosis of new problems.

Impact and quality control are two vital concepts in nursing today. Nurses are challenged to specify what they do that makes an impact on client care; they also are required to state how they contribute to client care. In addition, each nurse who is licensed as a professional has a legal responsibility for quality control; that is, there are variables in every nurse–client situation, and the nurse is responsible for helping the client make decisions that will best use the client's strengths to maintain or restore wellness to the extent possible. Using the concept of quality as perceived by the client, the nurse carries out the professional responsibilities of nursing. The nursing process provides a systematic means by which nurses can describe, explain, prescribe, and replicate those activities necessary to impact on human need fulfillment and to exercise a measure of quality control over the performance of client care. With human need theory and the nursing process providing the framework, research can proceed in an orderly systematic fashion to validate that *nursing makes a difference*.

REFERENCES

1. Wardell, S. *Acute intervention: Nursing process throughout the life span.* Reston, Va.: Reston, 1979, p. 380.
1a. Mundinger, M.D., & Jaron, G.D. Developing a nursing diagnosis. *Nursing Outlook*, February 1975, *23*, 94–98.
2. Harmer, B. *Methods and principles of teaching the principles and practice of nursing.* New York: Macmillan, 1926.
3. Yura, H., Ozimek, D., & Walsh, M.B. *Nursing leadership: Theory and process*, 2nd ed. New York: Appleton-Century-Crofts, 1981.
4. McCaffery, M. *Nursing management of the patient with pain.* Philadelphia: Lippincott, 1972, pp. 27–65.
5. Institute of Medicine. *Assessing quality in health care: An evaluation.* Washington, D.C.: National Academy of Sciences, 1976, p. 1.
6. *Ibid.*, p. 143.
7. Donabedian, A. Promoting quality through evaluating the process of patient care. *Medical Care*, 1968, *6*, 181–202.
8. Ridle, J.C. Quality assurance in ambulatory care. *Nursing Clinics of North America*, 1977, *12*, 583–593.
9. *Ibid.*
10. *Ibid.*
11. Planeuf, M. *The nursing audit: Self-regulation in nursing practice.* New York: Appleton-Century-Crofts, 1976.
12. Jelinek, R.C., Haussman, R.K.D., Hegyvary, S.T., & Newman, J.F. *A methodology for monitoring quality of nursing care.* Bethesda, Md.: U.S. Department of Health. Education and Welfare, Public Health Service. Health

Resources Administration, Bureau of Health Resources Development, Division of Nursing, 1974, p. 23.

13. Haussman, R.K.D., Hegyvary, S.T., & Newman, J.F. *Monitoring quality of nursing care.* Bethesda, Md.: U.S. Department of Health, Education and Welfare, Public Health Service. Health Resources Administration, Bureau of Health Manpower, Division of Nursing, 1976, p. 64.

14. Wandelt, M., & Ager, J. *Quality patient care scale.* New York: Appleton-Century-Crofts, 1976, p. 33.

15. Solomon, S.B. Quest for quality. *NLN Public Policy Bulletin.* Summer, 1986, IV (2).

16. *Quest for Quality.* Washington, D.C.: American Health Care Association, 1985.

17. *Maryland Appraisal of Patient Progress.* Baltimore: Department of Health and Mental Hygiene, Division of Licensing and Certification, 1982.

18. National Citizens' Coalition for Nursing Home Reform. *A consumer perspective on quality care: the residents' point of view.* Washington, D.C., 1985.

19. Committee on Nursing Home Regulation. Institute of Medicine. *Improving the quality of care in nursing homes.* Washington, D.C.: National Academy Press, 1986.

4

Application of the Nursing Process

The nursing process can be applied with clients in a variety of settings; it is flexible and adaptable, permitting the nurse to use judgment and creativity in caring for the client who is a person, a family, a community, in an organized, orderly, and systematic manner.

Nine client situations are presented in this chapter; seven relate to the client as a person, one to the client as a family, and one to the client as a community. Nursing care plans for each of the client situations are developed according to nursing's human need theory framework (Chapter 2) and the nursing process format presented in Chapter 3.

A model nursing care plan is presented for the readers' use and further development. A model nursing care plan is a representation of nursing efforts toward human need fulfillment, which apply to all clients displaying the target variables. A model presents the goal achievement efforts for the 35 human needs. It provides the nurse with an overview of the human needs for the client impacted by the target variables. The nurse then prepares an *individualized* nursing care plan for the client based on the possibilities presented in the model. The target variables may be medical diagnoses, gender, level of growth and development, and age. Multiple models may be developed for a single medical diagnosis that can occur throughout the life span; for example, the child with diabetes mellitus, the adolescent with diabetes mellitus, the young adult, the middle-aged adult, the elder adult, or the aged client with stage 1, stage 2, and/or stage 3 Alzheimer's disease. Model nursing care plans may be developed for each of the stages of the pregnancy experience or the presurgical, intrasurgical, and postsurgical experiences. Models are an efficient, ready reference for the nurse; they facilitate a client-centered focus within nursing's human need theory framework. Nurses in health care agencies are encouraged to determine the target variables common among the clients they serve, then develop the model nursing care plans reflecting these variables for easy access by nursing staff members. The models should be reviewed periodically to assure their viability and to incorporate relevant research outcomes. Accompanying the model should be a file of the available assessment tools of the human needs.

A model for the woman with Alzheimer's disease follows. In addition, selected human needs with nursing diagnoses are illustrated for the woman with acquired immune deficiency syndrome (AIDS) related complex (ARC). Readers are challenged to make any adaptations to the use of the model in the reader's practice.

The client situations illustrate (1) a variety of client health states, (2) a variety of clinical and environmental settings in which nursing's human needs framework and the nursing process can be used, (3) a person–family–community-centered approach to providing nursing service, and (4) the diversity, creativity, and flexibility inherent in nursing's human need theory framework and the nursing process. Study questions for the client situations are presented for the reader's enrichment and to provide an opportunity to add dimensions to the nursing care plan.

NURSING CARE PLAN 1
Teenager with Diabetes Mellitus
Developed by Patricia Frensky Orfini

Client Situation: Kathleen Krampitz

Three weeks ago Kathleen Krampitz, an attractive 17-year-old honor student, was told by Dr. Molinaire, her physician, that she had diabetes mellitus. She has been placed on a 2000-calorie diet and has begun taking 30 units of NPH insulin. She quickly learned to give her own insulin and is managing urine testing and coverage with regular insulin for spillover. Kathleen is the youngest of six children of John and Ophelia Krampitz and the only child at home. She is of Polish-American heritage and the favorite grandchild of her 86-year-old grandmother Anna, who resides with Kathleen and her parents. Anna has been a lifelong diabetic and suffered bilateral mid-thigh amputations ten years ago. Although her vision is failing, she continues to be a viable family member.

Kathleen has taken ballet since the age of seven and is an accomplished dancer. She won a full scholarship to the New York School of

Ballet as a result of her entrance in a dance competition. Her steady boyfriend, Basil, won a partial scholarship in the same competition. She planned to use the scholarship after she graduates next year. Initially Kathleen showed little reaction to the diagnosis of diabetes mellitus— until yesterday. Her mother found her in her room sobbing and when asked what was wrong she said: "How can I be a ballerina now? I won't be able to do anything but stay at home and watch that I don't injure my feet."

Nursing Care Plan for Human Need: *Wholesome Body Image*

Nursing diagnosis	Due to or related to	As evidenced by	Goal/expected behaviors
Unwholesome body image	Pathophysiologic impact of newly diagnosed diabetes mellitus Educational deficit regarding limitations imposed by diabetes Negative past experience with a person having diabetes	Sobbing, asks, "How can I be a ballerina now?" States she won't be able to do anything but stay at home and watch that she doesn't injure her feet	Client demonstrates wholesome body image • Resumes ballet lessons in 2 weeks • Verbalizes desire and ability to continue normal activities within 2 weeks • Continues to groom self and show concern for her appearance

Nursing Strategies and Frequencies

1. Assess Kathleen's perception of herself prior to diagnosis of diabetes and after learning diagnosis:

   - Were body changes of puberty difficult in terms of adjustment?
   - Adolescent body image problems? acne? weight concerns?
   - Have her describe how she looked prior to diagnosis. Compare to current description of her appearance.
   - Has she shared her diabetic condition with her friends?

   Talk to her parents about any changes they see in Kathleen's body image: activities, grooming, hygiene, concern for clothes, make-up.

2. Discuss with Kathleen her perceptions of and the details surrounding her grandmother's illness.

   - Was treatment made available for her grandmother immediately upon diagnosis? Was diagnosis made early? What was treatment years ago? Was it effective? If Kathleen does not know answers to these questions, encourage her to discuss these with her grandmother.

- Ask Kathleen to describe herself at 86. Is it an image of her grandmother? Is it favorable? Discuss the image and clear up any misconceptions.
- Ask Kathleen to describe herself in 5 years? Is this realistic or based on misconceptions about the disease?

Discuss with Kathleen.
Repeat the above discussion in 1 month.

3. Assess Kathleen's relationship with her grandmother. Is her grandmother increasing her fears?
4. Assess Kathleen's knowledge of her condition, especially as related to foot care. Does she understand the relationship between diabetes and foot problems? Can she list methods of prevention and treatment?
5. Based on assessment, review relationship between diabetes and foot problems.

- Explain the relationship between high glucose and lipid levels and early atherosclerotic changes (hardening and degeneration) in the walls of the large arteries.
- Describe how reduced blood supply to the feet is a result of atherosclerosis. Describe the manifestations of reduced blood supply and encourage her to report these signs.
- List ways to promote peripheral circulation:
    - Never use tobacco; explain reason.
    - Do not sit with legs crossed; explain reason.
    - Keep legs and feet warm; explain reason.
    - Do not use heat (hot water bottles, heating pads); explain reason.
- Explain possible reasons for Kathleen's grandmother's amputations in terms of pathophysiology.
- Stress importance of good foot and skin care to minimize foot infections or lesions.
- Teach Kathleen principles of good foot care:
    - Wash feet daily in lukewarm water with mild soap.
    - Dry the skin gently (do not rub) with special attention to area between and under toes.
    - Examine feet daily for such things as discoloration, cold temperature, reddened areas, disrupted skin integrity, and poor capillary refill.
- Explain how each of the following areas can be prevented or at least treated to prevent complications: dry skin, excessive sweating, corns and calluses, blisters, ingrown toenails, minor cuts and abrasions. Use article "What 'Foot Care' Really Means" by Graham

and Morley (*American Journal of Nursing*, July 1984, pp. 889–891) as a teaching guide.

- Have Kathleen demonstrate or describe her daily foot hygiene to you in 2 to 3 days.
- In 2 to 3 days, evaluate Kathleen's knowledge of care of foot/skin abrasions by having her describe what she would do in the situation. Do the same for other foot problems.

6. Emphasize importance of keeping glucose and lipid levels down through adherence to insulin therapy, blood glucose monitoring and diet therapy. Emphasize the fact that she can take control of the condition.

7. Allow Kathleen to ventilate her feelings about her disease, its effects on her aspirations, and her fears of amputation. Suggest that she join a support group and, if she is agreeable, make arrangements through the American Diabetic Association.

8. Discuss concept of body image with Kathleen.

9. Assess and discuss any other fears Kathleen may have (e.g., blindness). Teach Kathleen how to prevent the complications associated with diabetes.

Nursing Care Plan for Human Need: *Nutrition*

Nursing diagnosis	Due to or related to	As evidenced by	Goal/expected behaviors
Potential disturbance in nutrition	Pathophysiologic impact of diabetes mellitus	Poor eating practices typical of adolescent years	Client shows adequate nutrition
	Anxiety and fears of amputation	Incomplete data base	• Little fluctuation (+/−5 lb) in current weight (assuming current weight is acceptable to nurse and client and client is finished growth in terms of height)
			• Intake of a balanced 2000 calorie diet on any given day
			• Normal blood glucose level (60–120 mg/dl)
			• Verbalization by client of normal energy level

Nursing Strategies with Frequencies

1. Complete nutritional assessment and client knowledge assessment:

- Ask Kathleen to write down everything she ate or drank the previous day and at what times.
- Have Kathleen calculate the caloric intake (if she has difficulty assist her).
- See if Kathleen can assess the previous day's diet for balance, for ratio of proteins, fats, and carbohydrates. Discuss whether she was happy with this food intake and whether she felt hungry or lethargic. Assess whether she experienced any signs (symptoms) of hypo/hyperglycemia (hypoglycemia—[early symptoms]—hunger, increased pulse, increased respiratory rate, weakness; [later symptoms]—yawning, lethargy, increased difficulty in thought processes, irritability, belligerence; hyperglycemia—polydipsia, polyuria, fatigue, weight loss, dry skin, blurred vision, sore that is slow to heal, frequent yeast infections).

2. Using assessment data, review principles of diet therapy. Emphasize the positive and praise her for her knowledge and adherence to the diet. Make appropriate suggestions (keep in mind the foods teenagers like and the role of peer pressure). Elicit Kathleen's input as to ways she can improve her diet and/or eating habits.
3. Evaluate Kathleen's understanding of her disease in terms of the function of insulin, administration of insulin, signs of hyperglycemia and hypoglycemia, and processes of home urine and blood glucose testing.
4. Review any aspects of the disease, the insulin therapy, and the complications that Kathleen is unsure of or unaware of.
5. Explain relationship between stress, glucose use, and insulin therapy.
6. Discuss the relationship between exercise and insulin intake. Emphasize the need to eat additional food if excercising more than usual and to carry fast-acting sugars at all times to prevent hypoglycemia. Offer medic alert information. Help her to find a way of making this information readily available to others in case of emergency without affecting her self-image and relationship with her peers.

Nursing Care Plan for Human Need: *Confidence*

Nursing diagnosis	Due to or related to	As evidenced by	Goal/expected behaviors
Deficit of confidence: self-doubt	Pathophysiologic affront of diabetes mellitus and developmental tasks of later adolescence	Verbalized fear of failure as a ballerina Typical feelings of late adolescence	Client manifests confidence - Identifies feelings of self-doubt within 2 weeks

(continued)

Confidence (continued)

Nursing diagnosis	Due to or related to	As evidenced by	Goal/expected behaviors
		Emerging career choice	• Verbalizes belief in her ability to become a ballerina within 4 weeks

Nursing Strategies with Frequencies

1. Discuss feelings of self-doubt and lack of confidence with Kathleen. Help her to list reasons for these feelings. Explain that some degree of self-doubt is normal in late adolescence.
2. Discuss past accomplishments and successes. Emphasize these.
3. Discuss future goals and aspirations. Assess previous support persons for Kathleen and encourage her to call upon these people for encouragement again. Encourage her to verbalize any fears or anxieties she has regarding her scholarship to the New York School of Ballet: fears of failure, of leaving home, of being on her own.
4. Have Kathleen describe her relationships with and acceptance by her peers. Discuss any causes for self-doubt from this group.
5. Encourage Kathleen to share her feelings with her parents.

NURSING CARE PLAN 2
Toddler with Diabetes Mellitus
Developed by Patricia Frensky Orfini

Client Situation: Andrea Gillman

Andrea Gillman, aged 2 years, is in the process of being admitted to the endocrine/metabolic unit of Oceanside Children's Hospital. She is accompanied by her parents John (aged 20) and Brigid (aged 19) Gillman. John drives a delivery truck for Founder's Food Distributing Company and Brigid works part-time as a library aide. Her physician, Dr. Molinaire, a member of Oceanside Family Practice, a health maintenance organization holding the contract for the Founder's Company employee health insurance, completed the diagnosis of Andrea's diabetes mellitus during a recent office visit. Mrs. Gillman shared some of the problems encountered since the diagnosis was made with Primary Nurse Robin Blanchard: Andrea is not potty trained and it is difficult, if not impossible, to obtain a urine specimen; Andrea screams and "carries-on" when it is insulin time—the dosage of insulin given is questionable; Andrea picks at and plays with her food, often even refusing to eat for days at a time; and Andrea seems to be "sicker now than before she was diagnosed."

Nursing Care Plan for Human Need: *Nutrition*

Nursing diagnosis	Due to or related to	As evidenced by	Goal/expected behaviors
Undernutrition	Pathophysiologic affront of diabetes mellitus Developmental occurrence of inappropriate attention-seeking behaviors	"Picks at and plays with food" Refuses to eat for days at a time Mother's statement: "sicker now than before diagnosed"	Client demonstrates adequate nutrition • No weight loss • Eats in response to activity within 3 days • Accepts insulin injection without inappropriate attention-seeking behaviors within 2 weeks

Nursing Strategies with Frequencies

1. Assess the following about Andrea and her family from Mr. and Mrs. Gillman on first contact:

   - Typical daily routine of each family member; include sleep patterns.
   - Typical 24-hour dietary intake; food likes and dislikes; bottle or cup drinking; number of teeth; parents' reaction to lack of eating.
   - Prescribed insulin dosage, type, and time.
   - Favorite activities, toys, books, friends.
   - Result of urine glucose test when obtainable.
   - Has she experienced normal growth and development?
   - Has she remained in the same percentile for height and weight on growth charts since birth? language skills; social skills; fine motor and gross motor skills; feeding skills?
   - Signs and symptoms of hypoglycemia, hyperglycemia, or ketoacidosis; if so, is there any trend (e.g., always after a nap)?
   - Past medical/nursing problems; delivery problems.
   - Parents' attitude toward child.
   - Immunizations up-to-date.

2. Assess:

   - Blood sugar level
   - Vital signs, blood pressure

- Height and weight
- Urine glucose and acetone level, if possible
- Developmental milestones (e.g., runs fairly well, builds tower of 6 to 7 cubes, understands directional commands)
- Level of consciousness; alertness; activity/energy level
- Skin integrity

3. Review some of the characteristics of the toddler years with parents, particularly desire for autonomy, negativism, temper tantrums.

- Assess how the Gillmans currently deal with these topics.
- Acknowledge that the toddler years can be a confusing and trying time for parents.
- Offer suggestions as appropriate.

4. Explain that appetite and food preferences during the second year are normally sporadic. Point out that it is not unusual for a child to refuse food for 3 days in a row. Stress that toddlers typically have a lack of interest in food, decreased appetite, and go through food fads. Explain that erratic activity periods also occur in the second year normally, making diabetic control even more difficult.

5. Teach Andrea's parents that children with diabetes will easily eat in response to activity, except for times of lowered or elevated blood sugars. Explain that the child who plays with food, refuses to eat, or takes too long to eat may be using food as a means of getting attention. The more attention the parents give by force feeding, threatening, and cajoling, the less the child eats.

6. With parents and physician, plan to lower the insulin dosage so that there is no danger of hypoglycemia, then offer Andrea a plate of food. Plan for the meal to last 20 minutes and give attention to Andrea when she takes a bite of food (not necessarily praise her for eating, just talk to her). Ignore all other behaviors. After 20 minutes take food away without discussion of uneaten food. Stress the following points to the Gillmans:

- Continue this strategy for at least 1 week.
- This routine may require several days before results are seen.
- Mealtimes should be pleasant. It may be helpful for parents to eat at the same time.
- Offer food in small portions.
- A regular mealtime schedule and utensils help to meet the toddler's need for predictability and ritualism.
- Consistency is important; have parents explain plan to interim caretakers.

- Do not give any attention to disruptive or unacceptable behaviors; do not "beg" Andrea to eat any more than she wants.
- Give Andrea a "5-minute warning" before mealtimes so she can finish her current activity and have a smooth transition to eating. Offer food before she becomes so hungry that she loses control and is too cranky to eat.
- Do not use food as a sign of approval or as a reward.
- Encourage parents to try new food or "once rejected" foods in addition to favorites. "Once rejected" foods suddenly become favorites as fast as old foods become disliked.

If Andrea is drinking from a bottle, begin weaning by elimination of one or all of the bottles and/or by diluting milk or juice. Too much fluid consumed easily from a bottle will decrease appetite for and intake of solid foods.

7. Assess parents' understanding of and compliance with Andrea's prescribed diet. Have the Gillmans write down Andrea's food and fluid intake from the previous 24 hours. Make suggestions and offer praise for good choices. Encourage parents to keep a 24-hour diet diary along with daily records of urine/blood glucose records, insulin dosage and time, and activity. Use this record to find relationships between activity, food intake, and insulin therapy.

8. Explain how insulin injections are commonly used as attention-seeking devices. Encourage parents to make this a part of the daily routine. This may mean having to develop and follow a stricter routine that toddlers need (some toddlers more than others). The injection should become a habit, a normal part of the day. Specifically:

- Follow injection time with some preselected, positive attention (e.g., reading favorite book). Have parent do this same activity following each injection.
- Ignore screams and "carrying-on"; focus on the special time to come after the injection.

9. Review reasons for and action of insulin. Remind parents that insulin dosage frequently requires adjustment due to normal decreased growth and changes in eating during the second year.

- Have parents use diet/activity diary to observe activity and adjust food intake accordingly.
- Review signs and symptoms of hypoglycemia, hyperglycemia, and ketoacidosis.
- Provide medic alert information.
- Emphasize requirement to carry a fast-acting sugar and to offer carbohydrates during periods of increased activity.

10. Encourage parents to discontinue pressuring Andrea for a urine sample. Have them put her on the toilet (with catch cup attached to rim) before and after meals and at bedtime. Ask her to void; if no results within a few minutes, go on with another activity without reference to failure to void. Praise successful attempts. Teach parents how to use blood glucose monitoring (Dextrostix) to supplement or replace urine testing.

Nursing Care Plan for Human Need: *Structure, Law, Limits*

Nursing diagnosis	Due to or related to	As evidenced by	Goal/expected behaviors
Lack of structure, rules, and limits	Educational deficit on part of parents in regard to toddler needs	"Screams and carries on" at insulin time Picks at food	Client responds to appropriate limit setting, discipline, and structure • Parents verbalize understanding of principles of discipline for a toddler within 1 month • Andrea obeys two out of three rules on a given day within 1 month

Nursing Strategies with Frequencies

1. Assess discipline/limit-setting practices currently used by the Gillmans.
2. As appropriate, describe need for limit-setting and structure for a child (helps to establish routine and feelings of security for toddler in addition to encouraging socially acceptable behavior).
3. Explain principles of limit-setting:

   - Set decisive limits and plan to give consistent attention to them.
   - Begin with one new rule at a time.
   - Make sure it is reasonable, clearly defined, and understood by child.
   - Immediately correct errors in behavior and consistently enforce rules.
   - Ignore temper tantrums.
   - Praise compliance with the limits.
   - Offer reminders as necessary.

Nursing Care Plan for Human Need: *Autonomy*

Nursing diagnosis	Due to or related to	As evidenced by	Goal/expected behaviors
Potential deficit in autonomy	Pathophysiologic affront of diabetes Educational deficit about toddlerhood	Parents do not seem to be able to identify behaviors that are inappropriately attention-seeking Parents have limited understanding of normal developmental alterations of toddlerhood	Client incorporates appropriate autonomy • Andrea makes two choices/day within 3 weeks • Parents verbalize understanding of the role of autonomy for a toddler

Nursing Strategies with Frequencies

1. Assess the Gillman's knowledge of a toddler's need for autonomy.
2. Explain that acquiring a sense of autonomy and self-control is the most important psychosocial task of this stage.
3. Encourage parents to:

   - Give child freedom to be active in a safe, large area that is child-proofed (playpen is too limiting for a toddler).
   - Allow Andrea to make choices (e.g., do you want milk or juice?) throughout the day. Be sure you can abide by her choice (e.g., make sure milk and juice are available first).
   - Set up a flexible schedule/routine for Andrea. Share this routine with other caretakers. Explain that children lose control more easily and quickly when they are hungry or tired. Plan each day so as not to put off mealtimes and sleep periods.
   - Set limits and rules.
   - Provide toys, puzzles, games that the child can master with little assistance; praise for accomplishments.
   - Give small household tasks/responsibilities (e.g., put dirty clothes into hamper); acknowledge her helpfulness.
   - Allow child to decide on certain activities; try to say "yes" at least as many times as you say "no" to her suggestions/voiced wants.

Nursing Care Plan for Human Need: *Appreciation and Attention*

Nursing diagnosis	Due to or related to	As evidenced by	Goal/expected behaviors
Reduced appreciation, attention	Social and economic occurrence of mother working	Attention seeking behaviors:	Client demonstrates appreciation, attention

(continued)

Appreciation and Attention (continued)

Nursing diagnosis	Due to or related to	As evidenced by	Goal/expected behaviors
	part-time and father working full-time Incomplete data base	Screams, "carries-on" at insulin time; picks at and plays with food; refuses to eat for days at a time	• Accepts insulin injection without any fuss within 2 weeks • Eats some food at two out of three meals within 3 weeks

Nursing Strategies with Frequencies

1. Assess relationship between parents and Andrea; assess time spent with Andrea.

   - Activities done together?
   - Daily routine?
   - Loving relationship?
   - Is child left to entertain self?
   - Availability of toys, books?

2. As appropriate, using above information, demonstrate to the Gillmans appropriate activities for toddlers: games to play, things to teach their daughter, etc.

3. Discuss child care situation when Mrs. Gillman is working. Who cares for child? Location? Other children? Is this time a positive time for Andrea? What is her reaction to separation from her mother at this time? How does she appear and react when mother returns? Make suggestions about the situation carefully.

4. Discuss temper tantrums and other inappropriate attention-seeking behaviors with the Gillmans. Emphasize that the best approach is to ignore these behaviors. Encourage the Gillmans to praise and reward appropriate behaviors. Stress that it is entirely normal for a toddler or any person to seek attention; she must learn to do this in socially acceptable ways.

5. Suggest that parents engage in activities/games with Andrea where she will accomplish something or succeed (e.g., helping mommy sweep the floor, correctly sorting shapes) and then praise her for success. Encourage them to include her as much as possible in family activities. Give her choices during the day (e.g., peanut butter or tuna) and abide by these.

6. Deal with inappropriate attention-seeking behaviors at insulin time and mealtimes by following nursing prescriptions listed in items 6 and 8 of Nursing Strategies with Frequencies for Human Need: Nutrition.

Nursing Care Plan for Human Need: *Belonging*

Nursing diagnosis	Due to or related to	As evidenced by	Goal/expected behaviors
Potential diminished sense of belonging	Environmental affront of hospitalization	Typical toddler fear–separation	Client demonstrates sense of belonging
	Separation from parents and familiar territory		• Verbalizes time when parents will return within 2 days • Interacts with at least one or two others when parents are gone

Nursing Strategies with Frequencies

1. Encourage parents to spend as much time as possible with Andrea. Provide atmosphere and things they will require to stay with her. Be available to them for emotional support and teaching, in addition to helping them respond to Andrea's requirements.
2. If the parents must leave, have the primary nurse spend as much time with Andrea as consistently as possible. Allow her to cry (teach parents to expect protests, both verbal and physical). Voice understanding and emphasize the fact that the nurse will stay with her for a while. Encourage her to talk about her parents, their visit, where they must go. Stress that the parents will return. Use familiar times to describe return time (e.g., when it gets dark).
3. Orient Andrea to the unit and the people she will see daily. Repeat your name to her frequently. Repeat this explanation daily. Try to maintain a similar routine and familiar environment by having some favorite toys, blanket, etc.
4. Encourage play in the playroom at least twice daily where Andrea will probably feel secure and may work through her feelings.

Nursing Care Plan for Human Need: *Protection from Excessive Fear, Anxiety, and Chaos*

Nursing diagnosis	Due to or related to	As evidenced by	Goal/expected behaviors
Anxiety	Developmental alterations that occur during toddler years	Mother's voiced concern that Andrea is sicker now than before diagnosis	Client shows evidence of minimal anxiety

(continued)

Protection from Excessive Fear, Anxiety, and Chaos (continued)

Nursing diagnosis	Due to or related to	As evidenced by	Goal/expected behaviors
	Environmental affront of hospitalization Pathophysiologic impact of diabetes mellitus	Parent's implication that they have exhausted their knowledge and strategies in dealing with Andrea's behavior	• Lists new strategies for dealing with problems within 2 days • Verbalizes decreased anxiety within 4 days

Nursing Strategies with Frequencies

1. Encourage parents to ventilate feelings of anxiety and to list specific causes of their anxiety, if possible. Explain that it is much easier to deal with anxiety once specific stressors are defined.
2. Explain that the toddler age is a difficult stage for most parents to deal with. Encourage participation in a parent support group. Contact the local chapter of the American Diabetic Association, if parents are agreeable, to arrange participation in such a group.
3. Offer anticipatory guidance for meeting the needs and tasks of this age group.
4. Encourage them to use resource persons and support persons during this time (e.g., parents, clergy).
5. Discuss current problems and develop strategies for these problems as described in Nursing Strategies with Frequencies for Human Needs: Nutrition; Structure, Law, Limits; Appreciation and Attention.
6. Review strategies for effectiveness daily. Offer anticipatory guidance for future stages as appropriate. Recommend appropriate reading material on toddler years (White, Burton: *The First Three Years of Life.* New York: Avon, 1984).
7. Assure parents that you are available and open for questions. Give phone number prior to discharge and encourage them to call whenever necessary.
8. Assess for and help parents work through any feelings of guilt related to diabetes, mother working, etc.
9. Help parents to recognize body changes that indicate increased anxiety. Teach and demonstrate relaxation exercises.
10. Explain all procedures to the Gillmans and to Andrea. Answer all questions honestly.

NURSING CARE PLAN 3
Pregnant Woman with Diabetes Mellitus
Developed by Patricia Frensky Orfini

Client Situation: Annemarie Sokol-Velkie

Annemarie Sokol-Velkie just learned that she is in the 16th week of her pregnancy. Although she suspected she may be pregnant she could not be certain because of an erratic menstrual history. She decided to see Dr. Molinaire, a member of a Family Practice Group and primary physician for Annemarie because she has not felt well during the past month. She lost weight, felt nauseated, was inordinately thirsty, and complained of frequent urination. In addition to learning of her pregnancy, Mrs. Sokol-Velkie also learned she had diabetes mellitus. Annemarie is 30 years old and has been married 2 years to Paul Anthony Velkie, aged 40, a civilian hi-tech specialist with the Navy on maneuvers in the Mediterranean. He is expected back in 4 months and is not certain how long he will be home before being called out on assignment again. Mrs. Sokol-Velkie's diabetes will be controlled by diet (2200 calories) and NPH/regular insulin in the morning in a 2:1 ratio and equal doses of NPH and regular insulin in the evening. Annemarie will be followed in the Diabetic Clinic associated with the Birthing Center at Oceanside Medical Center headed by Dr. Molinaire in collaboration with Dr. Harley Rogers, obstetrician, and Marcie Falcone, MSN, certified nurse midwife.

Nursing Care Plan for Human Need: *Nutrition*

Nursing diagnosis	Due to or related to	As evidenced by	Goal/expected behaviors
Undernutrition	Pathophysiologic impact of diabetes mellitus Nausea related to pregnancy Increased nutritional needs related to pregnancy	Weight loss Nausea Diabetic symptoms (insulin requirements not met) Polydipsia Polyuria	Client experiences adequate nutrition • Gain weight of more than 1 kg/mo and not more than 3 kg/mo for second and third trimester • Have normal blood glucose level within 3 weeks • Have a total weight gain of approximately 27.5 lb

Nursing Strategies with Frequencies

1. Assess Mrs. Sokol-Velkie's feelings and knowledge about her pregnant state and her diabetic condition. Allow her to ventilate and

discuss her feelings. Emphasize that she is not alone in the situation; that you will be there to help her.

2. Depending on her knowledge and her emotional state, begin to present information about the pregnancy and diabetes in a simple manner. The first session must be directed toward equipping Mrs. Sokol-Velkie with initial "survival" techniques and knowledge. (Plan daily visits for a few days.)

   - Review basic information about pregnant condition.
   - Explain reasons for symptoms of pregnancy; emphasize normalcy of these symptoms/complaints.
   - Describe diabetic condition, importance of maintaining blood sugar levels within normal range for herself and her baby, and the role of insulin therapy and diet.
   - Answer all questions about infant and maternal complications honestly but do not offer this information at this time. Stress the fact that if there are no complications of pregnancy and diabetes is well controlled, her risks are the same as for any other woman. Acknowledge the incidence of risk factors and complications while stressing the control she can take over her condition and the outcome of her pregnancy.

3. Describe dietary needs in terms of both pregnancy and diabetic requirements.

   - Explain increased demands of pregnancy using four basic food groups.
   - Briefly review daily food plan (which should include meals, between-meal snacks, and bedtime snack) and sample meal plan (handout).
   - Calculate and describe to Mrs. Sokol-Velkie the distribution of proteins, fats, and carbohydrates in the diet.
   - Encourage her to review it that evening and plan to discuss this and distribution of protein, fats, and carbohydrates in greater depth the next day.
   - Emphasize that at no time should she go hungry or restrict caloric intake as this may result in ketonemia causing irreversible damage to fetus.

4. Instruct Mrs. Sokol-Velkie in insulin administration.

   - Explain purpose of insulin, type and action of NPH and regular insulins.
   - Describe and demonstrate techniques of storage and administration of insulin.

- Have Mrs. Sokol-Velkie practice techniques on an orange initially, then on self (may want to give injection to nurse before self) using saline solution for practice. Review available sites for injection.
- Continuously monitor her anxiety level, emotional status, etc.
- Positively reinforce often.

5. Describe and demonstrate the process of checking fractional urine sugar and acetone levels and of home glucose monitoring.

   - Have Mrs. Sokol-Velkie check her own freshly voided urine and interpret the result with her (trace to +1 glucose acceptable; +2 and up reported or covered with insulin).
   - Have Mrs. Sokol-Velkie obtain a drop of blood and test it on a glucose reagent strip (Dextrostix) to assess blood glucose levels. Explain how to record and when to report results.

6. Briefly describe symptoms of hyperglycemia, ketoacidosis, and hypoglycemia (handout) and treatment. Ask her to call with any symptoms that night or the next morning.

7. Review any material that is unclear; give Mrs. Sokol-Velkie your telephone number; encourage her to call anytime and set up a visit for the next day. Have her describe to you the dosage of insulin she will give herself that night and the next morning.

8. On visit 2 (next day):

   - Congratulate her on insulin injection.
   - Answer any questions; encourage her to describe and ventilate her feelings.
   - Assess blood sugar, vital signs, blood pressure, fetal heart rate, energy level, emotional status, anxiety level. Observe for signs or symptoms of hypoglycemia/hyperglycemia.

   a. Review basic information and provide more in-depth information regarding physiology of pregnancy, normal body changes, fetal growth and development.

      - Instruct on general health care (hygiene, rest and exercise, dental care, use of medications, sexual counseling).
      - Discuss current problems (nausea, urgency, and frequency of urination).
      - Offer treatment suggestions for nausea:

         - Avoid empty or overloaded stomach, offending odors, or foods that are hard to digest.
         - Maintain good posture to give stomach room.
         - Stop or decrease smoking.

- Eat dry carbohydrates on waking.
- Remain in bed till nausea subsides.
- Eat five to six small meals/day.
- Avoid spicy, fried, strong-smelling, greasy or gas-forming foods.
- Report any vomiting which persists.

Discuss (and initiate treatment, if necessary) problems common to the first and second trimesters. Address common questions such as bathing, swimming, clothing, employment, activity, travel.

b. Review previous information and provide more in-depth information regarding diabetic condition. Review signs and symptoms of hypoglycemia/hyperglycemia and treatment. Ask Mrs. Sokol-Velkie to describe what she would do if experiencing a certain set of symptoms. Assess response. Review as necessary. Discuss importance of good foot and skin care.

c. Review diet plan. Discuss distribution of proteins, carbohydrates, and fats in-depth. Ask her to write down everything she ate and when during the past 24 hours and assess it with her. Suggest use of "diet diary" to help her become aware of what and when she is eating. Plan to discuss it on the next and subsequent visits. Be sure she understands the importance of even distribution of calories throughout the day so that blood glucose remains constant and fetal equilibrium will be maintained without hyperglycemic/hypoglycemic episodes.

d. Review and discuss principles of insulin therapy in more depth. Emphasize importance of sterile techniques, cleanliness, and rotation of injection sites to prevent disruptions in skin integrity and infections. Discuss the increased risk of prenatal infection with diabetes. Instruct on signs of infection (redness, swelling, heat, pain).

e. Discuss results of home glucose monitoring and urine testing.
Assess how she felt about her ability to perform and interpret these tests.

f. Teach Mrs. Sokol-Velkie to keep a record of urine tests, insulin taken, exercise, and blood glucose levels. Explain how these can be used to help her recognize variations that affect her (such as the interaction between a favorite activity and her urine sugar level) and, therefore, can help her become better able to plan for herself.

    g. Eplain the importance of regular exercise and methods to adjust diet and insulin intake with changes in the exercise pattern. Explain that insulin requirements will change as pregnancy progresses and following birth.

    h. Decide with client whether next visit should be the following day or a few days later.

9. On visit 3:

    a. Assess weight, vital signs, blood pressure, urine, blood sugar, fetal heart rate. Observe for diabetic complications: hypoglycemia, hyperglycemia, and ketosis.

    b. Discuss any questions, problems. Briefly review all information and assess diet and insulin therapy.

    c. Develop and review plan of care:

- Schedule regular office visits (initially every week).
- Describe a routine physical examination including instructions for obtaining clean catch urine specimens and reason for this.
- Ask Mrs. Sokol-Velkie to remember when she first feels her baby move.
- Explain any upcoming tests/procedures (i.e., ultrasound, nonstress test, contraction stress test, estriol levels).

    d. Briefly address possible complications (dystocia, infections, pregnancy-induced hypertension) and possible consequences of fetal hyperglycemia and hyperinsulinism. Emphasize that the chance of the latter is minimized when blood sugar is kept within normal limits.

10. Carefully monitor weight, blood pressure, vital signs, urine and blood sugar, fundal height and gestational age, fetal heart rate and activity, edema on following visits. With physician, adjust insulin dose as necessary.

11. Prepare Mrs. Sokol-Velkie for labor and delivery during the third trimester. Suggest attendance at a childbirth education class with a significant other who can coach if husband is unavailable. Discuss husband's feelings with Mrs. Sokol-Velkie. Provide literature for her to send to him and possibly a recording of the baby's heart beat.

12. During intranatal period, add the following to routine intranatal care:

- Observe for hypoglycemia, hyperglycemia, and preeclampsia. *Hypoglycemia*—hunger, sweating, nervousness, weakness, fatigue, blurred or double vision, headache, pallor, clammy skin, shallow respiration, normal pulse.

Hyperglycemia—thirst, nausea, vomiting, abdominal pain, constipation, drowsiness, dim vision, increased urination, headache, flushed dry skin, increased respiration, weak rapid pulse, "fruity" breath.

Preeclampsia—[mild] hypertension with rise of 30/15 mm Hg or more (two separate readings at 6-hour intervals), weight gain more than 3 lb/week, slightly generalized edema, proteinuria; [severe] above symptoms plus hypertension of 160/110 or more (two separate readings at 6-hour intervals), proteinuria, oliguria, severe generalized edema, blurred vision problems; retinal arteriolar spasm on fundoscopy, epigastric pain or nausea/vomiting, irritability, emotional tension.

- Monitor urine for amount and presence of protein and glucose.
- Monitor blood sugar level.
- Monitor intravenous infusions: insulin, oxytocin.
- Culture urine after clean catch collection for asymptomatic urinary tract infection.

13. In addition to the normal postnatal care, provide the following care:

- Frequent fractional urine tests/blood glucose levels.
- Monitor food and fluids taken.
- Assess for clinical manifestations of hypoglycemia, hyperglycemia, and ketosis.
- Adjust insulin intake (regular) according to protocol prescribed. Progress to NPH according to physician prescription. Encourage Mrs. Sokol-Velkie to take over insulin injection when she desires.
- Instruct on breast-feeding if she desires. Explain how to adjust caloric and insulin intake. Counsel her about dietary requirements and the relationship between hypoglycemia and decreased milk supply.

Nursing Care Plan for Human Need: *Wholesome Body Image*

Nursing diagnosis	Due to or related to	As evidenced by	Goal/expected behaviors
Potentially un-wholesome body image	Personal occur-rence of pregnancy	16 weeks pregnant Loss of weight	Client manifests wholesome body image

(continued)

Wholesome Body Image (continued)

Nursing diagnosis	Due to or related to	As evidenced by	Goal/expected behaviors
	Pathophysiologic affront of diabetes mellitus	Normal changes of pregnancy Incomplete data base	• Verbalizes acceptance of body changes within 2 months • Continues to groom self and indicate concern for appearance

Nursing Strategies with Frequencies

1. Assess Mrs. Sokol-Velkie's perception of herself prior to learning diagnoses of pregnancy and diabetes and after learning diagnoses.
2. Listen to doubts, compliment on her appearance, provide information on prenatal exercises or classes where she will have the opportunity to keep some figure control and also have contact with other pregnant women.
3. Assist Mrs. Sokol-Velkie to acknowledge her altered body image. Help her to mentally draw a picture of her body and its relationship with others. Is it a positive one? Discuss perceived threats to current and future life-styles imposed by diabetes, pregnancy/motherhood.
4. Assist Mrs. Sokol-Velkie to focus on positive attributes and features.
5. Actively reinforce accomplishments, strengths, and positive attributes.
6. Discuss concepts of body image and self-esteem with Mrs. Sokol-Velkie. Emphasize that altered body image is a normal part of pregnancy.
7. Encourage Mrs. Sokol-Velkie to seek other support systems while husband is away. Encourage her to talk with other pregnant women and share feelings about body changes.

Nursing Care Plan for Human Need: Elimination

Nursing diagnosis	Due to or related to	As evidenced by	Goal/expected behaviors
Increased urinary elimination	Pathophysiologic affront of diabetes mellitus Personal occurrence of pregnancy	Frequent urination	Client able to accommodate increased urinary elimination • Verbalizes reason for increased urination within 3 days

(continued)

Elimination (continued)

Nursing diagnosis	Due to or related to	As evidenced by	Goal/expected behaviors
			• Lists signs of urinary tract infection within 2 weeks • Verbalizes understanding that urinary frequency and amount will decrease somewhat once diabetes controlled within 2 days.

Nursing Strategies with Frequencies

1. Explain to Mrs. Sokol-Velkie that increased urination will subside somewhat once diabetes is under control. Explain that some urinary frequency and urgency is likely because the bladder is compressed by the enlarging uterus. Also, vascular engorgement and altered bladder function due to hormones play a role.
2. Encourage Kegal exercises to strengthen pubococcygeal muscle and suggest limiting fluid intake before bedtime.
3. Discuss with Mrs. Sokol-Velkie the increased susceptibility of pregnant women to urinary tract infection (UTI) and the further risk of UTI due to diabetes. Explain the physiology to increase her understanding.
4. Teach Mrs. Sokol-Velkie the signs of UTI (pain and burning on urination, frequency, blood in urine, fever) and the importance of reporting these signs immediately.
5. Do routine clean catch urine testing each visit to assess for asymptomatic UTIs; explain that these can significantly change a woman's insulin requirement.

Nursing Care Plan for Human Need: *Sleep*

Nursing diagnosis	Due to or related to	As evidenced by	Goal/expected behaviors
Potential sleep disturbance	Personal occurrence of pregnancy Anxiety	Common problem during pregnancy Incomplete data base	Client experiences adequate sleep • Verbalizes rested feeling on waking with 3 weeks • Sleeps 7 to 8 hours/night without waking to void more than three times

Nursing Strategies with Frequencies

1. Assess prepregnancy and prediabetic sleep patterns and current sleep patterns.
2. Reassure the excessive sleep in first trimester is normal. Explain that insomnia is normal also, caused by a combination of physical discomfort, especially in last trimester, and a measure of anxiety at any stage.
3. Discuss past presleep rituals that helped Mrs. Sokol-Velkie to sleep, e.g., milk, music. Help institute these again. In addition do the following:

   - Suggest a sidelying position, which is the most comfortable position for many pregnant women.
   - Encourage foods high in tryptophan (milk, cheese, beans, peanut butter) before bed.
   - Discourage irritating foods, caffeine products, and drugs that interfere with sleep.
   - Have Mrs. Sokol-Velkie try a warm bath before sleep.
   - Teach Mrs. Sokol-Velkie relaxation exercises to be done before bedtime.
   - If she is especially lonely for her husband at this time, encourage her to write him a letter before bed or to read his last letter then.
   - Suggest that she begin a diary to record thoughts before sleeping (may or may not be shared with nurse).
   - Encourage short rest periods and naps during the day because extreme exhaustion can make sleep difficult.
   - Caution Mrs. Sokol-Velkie to avoid all sleep medications.

Nursing Care Plan for Human Need: *Activity*

Nursing diagnosis	Due to or related to	As evidenced by	Goal/expected behaviors
Potentially disrupted activity pattern	Pathophysiologic affront of diabetes and situational occurrence of pregnancy	Fluctuations in insulin and food requirements with different types of activity Incomplete data base	Client experiences normal activity pattern for a pregnant woman • Continues with prediabetic and prepregnancy activities except those discouraged within 4 weeks • Verbalizes way to meet needs during periods of strenuous exercise/activity within 1 week

Nursing Strategies with Frequencies

1. Assess prediabetic and prepregnancy daily routine and interests/activities.
2. Explain relationship between exercise, insulin, and glucose use to Mrs. Sokol-Velkie. Review onset, peak, and duration of action of NPH and regular insulin.

   - Stress that exercise/increased activity enhances use of glucose and decreases need for insulin.
   - Explain rationale for eating extra carbohydrates before strenuous exercise and the need to carry fast-acting sugars.

3. Using typical daily schedule and Mrs. Sokol-Velkie's records (urine and blood glucose levels, activity, insulin doses), help to alter food and/or insulin to meet requirements during times of increased activity.
4. Emphasize the importance of trying to keep meal/snack times on a fairly regular schedule, working activities around them.
5. Review the signs of hypoglycemia and help Mrs. Sokol-Velkie to recognize very early signs of low blood sugar levels.
6. Counsel Mrs. Sokol-Velkie to avoid very strenuous exercises that may reduce the blood supply to the placenta.

Nursing Care Plan for Human Need: *Adaptation to Manage Stress*

Nursing diagnosis	Due to or related to	As evidenced by	Goal/expected behaviors
Potential inability to manage stress	Pathophysiologic affront of newly diagnosed diabetes	Expectant bodily changes—first pregnancy	Client demonstrates ability to manage stress; has effective coping mechanisms
	Personal occurrence of newly diagnosed pregnancy	Nursing and medical surveillance	
	Situational occurrence of absence of husband, health care system participant	Absence of supportive presence of husband	• Lists stressors within 2 weeks
		Life-style changes—diet, insulin, nausea, frequent urination, experience of simultaneous multiple changes	• Elicits support of at least one nearby significant other within 1 week
			• Develops appropriate coping strategies within 4 weeks

Nursing Strategies with Frequencies

1. Assess Mrs. Sokol-Velkie's current coping mechanisms: long-term mechanisms and short-term mechanisms. Administer Effective

Coping Scale (Flynn, pp. 153–154).* Use data to explore coping status and opportunities.
2. Assess past coping strategies and support persons.
3. List current stressors. Explain to Mrs. Sokol-Velkie that the mere process of defining stressors relieves some of the anxiety they create because at least once listed they are "tangible" and can be tackled.
4. List those strategies that have the potential to be effective in dealing with these stressors.
5. Review those strategies that may appear useful in the short term but are ineffective for long-term crisis resolution (e.g., excessive sleep, denial, alcohol).
6. Encourage Mrs. Sokol-Velkie to employ one or two strategies per week and help her to evaluate their effectiveness.
7. Encourage Mrs. Sokol-Velkie to ventilate her feelings each visit. Provide support and encouragement.
8. Encourage Mrs. Sokol-Velkie to elicit the support of a nearby friend, relative. Look into the possibility of her joining a support group through the American Diabetic Association or a pregnancy related group (LaLeche League, etc.).

Nursing Care Plan for Human Need: *To Love and Be Loved*

Nursing diagnosis	Due to or related to	As evidenced by	Goal/expected behaviors
Diminished ability to love and to be loved	Situational occurrence of husband's absence	Husband away for 4 more months	Client experiences ability to love and feel loved.
		Unknown if husband will stay home for any extended length of time once home	• Continues to maintain relationship with husband via letters, phone calls, audio tapes
		Unknown if husband will be home for baby's birth	• Verbalizes feelings of loving others and being loved by other(s) within 1 month

Nursing Strategies with Frequencies

1. Encourage Mrs. Sokol-Velkie to continue relationship with husband by mail, phone calls, audio/video tapes. Provide her with information to send him regarding pregnancy, fatherhood, so she can share the event with him. If possible, obtain recording of baby's heart beat and picture from ultrasound to send to the father.

---

*Flynn, P. (1980). *Holistic health*. Bowie, Md.: Robert J. Brady Co.

2. Allow Mrs. Sokol-Velkie to ventilate any feelings of anger, loneliness, despair. Be supportive and understanding.
3. Encourage Mrs. Sokol-Velkie to become involved in a group where positive relationships are fostered (e.g., church group, support group).
4. Explore the possibility of obtaining a pet or having a friend live with her until husband returns. Suggest volunteer work in an area of interest (e.g., children's home).

NURSING CARE PLAN 4
Child with Diabetes Mellitus
Developed by Patricia Frensky Orfini

Client Situation: Jonathan Baselton

When Jonathan Baselton (aged 9 years) came home from his fourth grade class, he told his mother his teacher sent him to see the school nurse. His teacher thought his need to go to the bathroom so often during class time, his frequent trips to the water fountain, and his craving for sweets should be checked. The school nurse, Mrs. Bea Evans, learned from Jonathan that he is always thirsty and that he awakens three or four times a night to empty his bladder. During a preliminary health assessment, Mrs. Evans noted that Jonathan lost 5 pounds from the weight she recorded 3 months earlier. She noted he had a parenchymal infection on his index finger that, according to Jonathan, "doesn't want to go away, even with the salve my mother put on it." A test for urine sugar registered 4 +. Jonathan arrived home with a note from Mrs. Evans stating that sugar was found in his urine and Jonathan should be taken to see Dr. Molinaire as soon as possible. Mrs. Baselton was startled but immediately followed through with a call to Dr. Molinaire. Dr. Molinaire would see Jonathan and his mother in his office in 2 hours. Mrs. Evans followed up the note with a call to Mrs. Baselton. Mrs. Baselton stated she noted the water drinking behavior but thought Jonathan was following what he learned in health class about drinking eight full glasses of water daily. She also said that Jonathan seemed more irritable lately, had a few bed-wetting accidents, picked at his food, and seemed too tired to do much after school. Diabetes mellitus was verified by Dr. Molinaire who admitted Jonathan to Children's Hospital briefly for diagnosis and stabilization. Jonathan was placed on 20 units of NPH and 8 units of regular insulin at 7:30 A.M. daily and 10 units of NPH and 4 units of regular insulin at 4:30 P.M. daily. He was placed on a 2200 calorie diet consisting of three meals, three snacks, and food every 45 to 60 minutes during strenuous exercise. The Baselton family was referred to Mrs. Cynthia Baylor, a family nurse specialist in collaborative practice with Dr. Molinaire.

Nursing Care Plan for Human Need: *Nutrition*

Nursing diagnosis	Due to or related to	As evidence by	Goal/expected behaviors
Undernutrition	Pathophysiologic impact of diabetes mellitus	Weight loss "Picked at his food" Polydipsia Polyuria Glycosuria +4 Fatigue Irritability	Client experiences adequate nutrition • Blood glucose level 60 mg/dl to 140 mg/dl by 4th day • No glycosuria within 4 days • No further weight loss • Improved appetite (intake of approximately 2200 cal/day) within 1 week • Correctly selects food for 2 consecutive days within 2 weeks

Nursing Strategies with Frequencies

1. Assess Mr. and Mrs. Baselton's and Jonathan's perception of and knowledge of diabetes mellitus (previous experiences, friends, relatives, injections). Assess Jonathan's height, weight, vital signs, urine and blood glucose levels, activity/energy level, level of consciousness. Check for signs and symptoms of hypoglycemia/hyperglycemia every visit. (Hypoglycemia—[early symptoms] hunger, increased pulse rate, increased respiratory rate, weakness; [later symptoms] yawning, lethargy, increased difficulty in thought processes, irritability, belligerence; hyperglycemia—polydipsia, polyuria, polyphagia, fatigue, weight loss, dry skin, blurred vision, sores that are slow to heal.)

2. Describe simply, on first contact, the disease process, the purpose of insulin, and the necessity of diet therapy and administration of insulin to Mr. and Mrs. Baselton:

   • Expect and answer all questions regarding why and how their son acquired the disease, the implications for his future life and activities, and the limitations it will impose.

- Be honest, open, and empathic to establish a trusting relationship.
- Do not overwhelm with information; assess their psychological state/readiness to determine appropriate amount and complexity.
- Explain that you will be teaching them more about the disease in coming days and you are always available for questions.
- Provide written information.

3. Briefly name and describe diabetes mellitus to Jonathan. Explain basic concepts (i.e., he cannot get sugar into his cells without insulin) and the reasons for insulin injections and for following a specific diet. Be open and honest. The implied expectation should be that Jonathan will soon assume responsibility for self-management without difficulty. Provide with appropriate information from the American Diabetic Association.
4. Explain all procedures to Jonathan and his parents at all times. Keep teaching sessions with Jonathan short, no more than 15 to 20 minutes. Sessions with his parents should be periods of 45 to 60 minutes, longer if they desire. Gauge the amount and complexity of information daily by reactions, interests, questions, and anxiety.
5. Comprehensiveness of teaching depends on many factors: readiness, emotional status, acceptance of disease. Assess these and other factors. Give survival information first and continue rest of teaching later.
6. As soon as parents are ready, within the first day after diagnosis, begin to instruct on insulin administration. Briefly describe type and action of NPH and regular insulins.

- Teach strict aseptic technique for withdrawing and injecting insulin.
- Instruct on rolling bottle of NPH insulin between palm of hands until insulin thoroughly mixed.
- Describe and demonstrate steps for preparing NPH and regular insulins in one syringe.
- Stress importance of drawing up accurate dose(s).
- Emphasize importance of using correct syringe with correct insulin; use U100 insulin unless otherwise prescribed.
- Have parents practice drawing up with normal saline and injecting into an orange.
- Describe the injection sites available and the importance of rotation pattern.
- If desired, parents can practice giving each other or the nurse, or themselves an injection.

- Teach proper disposal of syringe and storage of insulin. To gain Jonathan's confidence, demonstrate injection techniques to Jonathan by giving the parents a saline injection and by having a parent(s) give an injection to the nurse or the other parent. One parent should give the next scheduled insulin dose.

7. After the parent gives Jonathan an insulin injection, teach Jonathan how to administer insulin (use same steps as in item 6). Use a doll instead of, or in addition to, an orange. Leave materials for practice. Have Jonathan give his own insulin dose when he is ready. Celebrate the event.

8. As soon as appropriate, sometime during first or second day of hospitalization, teach urine testing and blood testing procedures to parents and Jonathan.

   - Discuss reasons for testing and significance of results.
   - Teach and demonstrate techniques prescribed (Clinitest tablets, Ketodiastix, Dextrostix), interpret results (second voiding) and record results.
   - Supervise parents and Jonathan at next few testing times until accurate and confident.

9. As soon as appropriate, second or third day of hospitalization, review signs and symptoms and reasons for hypoglycemia, hyperglycemia, and ketoacidosis.

   - List precipitating factors for both.
   - Describe signs and symptoms for each (see item 1).
   - Outline management techniques.
   - Stress importance of carrying fast-acting sugar.
   - Explain importance of consuming extra carbohydrates before exercise and the importance of the bedtime snack.
   - Discuss when to seek medical care.
   - Give medic alert information.
   - Stress importance of maintaining and adjusting food, activity, and insulin at times of illness; have them notify physician about elevated blood sugar levels or urine glucose levels or vomiting.
   - Point out that illness, especially infection, vomiting, and diarrhea, may precipitate ketoacidosis.
   - Explain that hyperglycemia resulting from growth is to be anticipated and insulin doses may be increased accordingly.

10. As soon as appropriate, second or third day of hospitalization, have dietitian (with reinforcement from nurse) discuss the following with the parents and Jonathan:

- Teach role diet plays in disease management.
- Assess current dietary habits and develop prescribed diet managment within this framework.
- Discuss terms such as calories, carbohydrates, protein.
- Guide family in reading labels for nutritional value of foods.
- Discuss situations a child might encounter in the classroom and in the cafeteria. Role playing may help to assess understanding.
- Have Jonathan keep a "food diary" and then assess his diet with him and his parents.

11. Before hospital discharge (third day or so), discuss with Jonathan and his parents the importance of good foot and skin care. Gear initial discussion to Jonathan's level of understanding:

- Washing and drying daily.
- Avoidance of temperature extremes.
- Importance of wearing shoes at all times.
- Notify parents and care for a cut, sore, lesion immediately.

Continue discussion alone with parents covering:

- Toenail trimming.
- Treatment of corns, calluses, blisters, ingrown toenails.
- Treatment of abrasions of skin; when to seek medical/nursing care.

Teach Jonathan to keep a record of urine results, blood glucose levels, insulin taken, and activities. Explain to Jonathan and his parents how these can be used to help recognize variations that affect him (e.g., interaction between a favorite activity and urine sugar level).

12. Before discharge, discuss exercise considerations with Jonathan and his parents. (see Nursing Diagnosis for Disruptions in Activity)
13. If agreed to, arrange for family attendance at a diabetic education class in a few weeks. Give address for the American Diabetic Association (1 W. 48th Street, New York, New York 10020). Give address and phone number for the local chapter of the American Diabetic Association.
14. Plan for a telephone call to family in the evening (arrange time beforehand) on the day of discharge to assess adaptation. Give telephone number and encourage them to call at anytime with questions.
15. Plan for a visit 1 week after discharge with Jonathan. Assess:

- Attitude toward disease, insulin administration, diet.
- His records (discuss these together).

- The previous day's diet in terms of compliance, how he liked it, nutritional value.
- Injection procedure.
- Overall state of health, feeling of well-being, problems.

Answer any questions and review pertinent information. Check vital signs, urine glucose and blood glucose, weight, activity level.

16. Plan for a visit in 1 week with parents. Assess their attitude toward Jonathan's condition, the insulin administration and diet prescription, and their impression of their son's physical and emotional state. Review all previous teaching in greater depth now that anxiety state is somewhat lessened. Either at this visit or a future one, discuss possible complications of diabetes: neurologic changes, eye problems, kidney disease, arteriosclerotic changes, etc. in a tactful, clear, and nonfearful manner.

17. Arrange for visit 2 weeks after this visit (3 weeks after discharge) to again assess nutritional status, review all material, and answer questions. Assess blood sugar, vital signs, records, activity level, emotional status, signs of hypoglycemia, hyperglycemia or ketoacidosis and determine if control has been achieved.

18. Schedule future visits accordingly.

Nursing Care Plan for Human Need: *Wholesome Body Image*

Nursing diagnosis	Due to or related to	As evidenced by	Goal/expected behaviors
Potentially unwholesome body image	Pathophysiologic impact of diabetes mellitus	Changed body perception with chronic disease	Client experiences wholesome body image
		Potential feeling that he is different, sick, bad	• Verbalizes recent achievements and successful competitions signifying a functional body within 1 month • Parents verbalize his continued acceptance in peer group and no change in his normal activities within 1 month

Nursing Strategies with Frequencies

1. Assess preillness and current body image status.

- Sense of industry?
- Enjoyment in achieving things?
- Gains recognition from peers?
- Feelings of inferiority? inadequacy?

2. Assess parent's perception of Jonathan's diabetic condition and of their son's body image. Discuss any misconceptions or poor perceptions. Show how their perceptions can be perceived and internalized by Jonathan. Explain the importance of fostering positive view of self and wholesome body image in the school child dealing with industry versus inferiority tasks.

3. Encourage parents to emphasize the fact that his diabetic illness can be controlled, that activities will not need to change, that he is loved as before. Discourage the use of words, such as "different" or "sick," in describing Jonathan or his normal state of health.

4. Have parents encourage activities outside the home with peers soon after discharge. Have them encourage participation in activities/ sports where he will be successful, attain a feeling of mastery, and gain recognition from peers and family.

5. Suggest that parents delegate responsibilities suited to his abilities that contribute to the well-being of all the family.

Nursing Care Plan for Human Need: *Skin Integrity*

Nursing diagnosis	Due to or related to	As evidenced by	Goal/expected behaviors
Disrupted skin integrity	Pathophysiologic impact of diabetes mellitus—required multiple daily injections and infection of index finger	Persistent infection of index finger Multiple daily injections and "sticks"	Client maintains skin integrity aside from daily injection • Infected index finger healed in 4 weeks • No future infections • Verbalizes treatment methods for abrasions within 2 weeks • Demonstrates rotation of injection sites in 1 week • Verbalizes signs and symptoms of infection in 2 weeks

Nursing Strategies with Frequencies

1. Assess index finger: size of lesion, drainage (color, amount), color of lesion, pain.
2. Assess current treatment method.
3. Explain the increased susceptibility of persons with diabetes to infections and the reasons for poor healing.
4. Refer to physician for evaluation and possible antibiotic cream.

5. Teach Jonathan and parents the care of infected finger. Reassure that healing will be faster once blood sugar levels are controlled.
6. Emphasize the need to prevent and treat infections and skin injuries because of increased risk, slower healing, and increased requirement for insulin caused by infections along with the greater risk of ketoacidosis.

   - Stress that even slight injuries can become infected, i.e., scratches, splinters, and blisters.
   - Teach to carefully clean areas with soap and water and dry.
   - Avoid use of antiseptics that contain phenol, bichloride of mercury, oil of mustard, cantharidin, or salicyclic acid because these substances tend to burn the skin. (Luckman and Sorenson, p. 1575).*
   - After cleansing, apply a sterile gauze bandage. Avoid using adhesive tape that irritates skin.
   - Report serious injuries, infections to physician immediately.
   - Teach Jonathan and parents the signs of infection.

7. Assess routine for and compliance with rotation of injection sites.
8. Describe the lipodystrophies to parents. Identify ways to prevent these to maintain normal insulin absorption at the injection site.

   - Use insulin at room temperature.
   - Rotate sites systematically.
   - Inject insulin into pocket between fat and muscle.

9. Emphasize need for sterility during injection procedure and home glucose monitoring.

   - Use only sterile syringes and needles.
   - Always clean top of insulin bottle with alcohol before inserting sterile needle.
   - Clean skin with alcohol prior to injection

Nursing Care Plan for Human Need: *Freedom from Pain*

Nursing diagnosis	Due to or related to	As evidenced by	Goal/expected behaviors
Pain	Insulin injections and blood sugar monitoring related to pathophysiologic affront of diabetes mellitus	Insulin injections two times daily Daily blood sugar tests Inadequate data base	Client demonstrates ability to cope with discomfort • Tolerates brief

(continued)

*Luckmann, J., & Sorensen, K. (1980). *Medical–surgical nursing*. Philadelphia: W.B. Saunders.

Freedom from Pain (continued)

Nursing diagnosis	Due to or related to	As evidenced by	Goal/expected behaviors
			discomfort willingly (no crying, kicking, etc.) in 2 weeks • Verbalizes understanding of reason for injections and blood glucose testing in 3 weeks

Nursing Strategies with Frequencies

1. Assess Jonathan's response to injection and blood glucose sticks. Assess his parents' response to his getting the injection and their response to his response.
2. Review the purpose of insulin therapy and blood glucose sticks; present the injections as the good thing that prevents irritating symptoms.
3. Explore with Jonathan different methods and areas for injection that are less painful than others. Encourage that he use these.
4. Assess Jonathan's level of anxiety about the injection. Explain how the muscle tension associated with sympathetic responses to anxiety may exacerbate the pain. Relieve anxiety. Discuss his feeling about the daily injections.
5. Teach Jonathan to use distraction to reduce the discomfort of injections and "sticks."
6. Limit blood glucose monitoring to as little as possible; supplement with urine testing for glucose.

Nursing Care Plan for Human Need: *Activity*

Nursing diagnosis	Due to or related to	As evidenced by	Goal/expected behaviors
Disruptions in activity Diminished activity	Pathophysiologic affront of diabetes mellitus	Fatigue after school Less activity after school	Client resumes normal activity • Denies fatigue until bedtime within 2 weeks • Engages in school activities and after school activities within 4 weeks • Blood sugar normal in 1 week

(continued)

Activity (continued)

Nursing diagnosis	Due to or related to	As evidenced by	Goal/expected behaviors
			• Verbalizes methods to meet requirements during strenuous exercise within 4 weeks

Nursing Strategies with Frequencies

1. Assess preillness typical daily schedule and interests/hobbies.
2. Explain relationship between exercise, insulin, and glucose use to Jonathan and his parents. Review onset, peak, and duration of action of NPH and regular insulins.

   - Stress that exercise enhances use of glucose and decreases requirement for insulin.
   - Explain rationale for eating extra carbohydrates before strenuous exercise and the requirement to carry fast-acting sugars.

3. Using typical daily schedule (item 1) and Jonathan's records, help Jonathan and his parents alter food and/or insulin to meet requirements during times of increased activity. Review signs and symptoms of hyperglycemia and hypoglycemia. Help Jonathan to become aware of the onset of these signs and to react appropriately.
4. Explain that food intake often needs to be increased in summer when children are more active and decreased on return to school.
5. If Jonathan is on a sports team, stress the requirement for increased food intake on the days of activity and maybe even more on days of competition/races.
6. Inform family that if increased food is not tolerated, decreased insulin is the next step (to be discussed with physician).
7. Explain that if timing of exercise is changed so that supper meal is delayed, the insulin in the second dose may be moved back to precede mealtime.

Nursing Care Plan for Human Need: *Elimination*

Nursing diagnosis	Due to or related to	As evidenced by	Goal/expected behaviors
Disturbance in urinary elimination pattern	Pathophysiologic affront of diabetes mellitus	"Awakens three to four times a night to void"	Client returns to normal urinary elimination pattern

(continued)

Elimination (continued)

Nursing diagnosis	Due to or related to	As evidenced by	Goal/expected behaviors
		"A few bed-wetting accidents"	• Awakens to void no more than one time per night within 2 weeks • No enuresis within 4 weeks

Nursing Strategies with Frequencies

1. Assess preillness urinary eliminaton pattern; adjust expected behavioral outcomes accordingly.
2. Explain the relationship between polyuria, nocturia, and diabetes mellitus.
3. Reassure that polyuria, nocturia, and enuresis will stop once control of diabetes is achieved.
4. Caution parents against scolding or shaming for enuresis.
5. Discuss enuresis with Jonathan, relieving him of any feelings of shame, guilt, or parental disapproval.
6. Suggest that restricting or eliminating fluids after the evening meal may help to reduce sleep disruption due to nocturia.
7. Stress need to replace fluid during times of polyuria.

Nursing Care Plan for Human Need: *Protection from Excessive Fear, Anxiety, and Chaos*

Nursing diagnosis	Due to or related to	As evidenced by	Goal/expected behaviors
Potential anxiety and fear	Environmental affront of hospitalization Medical, pharmacologic, nursing therapies	Decreased self-control Pain associated with procedures Strange environment and people	Client experiences minimal anxiety without fear • Verbalizes fear by second day • Explores unit, interacts with others by second day

Nursing Strategies with Frequencies

1. Encourage one or both parents to stay with Jonathan to increase his security and relieve him of any separation anxieties.
2. Assess for and discuss feelings of loneliness, boredom, isolation, and depression.
3. Help Jonathan to maintain his usual routine by continuing some school lessons, telephone calls, and visits by friends.
4. Thoroughly orient him to his room, the unit, the people he can expect to see, and the hospital routine (shift changes, mealtimes).

5. Explain all procedures beforehand (not too far beforehand to cause anxiety) and allow Jonathan to be as involved as possible in them.
6. Discuss typical school-age fears, such as fear of death, abandonment, permanent injury, loss of peer acceptance, lack of productivity (industry versus inferiority), inability to cope with stress/pain according to cultural expectation ("act like a man"), with Jonathan's parents and with Jonathan as appropriate.
7. Encourage increased sense of control by encouraging Jonathan to make his bed, choose his activities, assist in procedures, and make choices throughout the day.
8. Be honest and factual in answering questions or presenting information. Seeking information is one way children maintain a sense of control.
9. Encourage Jonathan's parents to bring familiar articles from home if he desires.

Nursing Care Plan for Human Need: *Adaptation, to Manage Stress*

Nursing diagnosis	Due to or related to	As evidenced by	Goal/expected behaviors
Potential inability to manage stress	Pathophysiologic affront of chronic illness Environmental affront of hospitalization	Mother "startled" Sudden onset of a chronic illness Stressors in hospital environment	Client demonstrates ability to manage stress; effective coping mechanisms • Lists stressors within 2 days • Uses effective coping mechanisms within 3 days • Ventilates feelings within 1 day

Nursing Strategies with Frequencies

1. Assess the parents' current coping mechanisms—long-term and short-term mechanisms. Administer Effective Coping Scale (Flynn, pp. 153–154).* Use data to explore coping status and opportunities.
2. Assess the parents' past coping mechanisms and resource support persons. Assess family factors: other children, ages, health; proximity of home to hospital; extended family nearby; past experiences with illness; relationship between parents; age of parents; health of parents.
3. List current stresses that potentially contribute to crises for the parents (e.g., caring for other children while at hospital).

*Flynn, P. (1980). *Holistic health*. Bowie, Md.: Robert J. Brady.

4. List those strategies that have the potential to be effective in dealing with crises for Jonathan's parents (e.g., maternal grandparents stay with children, hire a nanny, have friends care for children).
5. Reinforce past coping strategies that have the potential to be effective with current stresses/crises (e.g., ventilating feelings, seeking out new information).
6. Review those strategies that may appear useful in the short term but are ineffective for long-term crisis resolution (e.g., alcohol, denial).
7. Allow parents to ventilate their feelings about the situation. Provide support and encouragement.
8. Discuss any guilt feelings. Watch for signs of overprotectiveness that result from guilt feelings and feelings of the unknown. Watch for neglect, which is a mechanism to provide relief from guilty feelings.

NURSING CARE PLAN 5
Mature Woman with Diabetes Mellitus
Developed by Gaie Rubenfeld

Client Situation: Monique Morales

Monique Morales, a 65-year-old Mexican immigrant who just became an American citizen, was taken to the Emergency Room by her daughter Maria after suffering a "fainting spell" at home. Monique and Maria (newly widowed) share a two-bedroom apartment in the Spanish section of the city. Both Monique and Maria earn a living doing housework in the affluent section of the city, about 5 miles away by bus. Both salaries are needed to manage expenses since Maria's husband died a month ago. Prior to his death, Monique maintained the apartment, cooked, washed, and cleaned, and on occasion relieved Maria when she wanted a day or two off.

Monique was diagnosed as having diabetes mellitus 5 years ago and in the past was maintained on a diet ranging from 1800 to 2200 calories and NPH insulin, 20 to 40 units, at different times. She faithfully attends Diabetic Clinic at the hospital nearby and prior to her fainting spell was on a 2000-calorie diet and 35 units of NPH insulin. Dr. Molinaire, who services the Diabetic Clinic, was called to see Monique Morales by the Emergency Room nurse. On admission Monique was flushed, had a fruity odor to her breath, was breathing heavily, and seemed lethargic. It was difficult getting a coherent response from her. Emergency intervention averted the hyperglycemia and ketoacidosis.

Monique was transferred to a medical nursing unit for a 2-day stay for surveillance and follow-up.

Nursing Care Plan for Human Need: *Adaptation, to Manage Stress*

Nursing diagnosis	Due to or related to	As evidenced by	Goal/expected behaviors
Ineffective physiological adaptation	Excessive physical and emotional stress Physiologic effects of diabetes	Fainting spell Breathing heavily Lethargic Incoherent Fruity odor to breath Usual diabetes treatment now ineffective	Client has a plan to adapt to stressors by the time of discharge • Lists her present life stressors • Identifies the relationship of stress to diabetes control • Identifies coping mechanisms to assist her with present stressors

Nursing Strategies with Frequencies

1. Assess Monique's perceptions of her present stressors.
2. Help her list those stressors; consider grief response, fears about financial situation, increased work load, level of fatigue, age-related stressors, less time at home, and others.
3. Explain the body's stress response and show how emotional and physical stress cause diabetic instability.
4. Ask Monique to list previously used coping mechanisms during times of excess stress in her past.
5. Ask her to identify those coping mechanisms that might be effective now.
6. Suggest additional coping mechanisms specific to the present stressors:

   - Consider the possibility and feasibility of working fewer hours and closer to home.
   - Consult with social worker to explore financial aid options.
   - Suggest a discussion with her pastor or a counselor to assist her with her grief response if needed.
   - Plan relaxation time and activities into her daily activity schedule, such as an afternoon rest period to break up the work day.

7. Teach Monique how to monitor physiological responses and intervene to avoid crises (see Human Need for Safety).

Nursing Care Plan for Human Need: *Safety*

Nursing diagnosis	Due to or related to	As evidenced by	Goal/expected behaviors
Potential for injury	Altered sensory status secondary to unstable diabetes, to excessive work and personal stressors	Hospitalized for fainting episode and symptoms of ketoacidosis	Client experiences physiological safety by time of discharge from hospital and thereafter
		Required insulin and dietary changes in past for control of diabetes	By day 1 after immediate health crisis is controlled, Mrs. Morales:
		Travels by bus 5 miles to work	• Lists signs and symptoms of hyperglycemia and ketoacidosis
		65 years old	• Demonstrates technique for testing urine for sugar and acetone
		Employment—housework (probable that she would be alone during work day)	• Identifies actions for treatment of hyperglycemia or ketoacidosis
		Mexican immigrant (English is second language)	• Lists signs and symptoms of hypoglycemia
		Needs to work for financial reasons	• Identifies actions for treatment of hypoglycemia
		Increased work load in past month	By day 2:
			• Identifies factors that increase safety hazards
			• Plans actions to decrease safety hazards
			• Has a written emergency action plan to carry at all times

Nursing Strategies with Frequencies

Day 1

1. Plan joint sessions with Monique and Maria.
2. Assess present level of knowledge of emergency care for hazards associated with diabetes.
3. Teach the signs and symptoms of hyperglycemia and/or ketoacidosis in terms that are simple and can be remembered easily:

increased thirst; dry, flushed face; elevated temperature; nausea, vomiting; *air hunger or difficulty breathing; *fruity breath odor; dim vision; lethargy; sugar and/or ketones in urine. If symptoms are starred (*), call physician immediately.

4. Write these on a card and translate into Spanish if necessary. Have Monique read and explain each one.

5. Review steps of checking urine for sugar and ketones; have Monique demonstrate this.

6. Review the times when urine should be tested: before meals, at bedtime, and whenever she experiences any of the symptoms listed on the card.

7. List actions to be taken when symptoms occur: if starred (*) symptoms on card occur, call physician immediately; have back-up emergency number to call if physician is unavailable (hospital, ambulance, or daughter). If other symptoms, check urine first; if sugar and ketones present, call physician.

8. Coordinate teaching plan with physician's instructions for other actions such as insulin coverage.

9. Teach signs and symptoms of hypoglycemia: nervousness, irritability, weakness, perspiration, confusion, trembling, headache, blurred or double vision, tachycardia or palpitations, numbness of lips or tongue, incoherent speech.

10. Write these on a card in Spanish, if necessary.

11. Explain cardinal differences between hyperglycemia and hypoglycemia attacks:

	Hypoglycemia	Hyperglycemia
Onset	Rapid (minutes)	Slow (days or weeks)
Thirst	Absent	Increased
Nausea/vomiting	Absent	Frequent
Vision	Double	Dim
Respirations	Normal	Difficulty
Skin	Moist, pale	Hot, dry, flushed
Tremors	Frequent	Absent

12. List actions to be taken for treatment of hypoglycemia: eat high carbohydrate food immediately; give examples: fruit juice, cola, graham crackers. If symptoms persist 5 to 10 minutes after eating, eat again.

13. Tell Monique and Maria to call physician if several hypoglycemic attacks occur within 1 week.

Day 2

1. Plan joint session with Monique and Maria.
2. Explore daily activities to identify safety hazards. Assess for: diabetes identification bracelet or tag (consider the necessity of one in Spanish and one in English); daily meal schedule; financial ability to buy food and medicine; times when Monique is alone; ability to communicate needs.
3. After identification of hazards, make plans with Monique and Maria to decrease hazards. Emphasize that Monique must:

   - Always have diabetic identification with her.
   - Always carry high carbohydrate food.
   - Have telephone numbers of physician, Maria, hospital, and another resource person readily available.
   - Always have in writing, the address of the house where she is working.
   - If possible, make sure regular bus driver knows her and of her diabetic condition.

NURSING CARE PLAN 6
Young Adult Man with Diabetes Mellitus
Developed by Gaie Rubenfeld

Client Situation: Vincent Valentino

Vincent Valentino, age 26, was sworn in as a new law partner in the firm of Smith, French, and Rodale—a firm of very successful criminal lawyers. Vincent scored the highest in the state in the bar examination and was sought after by numerous firms. His acceptance of the Smith, French, and Rodale offer was viewed by his professional friends and colleagues as an excellent decision with an expectation of a brilliant future. Vincent and his fiancé, Christina, will be married in 2 weeks, and an old-fashioned Italian wedding is planned. Three-hundred relatives will convene. Christina is 2 years older than Vincent and is becoming increasingly known for her fashion designs that have caught the eyes of celebrities. A dual career marriage has been decided.

As part of the formal appointment to the law firm, a complete physical examination was done 2 days ago by Dr. Molinaire, the family's physician. A blood sugar of 350 mg and a 4+ urine sugar were found. Vincent was immediately scheduled for a glucose tolerance test that verified diabetes mellitus. Vincent was devastated by the news as was

Christina. They questioned family members about a history of diabetes mellitus and no prior history could be determined for Vincent but Christina learned that her great-grandmother was suspected to have had diabetes. There was never a formal diagnosis due to an absence of medical care. Dr. Molinaire hoped to maintain Vincent's diabetes mellitus by diet alone. Initially he ordered a 2000-calorie diet.

Nursing Care Plan for Human Need: *Adaptation, to Manage Stress*

Nursing diagnosis	Due to or related to	As evidenced by	Goal/expected behaviors
Potential for ineffective coping with stress	Excessive personal, physiologic, and situational changes	New, high-stress job in criminal law firm	Client exhibits effective coping with stress
		Marriage in 2 weeks	• Expresses intent to adhere to 2000-calorie diet today
		Large wedding (implying much planning)	• Communicates his feelings and concerns to Christina today and plans to continue this daily
		Newly diagnosed diabetes mellitus	
		Blood sugar 350 mg	• Delegates responsibility for all but essentially his wedding plans to other family members and friends within this week
		4+ urine sugar	
		Newly-ordered 2000-calorie diet	
		Devastated by news of diabetes diagnosis	• Identifies a work schedule that allows time for eating meals, resting, and relaxing on a regular, daily basis, within 1 week of starting work
			• Has blood sugar in normal range within 1 month

Nursing Strategies with Frequencies

Session 1

1. Plan joint sessions with Vincent and Christina, if possible.
2. Assess communication patterns of couple.
3. Encourage them to express their concerns to each other.
4. Ask them to identify coping mechanisms used in the past. Assist process by helping each of them think of high-stress situations in

the past, then identify outcomes and mechanisms that were effective in reducing stress.

5. Reinforce their use of coping strategies that worked in the past, and remind them of their combined resources as a couple.

6. Teach new strategies, specific to the present stressors: diet strategies (in Human Need for Nutrition).

7. Have Vincent and Christina make lists of wedding plans that can be implemented by others.

8. Acknowledge any problems they may have relinquishing control of wedding activities, because they are both high achievers and likely to have strong needs to control.

9. Teach them the relationship between stress and blood glucose levels; emphasize the necessity for Vincent to work at controlling his diabetes immediately.

10. Set up an appointment with them for 1 week after they are back at work.

Session 2—1 week after return to work

1. Assess compliance with prescribed diet and reinforce previous teaching as needed.

2. Encourage Vincent and Christina to discuss work schedules and list plans for meal times, recreation, and relaxation.

3. Remind Vincent that his perfection as a new law partner can be used as a strength to assert his schedule needs.

4. Assess their requirement for learning new stress management techniques; teach as necessary.

5. Check blood sugar results and discuss the significance of them.

Nursing Care Plan for Human Need: *Nutrition*

Nursing diagnosis	Due to or related to	As evidenced by	Goal/expected behaviors
Potential disturbance in nutritional pattern	Lack of effective meal planning	2000-calorie diet prescribed	Client experiences adequate nutrition
	Pathophysiologic impact of diabetes mellitus	Dual career couple with new careers (implies busy schedule and high potential for frequently eating in restaurants)	• Maintains weight appropriate to age, height, and gender • Acknowledges the necessity to adhere to a 2000-calorie diet
		Busy schedule predisposes couple to lack of time for meal planning	• Correctly plans a menu using American Diabetic Association guidelines

(continued)

Nutrition *(continued)*

Nursing diagnosis	Due to or related to	As evidenced by	Goal/expected behaviors
		Italian heritage (potentially strong link to ethnic eating patterns)	• Shows how his favored ethnic foods fit into prescribed diet
		Weight change	• Lists those foods he should not eat
			• Plans meals he can carry with him and eat "on the run"
			• Plans meals from restaurant menus that are consistent with prescribed diet

Nursing Strategies with Frequencies

1. Determine pattern of body weight and establish baseline weight.
2. Schedule teaching session with Vincent and Christina together, if possible.
3. Assess readiness to learn; assess level of stress and possible interferences to learning (see plan for Human Need for Adaptation to Manage Stress).
4. Explain relationship between dietary intake and diabetes control.
5. Acknowledge their life-style and reassure them that 2000-calorie diet and eating habits can be compatible.
6. Provide literature to assist them to plan spoil-proof lunches that can be prepared and carried in one's briefcase.
7. Provide sample restaurant menus with calories calculated.
8. Calculate calories in favorite ethnic foods.
9. Focus on the positive aspects of foods he can eat but acknowledge those foods he should not eat, such as concentrated sweets.
10. Give address and telephone number of the local American Diabetic Association and explain their services.

Nursing Care Plan for Human Need: *Sexual Integrity*

Nursing diagnosis	Due to or related to	As evidenced by	Goal/expected behaviors
Potential sexual dysfunction	Physiologic changes associated with diabetes mellitus	New diagnosis of diabetes Fasting blood sugar 350 mg	Client and spouse have a satisfying sexual relationship

(continued)

Sexual Integrity (continued)

Nursing diagnosis	Due to or related to	As evidenced by	Goal/expected behaviors
	High stress New marriage Possible fears of passing diabetes to offspring Psychological and genetic impact of diabetes mellitus	4+ urine sugar Marriage in 2 weeks Large wedding planned New job as law partner Vincent and Christina devastated by news of diabetes Christian's great-grandmother suspected to have had diabetes	Prior to their wedding, Vincent and Christina: • Voice any concerns about their sexual integrity • State the possible effects of diabetes on sexual response • Acknowledge the importance of diabetic control on optimum sexual functioning • Plan actions to take if sexual dysfunction occurs • Have a resource for genetic counseling to use if and when they plan to have children

Nursing Strategies with Frequencies

1. Plan one counseling session with Vincent and Christina together (unless Vincent prefers a session alone) before their wedding, if possible.
2. Acknowledge any discomfort they may have in discussing their sexuality, but encourage open communication.
3. Present findings about effects of diabetes on sexual function.*

   - Note that in men, impotence is sometimes a problem caused by physiologic or psychological factors.
   - Emphasize that sexual problems do not arise in many persons with diabetes, especially in those whose disease is well controlled.
   - Reassure them that, although the physiological causes of sexual dysfunction are not always clear, there are treatments that are effective in correcting the problems.
   - Acknowledge to them that psychological stressors causing impotence can also be overcome. Note examples of possible stressors: fear of transmitting diabetes to offspring, fear that having diabe-

---

*Suggested reference: Hogan, R. (1985). *Human sexuality: A nursing perspective*, 2nd ed. (Chapter 26, Impaired Hormonal Function). Norwalk, Conn., Appleton-Century-Crofts

tes makes one "less of a man," career pressures, or busy schedules.

4. Make a strong point that knowing problems could occur does not mean they will occur.
5. Stress the importance of open communication between them as the best prevention for sexual dysfunction.
6. Review the essentials of diabetes control, especially dietary control to keep blood glucose levels normal (see other nursing care plans).
7. Give them resources for aid if they have future questions or sexual problems: Vincent's physician, an endocrinologist, sex therapist, American Diabetic Association.
8. Assess their plans for having children; suggest that they might want genetic counseling if they plan to have children, as there is diabetes in both of their families.
9. Provide a resource for genetic counseling such as an endocrinologist or a geneticist.
10. Considering their present stress levels, encourage them to return for more discussion after their wedding to review this information.

NURSING CARE PLAN 7
Middle-Aged Man with Diabetes Mellitus
Developed by Gaie Rubenfeld

Client Situation: Christopher Harrell

Christopher Harrell is a 40-year-old Professor of African Studies at Mylanta University. He has received numerous awards for his research on African literature and is sought after as a lecturer nationally and internationally. His African–American heritage has been particularly useful in his research and bilingual fluency in French as well as English facilitates his presentation to a wide range of audiences. He is newly divorced and is establishing himself after 20 years of marriage as a single head of household. He was diagnosed as having diabetes mellitus 10 years ago and has been controlled by diet alone through the years. Prior to and during the divorce proceedings he noted an exacerbation of symptoms despite his efforts to stick to his diet. Symptoms were severe enough to warrant hospitalization for stabilization of his diabetes. His physician, Dr. Molinaire, believes a 2000-calorie diet with 30 units of NPH insulin plus regular insulin coverage for spillover based on urine testing is the treatment of choice for the present. Mr. Harrell must be taught to give himself insulin before he can be discharged. He has expressed great concern about taking insulin and being tied down by having to inject himself one or more times daily. He has refused all attempts by the nursing staff to teach him to inject himself.

Nursing Care Plan for Human Need: *Self-Control, Self-Determination, Responsibility*

Nursing diagnosis	Due to or related to	As evidenced by	Goal/expected behaviors
Diminished self-control, self-determination, responsibility	Nonacceptance of altered body requirements and diabetic role Pathophysiologic impact of diabetes mellitus	Unstable diabetes Prescribed treatment: 30 units NPH insulin and regular insulin coverage Expresses concern about taking insulin Expresses perception of being tied down by insulin injections Refuses insulin injection, teaching sessions Recently divorced (probably no other person to do insulin injections for him)	Client assumes self-control and responsibility regarding his diabetes. • Accepts the role of diabetes manager for himself by end of session 1 • Accepts the necessity of self-injection by the end of session 1 • Demonstrates the correct technique for insulin injection by the end of session 2 • Plans meals that are compliant with 2000-calorie requirement by the end of session 3 • Verbalizes a plan for incorporating diet and injections into his daily life events by session 4 • Has a blood sugar in normal range 1 week postdischarge

Nursing Strategies and Frequencies

Plan several sessions with Mr. Harrell, each having well-defined goals.*

Session 1: Role acceptance

1. Have Mr. Harrell list his various roles—professor, researcher, lecturer, African-American, linguist, divorcee, and others.

---

*Plan based on concepts from model by Dracup, K.A., & Meleis, A.I. (1982). Compliance: an interactionist approach. *Nursing Research, 31* (1), 31–35.

2. List accomplishments, tasks, and responsibilities that accompany these roles.
3. Explain how being a person with diabetes constitutes a role ascribed to him, and compare the tasks and responsibilities of this role to those of other roles.
4. Focus on Mr. Harrell's strengths and successes in his roles.
5. Have him state: "I am a diabetic; this role has certain responsibilities. These responsibilities are giving myself insulin injections and eating a 2000-calorie diet."
6. Encourage Mr. Harrell to list coping mechanisms he used for other role responsibilities that could be used in this new role as insulin-dependent diabetic.
7. Tell him that you will return for session 2 with knowledge that he can use to implement his role requirements.

Session 2: Knowledge for role enactment—insulin injection

1. Ask Mr. Harrell to repeat his statement of acceptance of the diabetic role.
2. Remind him of his intellectual accomplishments and ask him to assume a student role.
3. Review the objectives for this teaching–learning session.
4. Explain the procedure for preparing insulin dose and steps of injection procedure.
5. Ask Mr. Harrell to repeat back to you the steps of the process.
6. Have him demonstrate the correct procedure of injecting himself at the scheduled time for his NPH insulin.
7. Teach Mr. Harrell the steps for checking urine for sugar and acetone.
8. Have him prepare regular insulin for coverage of spillover based on urine testing.
9. Have him demonstrate correct procedure for injection of regular insulin.
10. Give him a "grade" on his learning.

Session 3: Knowledge for role enactment—dietary management

1. Ask Mr. Harrell to repeat his statement of acceptance of diabetic role.
2. Ask him to assume a student role.
3. Review the objectives for this teaching–learning session.
4. Review principles of diet management, reinforcing correct dietary techniques used in the past 10 years when his diabetes was controlled by diet alone.
5. Explain how insulin treatment affects dietary intake and vice versa.

6. Explain the peak actions of both types of insulin (regular, 2 to 4 hr; NPH, 8 to 12 hr) and how this relates to time of scheduled meals.
7. Have Mr. Harrell plan menus from the American Diabetic Association diet lists that meet 2000-calorie requirements.
8. Give him a "grade" on his learning.

Session 4: Counter-roles—incorporating new role into usual life-style

1. Ask Mr. Harrell to repeat his statement of acceptance of diabetic role.
2. Review the objectives for this session.
3. Ask him to describe his usual schedule for a typical month.
4. Ask him to pick out significant counter-roles in his usual interactions—students, those who invite him to lecture, colleagues, friends, family members, physicians, nurses, others.
5. Ask him to indicate which of these counter-roles and situations will help and which ones will hinder his adherence to his diabetic role.
6. For those roles and situations that interfere with his diabetic role, ask him to plan coping mechanisms. Help him plan "what if" scenarios:

   - What if you are traveling in a plane and are required to check urine and give yourself regular insulin? (Tell stewardess your requirement, always carry insulin and urine testing equipment in your hand luggage.)
   - What if you are traveling and your plane is late and you have to eat? (Carry food at all times in hand luggage.)
   - What if you must eat in restaurants frequently? (Carry diet exchange lists in your pocket; ask waiter for food prepared without unknown sauces.)

7. For those roles and situations that help with his diabetic role, encourage Mr. Harrell to enlist the aid of helpful persons. Reinforce the fact that he can be open about his disease and his needs.
8. Teach Mr. Harrell safety-enhancing measures:

   - Wear diabetic identification tag or bracelet.
   - List signs and symptoms of hyperglycemia and hypoglycemia.
   - List emergency treatments for hyperglycemic and hypoglycemic episodes.

Session 5: One week after discharge—evaluation and feedback

1. Ask Mr. Harrell to repeat his statement of acceptance of diabetic role.
2. Ask him to report on his activities in the past week.

3. Check insulin injection sites for any signs of inflammation or discomfort.
4. Check glucose level.
5. Ask for any need to review information from any previous teaching session. Review material as needed.
6. Provide positive feedback for actions that indicate proper diabetic control.
7. Plan for subsequent appointments.
8. Compliment Mr. Harrell on his new role accomplishments.

NURSING CARE PLAN FOR THE FAMILY
Developed by Kathryn Caufield

Family Situation: The Lily Lawson Family

Mrs. Lily Lawson is a 78-year-old woman with a 15-year history of insulin-requiring diabetes mellitus. She is a small, thin woman who had lived alone since the very sudden death of her husband Andrew from a heart attack 6 years ago when he was 75 years old. Prior to his death, he had been a healthy, robust, and energetic man, who had never been sick "a day in his life." Since her husband's death, Mrs. Lawson's health had gradually deteriorated as had her enjoyment of her other activities such as cooking, gardening, needle work, reading, and watching television. In recent years she has also experienced decreased visual activity because of mild open angle glaucoma and cataracts. These conditions have contributed to her decline in activity as well. She gets little or no exercise.

Mrs. Lawson owned a comfortable two-story home about a 20-minute drive from her daughter, Mary (Lawson) Boulder. She had two close friends in the neighborhood. Mrs. Lawson was picked up about three times a week to have dinner with her daughter, son-in-law Joseph, and 15-year-old granddaughter, Jackie. On the other days, her daughter would telephone. Recently, however, Mrs. Lawson would not always hear the phone because of an increasing hearing impairment. When this happened, Mary would drive over to check on her mother. Mrs. Lawson tended to eat poorly, test her urine for glucose irregularly, overextend herself, and be somewhat fearful of being alone.

Mrs. Lawson was discharged from Glendale General Hospital 2 weeks ago after a 12-day hospitalization for a severe urinary tract infection and a subsequent episode of mild diabetic ketoacidosis. Both problems had been resolved enough for her to be discharged. The difficult decision that she live with her daughter and son-in-law was made collaboratively, though reluctantly, by them and the family physician during the hospitalization. It was the consensus that Mrs. Lawson required closely supervised care to more diligently monitor her diabetes and prevent a recurrence of the recent problems. They also concluded that the upkeep of her home was too strenuous and expensive for her on her fixed income. She is now taking 30 units of NPH insulin each morning and is on a 2500-calorie diet. Five units of regular insulin are given before each meal. Her daughter was taught to perform home blood glucose monitoring, to be done four times a day, before meals and at bedtime.

The Boulders live in a fairly large comfortable home. Mary is 55 years old, has been obese "for years," but otherwise describes herself to be in good health. She has not seen a doctor for over 10 years. Her husband, Joseph, is 60 years old, also has long-standing obesity, and had to retire last month due to a heart condition. He had a heart attack 7 years ago and now has frequent episodes of angina. He is under the care of a cardiologist and takes digitalis and a diuretic daily and nitroglycerine as needed. His father died of pneumonia at age 26. His mother died of congestive heart failure at age 75. Jackie is the youngest of 5 children (3 girls aged 15, 22, 29, and 2 boys aged 18 and 26) and the only one living at home on a permanent basis. During holidays and summers, two of the other children live at home. Jackie has always been a healthy child.

The oldest daughter (aged 29) has an obesity problem and is newly diagnosed with diabetes mellitus and is controlled by diet. Prior to her husband's retirement, Mrs. Boulder had the house to herself most of the day. Mrs. Boulder had been active in church activities—Altar Society and Choir, but gave these up when Joseph retired "to keep him company."

During his later working years Joseph, with his wife, made frequent weekend trips to the mountains or went cruising on their sailboat. They sold the sailboat recently because of Joseph's illness and the increasing maintenance costs. He describes his retirement as "boring." Neither Mary nor Joseph Boulder get any exercise to speak of.

The home care nurse from Glendale General Hospital, Ms. Evans, comes to make a family assessment and to see how Mrs. Lawson and the Boulders are adjusting to their changed family situation. Ms. Evans is speaking with Mary and Joseph Boulder in the kitchen and can see Mrs. Lawson sitting in the den reading a book. While they are speaking, Jackie returns from school with three girlfriends. They pause momentarily at the doorway of the den when they see Mrs. Lawson. One of the girls turns and abruptly leaves. The other girls go into the den and turn on the television set, chatter about school, and begin to play a game of Trivial Pursuit.

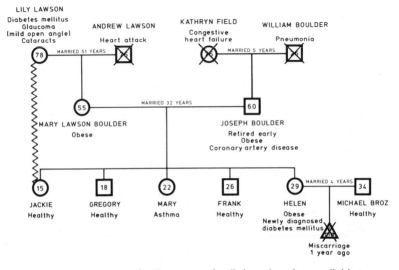

Figure 4–1. Genogram for the Lawson family based on data available to date (numbers within symbols refer to present ages).

Mrs. Lawson gets up, turns up the volume of the television set, and sits close to the girls to watch their game and suggest some answers. Within 15 minutes Jackie's other girlfriends leave. Jackie slams the door of the den as she leaves to go to her room.

Ms. Evans also learns that Mrs. Lawson has lost weight (5 pounds in a week) and she is having elevated blood glucose levels almost continuously and occasional trace to 1 + ketones in the urine. From the available data Ms. Evans developed a genogram (Fig. 4–1) and a family nursing care plan using the human need theory framework and the nursing process.

Family Nursing Care Plan for Survival Human Need: *Nutrition*

Family nursing diagnosis	Due to or related to	As evidenced by	Goal/expected behaviors
Disturbed family survival needs: nutrition	*Physiologic—* Pathophysiologic state of diabetes mellitus of Lily Lawson (characterized by inappropriate/inadequate uptake, utilization, metabolism of carbohydrates, fats, proteins) requiring special diet	Lily Lawson's requirement for insulin and special diet	All family members demonstrate adequate nutrition
Nutritional deficits (Mrs. Lily Lawson)		States she was eating poorly when living alone. Lost 5 lb	• Mrs. Lawson takes in a well-balanced diet of 2500 calories daily within 1 week
Excess nutrition (Mary and Joseph Boulder)			
Potential for disturbed nutritional patterns (Jackie Boulder)		Lily Lawson gets little or no exercise	

(continued)

Nutrition (continued)

Family nursing diagnosis	Due to or related to	As evidenced by	Goal/expected behaviors
	Diabetes inadequately controlled at present time	Has elevated blood sugar and 1+ ketones in urine	• Demonstrates a normal range of blood sugars throughout the day by end of 2 weeks
	Situational—Physiologic stresses of recent illness aggravated by diabetic state	Long-standing obesity of Mr. and Mrs. Boulder. Both get virtually no exercise	• Gains at least 3 lb in the next 3 weeks
	Personal/family—Possibly (due to) lack of family knowledge of changes needed in family nutritional patterns to accommodate Lily Lawson's caloric requirements and need for appropriate balance of carbohydrates, proteins, fats.	29-year-old daughter—obese—recent diagnosis of diabetes mellitus	• Mr. and Mrs. Boulder identify eating patterns that contribute to weight gain by follow-up visit in 3 days
		Jackie—15-year-old-girl, youngest of 5 children. Only child living at home on a permanent basis. Healthy child. Eats with family (usually). Family history of diabetes and obesity. Incomplete data base	• Describe the relationship between activity level and weight gain/loss at follow-up visit in 3 days
	Personal/family—Traditional family eating habits, consisting of intake greater than body requirements in relation to energy/activity expenditures for Mr. and Mrs. Boulder	Weight in normal range for height and age	• Experience a 2-pound weight loss per week through a combination of increased activity and decreased food intake beginning in 1 week
	Physiologic—The maintenance of nutritional patterns that meet the growth and developmental needs of an adolescent girl (Jackie)		• Jackie consumes a diet adequate to meet her individual growth and developmental needs, as determined, within 4 weeks

Nursing Strategies with Frequencies

1. **a.** Further nutritional assessment for Mrs. Lily Lawson (gather data from Mrs. Lily Lawson and M. and J. Boulder):

   • 24-hour dietary recall, include snacks.
   • Food preferences.

- Past eating habits, such as time of meals, where eaten, how food was prepared.
- Compare with present family eating patterns.

   b. Encourage Mrs. Lawson to keep a 24-hour log of food intake and activity. Mrs. Boulder will also keep 24-hour log of foods served at each meal.

   c. Evaluate logs with Mrs. Lawson and Mrs. and Mr. Boulder at next visit in 3 days. Discuss areas where modifications are needed.

   d. Teach family members to recognize the unique nutritional needs of Mrs. Lawson, i.e., the importance of regular well-balanced meals with appropriate snacks. Explain food exchanges and calorie requirements necessary for Mrs. Lawson's diet.

   e. Plan sample menus with Mrs. Boulder that will meet the nutritional requirements of Mrs. Lawson, incorporate food preferences of all family members as well as provide all family members with a nutritionally sound diet. Assist with ongoing meal planning as needed.

2. a. Perform a brief health assessment on Mrs. Lawson at each home visit to evaluate for subtle changes in overall health status.

   b. Within 3 days review with Mrs. Lawson and Mrs. Boulder technique being used for monitoring blood glucose. Observe technique. Reinforce where needed.

   c. Review technique for testing urinary ketones. Establish a pattern for daily testing of urinary ketones by 3 days.

   d. Review with Mrs. Lawson and Mrs. Boulder and observe: care of insulin, technique for drawing it up, injection technique, and site rotation.

   e. Assist Mrs. Lawson to record blood glucose values and ketone readings. Provide forms/booklets for recording purposes. Review recordings at each follow-up visit.
Stress importance of always bringing record to physician's office visits.

   f. Review technique of insulin injection with Mrs. Lawson. Plan with and instruct a family member how to give insulin injections in the event Mrs. Lawson becomes incapacitated and cannot give her own insulin.

   g. Encourage independence for Mrs. Lawson in the above areas.

   h. Within 1 week consult with Mrs. Lawson's physician about possible restrictions on physical activities. Based on this, devise a planned progressive program of exercise for Mrs. Lawson.

   i. Determine family informational needs concerning diabetes mellitus, insulin reactions (hypoglycemia), hyperglycemia.

   j. Plan with family how to handle an emergency associated with Mrs. Lawson's diabetes mellitus by 2 weeks.

   k. Instruct family when to call the physician about Mrs. Lawson, e.g., continued persistent elevation in blood glucose, persistence of ketones in urine, signs of infection, vomiting, diarrhea, change in mental status, loss of appetite.

   l. Explore feelings of family members regarding recent diagnosis of diabetes in oldest daughter by 1 week.

   m. Instruct family members in the above areas as requirement is determined. Supply printed materials about diabetes mellitus to promote understanding and reinforce teaching. Provide material about community resources within 2 weeks.

3. The strategies 1a through e and 2a through i promote a diet adequate for specified weight gain, that incorporates variety, food preferences, and established requirements as well as satisfactory control of diabetes mellitus for Mrs. Lawson.

4. a. Assess for factors that may contribute to overeating:

   - Stress response.
   - Lack of basic knowledge about nutrition.
   - Sedentary life-style.
   - Others.

   b. Request that Mr. and Mrs. Boulder each write down all food eaten for the past 24 hours.

   c. Instruct them to keep a diet diary for the next 3 days to include:

   - What was eaten, when, where and why.
   - Other activities at the time of eating.
   - How they felt just before eating.
   - Other persons present at mealtimes.

   d. At follow-up visit in 3 days, review diet diary with them to point out patterns of food intake.

5. a. At 3-day follow-up visit, explain simply the relationship between activity level and calories burned—weight loss or weight gain.

   b. Show clients sample table of common foods, listing caloric value and the amount/type of activity needed to burn that amount of calories. (Example: fried egg = 100 calories, requires approximately 30 minutes of moderately fast walking to burn.)

   c. Assist them to identify activities they could implement that would increase their energy expenditures.

   d. Explain benefits of exercise, not only consumes calories, but reduces stress, may increase self-esteem, feelings of control, etc.

6. a. Set realistic weight loss goals with Mr. and Mrs. Boulder, i.e., 2 pounds per week. This would require a decreased daily intake of 500 calories.

b. Assist them to plan balanced acceptable meals incorporating considerations for Lily Lawson, cultural/personal preferences, choices, etc.

c. Suggest community resources/support groups such as Weight Watchers and Overeaters Anonymous.

d. Combine above dietary changes with behavioral modification techniques that emphasize identification and elimination of inappropriate eating habits such as:

- Eat only at specified times.
- Eat only in a specified place.
- Do nothing else while eating, such as watching television, reading, talking on the phone.
- Prepare acceptable foods in an attractive manner.
- Avoid puchasing problem foods.
- Slow pace of eating.
- Use smaller plates to make amount of food seem larger.
- Leave a small amount of food on plate.

e. Suggest methods other than eating to be used to deal with emotional stress, boredom, fatigue. Substitute other activities for eating in response to these feelings to help divert attention from food: crocheting, working at hobby, taking a short walk.

f. Plan a structured, progressive exercise program for both Mr. and Mrs. Boulder. Advise them both to consult the family physician before increasing activity level.

g. Instruct to begin increasing activity level with a daily walking program and gradually increase rate and length of walk.

- Include Mrs. Lawson in walking program.
- Progress slowly.
- Avoid pushing too hard or becoming overly fatigued.
- Start out at 5 to 10 blocks (1/2 to 1 mile) per day, increase 1 block or 1/10 mile per week.

h. Instruct to stop activity immediately if any symptoms of lightheadedness; chest pain, severe; sudden breathlessness; dizziness, nausea, loss of muscle control.

i. Instruct each to weigh self weekly and keep a record.

j. Give each other positive reinforcement for accomplishments. Use tangible, nonfood rewards— an overnight trip, new clothes.

7. a. Meet with Jackie if possible within the next 2 weeks to review her dietary intake by a 24-hour recall, also using information

from Mr. and Mrs. Boulder about family nutrition patterns.
  b. Based on above assessment, evaluate adequacy of her diet for her height, weight, gender, and age.
  c. Recommend appropriate dietary alterations, if necessary.

Family Nursing Care Plan for Survival Human Need: *Elimination*

Family nursing diagnosis	Due to or related to	Evidenced by	Goal/expected behaviors
Disturbed family survival needs: elimination Disturbed patterns of urinary elimination (Mrs. Lily Lawson)	*Pathophysiologic—* Pathophysiologic state of diabetes mellitus Recent severe urinary tract infection Present inadequate control of diabetes mellitus	Recent hospitalization for severe urinary tract infection and accompanying mild ketoacidosis Occasional ketones in the urine Frequent elevated blood glucose levels by home blood glucose monitoring (increasing her susceptibility to recurrent infection)	Family members experience normal patterns of urinary elimination • Mrs. Lawson will have ketone-free urinary output by the end of 2 weeks • Mrs. Lawson will remain free of signs and symptoms of urinary tract infection at weekly visits
Potential for excess urinary elimination (Joseph Boulder)	*Pharmacologic—* Effect of diuretic therapy	Takes diuretic for heart condition Data base incomplete	• Mr. Boulder experiences excessive urinary output only during waking hours within 1 week

Nursing Strategies with Frequencies

1. a. See strategies under Nursing Diagnosis of Nutritional Deficits related to bringing Mrs. Lawson's diabetes mellitus under good control.
   b. Review chart of urinary ketone reading within 1 week. Based on recorded results, reinforce teaching as needed.
2. a. At weekly visits, elicit information about urinary output: quantity, color, cloudiness, frequency, symptoms urgency, burning on urination, or abdominal or back pain.
   b. At each visit, palpate abdomen for distended bladder, tenderness. Check for costovertebral angle tenderness.
   c. Obtain fresh urine specimen from Mrs. Lawson. Observe color and clarity. Measures specific gravity, glucose, ketones, blood, nitrates, and leukocytes weekly. If any abnormalities are detected, contact physician or consult protocol for urinary tract infection.
   d. Determine informational needs, e.g., urine surveillance.

   e. Determine location of bathroom and safety measures instituted to facilitate Mrs. Lawson's trips to the bathroom at night. Install night light in hallways and bathroom immediately.

   f. Review hygienic procedures regarding proper wiping, cleansing to prevent irritation and possible infection.

3. Ask Mr. Boulder to keep a record of urinary output, time of voiding day or night, quantity, for 1 week. Review urinary output record. Review Mr. Boulder's intake of diuretic therapy and relationship to urinary output. Refer to physician for diuretic adjustment if urinary output diminished, if swelling, congestion noted or if urinary output is highest at night disturbing Mr. Boulder's sleep despite his taking the diuretic early in the day.

Family Nursing Care Plan for Survival Human Need: *Sensory Integrity*

Family nursing diagnosis	Due to or related to	As evidenced by	Goal/expected behaviors
Disturbed family survival needs: Sensory integrity Partial sensory deprivation (Mrs. Lily Lawson)	*Pathophysiologic*— Visual changes and hearing impairment (of Mrs. Lily Lawson)— glaucoma (mild open angle) and cataracts	Decreased visual acuity, contributing to diminished enjoyment of activities. Previously enjoyed cooking, gardening, needle work, reading, watching television Not always hearing phone because of increasing hearing impairment. Requires increasing volume on television	All family members experience sufficient and meaningful sensory input • Mrs. Lawson experiences optimal visual acuity (within existing limitations) by 2 weeks • Verbalizes satisfactory adaptation to visual limitations within 4 weeks • Experiences optimal auditory acuity within 3 weeks • Mrs. Boulder verbalizes no indications of sensory overload within 3 weeks
Potential for sensory overload (Mary Boulder)	*Situational*—Recent changes in family living situation	Over the past 1 month, husband and mother are now around the house all day long, whereas before, Mrs. Boulder had the house to herself much of the day. Mrs. Lawson requires high volume on television	

Nursing Strategies with Frequencies

1. a. Test Mrs. Lawson's near and far vision for gross estimate of present visual acuity. Test with glasses on, each eye separately, by next visit.

    b. Review with Mrs. Lawson the proper use of her eye medications.

    c. Assist family to make appointment with Mrs. Lawson's ophthalmologist for a re-evaluation of her glasses, glaucoma, and cataracts. Suggest they discuss with him or her the feasibility, risks, benefits of surgery to remove cataracts.

2. a. Explore community resources available for the visually impaired. Suggest library books with large print and subscription to large-print Reader's Digest.

    b. Review with Mrs. Lawson the importance of proper lighting when reading or watching TV to avoid eye strain.

    c. Remind family members to be sensitive to Mrs. Lawson's visual limitations.

3. a. At next visit, examine ears using otoscope to determine presence of cerumen that may contribute to a conduction hearing loss. Observe tympanic membrane for intactness, presence of fluid, or inflammation.

    b. Suggest testing of Mrs. Lawson for improvement with a hearing aid. Explain to her and family that many people are resistant to using hearing aids because of matters of pride. Explore feelings about this. Provide reassurance. Explain that many famous people use hearing aids.

    c. Suggest contacting phone company for an attachment appliance for the hearing impaired.

    d. Demonstrate ways to facilitate communication with Mrs. Lawson, e.g., standing in front of her when speaking, enunciate with lip movement, eliminate extraneous sounds when conversing such as radios. Avoid calling her from another room.

4. a. Assess with Mrs. Boulder possible perceived sensory overload related to changed family situation by 1 week.

    b. Recommend to Mrs. Boulder some private time away from the increased and louder conversations and house noises that were not part of the household previously until she can adapt and problem solve some of the excess.

Family Nursing Care Plan for Survival Human Need: *Rest, Leisure*

Family nursing diagnosis	Due to or related to	As evidenced by	Goal/expected behaviors
Disturbed family survival needs: rest and leisure	*Pathologic*—Limitations of chronic illnesses of Lily Lawson and Joseph Boulder	*Mrs. Lawson*—Pathophysiologic changes associated with diabetes mellitus. Visual and hearing deficits, decreased participation in activities.	All family members participate in diversional/leisure activities on a regular basis.
Potential for loss of leisure time and activities for family members			

(continued)

Rest and Leisure (continued)

Family nursing diagnosis	Due to or related to	As evidenced by	Goal/expected behaviors
	Situational—Care demands of her mother and husband for Mrs. Boulder	Possible incomplete grief related to husband's sudden death	• Family members verbalize their recognition of the need for leisure/diversional activity by 1 week
	Enforced retirement of Joseph Boulder affecting all family members	Joseph Boulder—Physical limitations imposed by coronary artery disease. Physically unable to work. Decreased income related to retirement. Finds retirement "boring"	• Each family member engages in one preferred diversional activity (individually or together) by the end of 3 weeks
		Mrs. Boulder—Additional time and attention needed to supervise and assist in the care of Mrs. Lawson.	• Family engages in one family group activity by the end of 1 month
		May be unwilling to leave her mother	• Family begins long-range plans for summer vacation activities that include all members by end of 6 weeks
		Prior to recent retirement, Mary and Joseph Boulder made frequent weekend trips to the mountains or went cruising on their sailboat. Recently sold sailboat because of Joseph's illness and increasing maintenance costs	
		No data available on Jackie's leisure time/activities	

Nursing Strategies with Frequencies

1. a. Meet with family members to discuss feelings/attitudes about leisure/recreational activities by next visit.

   b. Explain principles related to the importance of rest/leisure/recreation as a human need.

      • In the adult, lack of stimulation can result in boredom and depression.

- Boredom paralyzes an individual's productivity, causes feelings of stagnation, introspective feelings of being oppressed and trapped, which can give rise to conscious or unconscious anger or hostility.
- Being aware that one is bored or feeling deprived of leisure time allows one to redirect activities to increase stimulation.
- Taking responsibility for doing something about a boring situation is a positive means of dispelling boredom.

   c. Explain the benefits that accrue for the person and the group from engagement in satisfying leisure activities.

2. a. Assist each family member to verbalize activities in which he or she would like to engage.

   b. Contract with each member individually that he or she will engage in one preferred activity by the end of 3 weeks.

   c. Encourage Mrs. Lawson to call each of her two close friends from her former neighborhood within the next 2 weeks.

   d. Refer her to the local senior citizen center. Suggest she plan spending a specified period of time weekly (for example one or two mornings) at the center to increase her social contacts and provide some diversional activity.

   e. Explore possible household projects that Joseph Boulder may enjoy.

   f. Encourage Mary and Joseph Boulder to periodically engage in sailing activities with friends.

   g. For Mary and Joseph Boulder, suggest weekday trips rather than weekend to take advantage of cheaper rates. Explore reduced rates for leisure activities for older citizens.

   h. Assist in the arrangement of care services for family members requiring care and supervision when family members are away.

   i. Explore with Jackie her leisure activities and assess their adequacy for meeting her needs for rest and leisure.

   j. Encourage individual family members to use strengths and energy to help self and others. Acknowledge efforts made. Encourage the person to challenge him or herself by learning a new skill or pursuing a new interest.

3. a. Encourage the family to plan specific times for leisure activities by 1 week.

   b. Explore affordable group activities. Make suggestions (light dinner and a movie, outing in a park, tour a museum, shop for a needed household item, visit a historic site, go to church together, etc.).

4. a. Encourage long-range planning. Suggest use of travel agency as appropriate, to facilitate planning.

   b. Emphasize importance of appropriate budgeting in advance.

   c. Follow up on these plans regularly and provide support as needed.

Family Nursing Care Plan for Survival Human Need: *Adaptation to Manage Stress*

Family nursing diagnosis	Due to or related to	As evidenced by	Goal/expected behaviors
Disturbed family survival needs: adaptation, to manage stress Ineffective family adaptation, to manage stress	*Situational*—Recent transitional/situational and developmental changes in the family unit and resulting stressors • Chronic illness of two members • Retirement • Territorial changes • Decreased income • Arrival of an additional family member who is aged • Three generations of family members	Mrs. Lawson's chronic illness and recent acute illness and hospitalization, incomplete recovery now requiring supervision for daily living, loss of independence, and new living environment. Poor control of diabetes mellitus Joseph Boulder's chronic illness and early forced retirement. His incapacitating heart condition, increased dependency, and changed responsibilities Mrs. Boulder's added responsibilities of care for her ailing mother and husband, loss of privacy, and personal space Jackie's reactive behavior, loss of privacy and control over specific territory	Family members establish a functional system of coping and mutual support to facilitate management of family stress, within 1 month Family members are able to: • Identify effective coping mechanisms that have been used in the past by 1 week • Identify factors present in the current family situations that may be causing and/or contributing to family stress by 1 week • Evaluate whether coping mechanisms used in the past are adaptable to present situations by 2 weeks • Devise five new strategies for reducing family stress by 3 weeks • Verbalize satisfaction with newly devised coping systems by 1 month

Nursing Strategies with Frequencies

1. a. Meet with all household members if possible. Assist them to identify one or two family problems that have occurred in the past and explain how they were solved. Point out what might have been dysfunctional responses to the problem (denial, threats, violence, neglect, scapegoating, authoritarianism—no negotiation).

    b. Focus on the functional/constructive coping strategies that were used. (For example: family group reliance, use of humor, increased sharing together of thoughts and feelings, increased communication, accurate appraisal of the problem, controlling the meaning of the problem, joint problem solving, role flexibility, seeking knowledge, using community resources, and other social and spiritual support systems.)

    c. Acknowledge these as strengths that the family has and has used effectively in the past. Praise these abilities/strengths.

2. a. Assist family members to identify factors in the present family situation that they feel are causing problems. See section As Evidenced By. Share own observations about the situation. Assist them to accurately appraise the problems and their meaning to the family.

    b. Explain effects of excessive stress on family members, particularly Mrs. Lawson and Joseph Boulder who have chronic illnesses. Reinforce on subsequent visits. Relate subjective and objective data, such as increased pulse and respiratory rates, hyperglycemia, frequent episodes of angina, fatigue, that can be attributed to increased stress.

3. a. Assist family members to adapt past constructive coping mechanisms to present situations. Specify the strategies that they might use.

4. a. Explore and explain additional effective family coping strategies (as listed under 1b) that are available to them. Describe them, explain what they mean, and how they might be implemented. Emphasize especially communication—sharing of feelings and thoughts, promotion of each member's individuality, use of support systems.

    b. Concerning ill family members, emphasize importance of all members fostering independence, accepting residual disability and making necessary accommodations, adapting to new living situation, and recognizing depression and anxiety in ill family members as wellness–illness patterns fluctuate.

    c. The family must return to normalcy by returning to previous activities as much as possible and incorporating ill members into the flow of family activities and responsibilities.

5. a. Provide ongoing support for progress made. Acknowledge success. Assist family to evaluate progress toward goal.

    b. Initiate teaching/counseling and referrals as necessary.

Family Nursing Care Plan for Closeness Human Needs: *Personal Recognition, Esteem, Respect*

Family nursing diagnosis	Due to or related to	As evidenced by	Goal/expected behaviors
Disturbed family closeness needs: personal recognition, esteem, respect Potential for disturbed self-esteem (Joseph Boulder and Lily Lawson)	*Situational*—Joseph Boulder: inability to work, early retirement, career prematurely terminated, decreased income	Job loss; forced retirement; possible perceived increase in dependency. Situational loss of "provider" status for family at a time when an additional family member is added. Possible fear of being unneeded. Describes retirement so far as "boring"	Joseph Boulder and Lily Lawson experience enhanced self-esteem • Joseph Boulder identifies strengths that he can use to contribute to his own personal development and others by 2 weeks • Participates in home and community activities that are personally fulfilling by 1 month • Relates feelings of improved self-esteem and productivity by 6 weeks
	Situational—Lily Lawson: increased dependency and other losses associated with chronic illness and advancing age	Possible unresolved grief. Decline in activities, loss of independence—loss of own home, moving in with daughter's family, physical limitations, fixed income, possible feelings of being rejected by Jackie and her friends	• Mrs. Lawson verbalizes feelings about husband's sudden death within 2 weeks • Actively assumes some household responsibilities as a participating family member within 2 weeks • Engages in one personally satisfying, productive activity within 2 weeks • Verbalizes confidence in her ability to accomplish the above and be a productive family member within 2 months

Nursing Strategies with Frequencies

1. **a.** Explore with Joseph Boulder the impact of his illness and early retirement on his self-esteem, role functions, and personal iden-

tity to assess presence or degree of disturbed self-esteem by 1 week.

b. Review his past job responsibilities, leadership, and organization abilities and how they could be applied to community agencies that require these skills.

c. Review technical skills and hobbies he developed over the years that could be used to increase his productivity at home and outside the home, now that he is retired.

2. a. Assist Mary and Joseph Boulder in their plans to review some long neglected household projects that Joseph can undertake on his own as well as those they can do together, appropriate to his capabilities by 2 weeks.

b. Suggest that Joseph Boulder explore community agencies or organizations that need member support.

c. Encourage the plan of the Boulders' to hold a garage sale for next weekend. This is to be a family project. Encourage Jackie and her grandmother to participate.

d. Encourage Mr. Boulder's interest and efforts to join the civic association and to accept the nomination of Chairman, Task Force on Community Security Improvement for the Civic Association.

3. Elicit feedback from Joseph Boulder about satisfaction with the above activities.

4. a. Explore with Mrs. Lawson her feelings about the sudden death of her husband 6 years ago within 1 week.

b. Assess contributing factors that might have delayed the resolution of her grief (denial, shock, anger, depression, guilt, fear, dependency, nature of the relationship) by 1 week.

c. Reduce contributing factors, if possible, by: promoting feelings of self-worth through productive activity (see below), consider referral for individual and/or group counseling to assist her through the grief process. Encourage family to offer support and reassurance.

Encourage family communication about the loss of Mr. Lawson, especially the feelings of other members about the loss.

Demonstrate respect/acceptance for Mrs. Lawson's feelings of loss, but at the same time emphasize the importance of her seeking assistance to work through it.

d. Provide ongoing support and referral as indicated.

5. a. Explore with Mrs. Lawson and Mary Boulder some household responsibilities that Mrs. Lawson could take on as a regular responsibility. Evaluate likes and dislikes regarding household tasks. Encourage choosing an activity that Mrs. Lawson is good at and enjoys, feels some expertise in, and is a significant contribution to the family (examples: seeing that family

clothing is washed, dried, folded, preparing salads or other specialty dishes, taking charge of the care of all household plants).

   b. Review activities that may not be safe for her (example: ironing, cleaning bathtubs, anything involving climbing, balance).

   c. Encourage family to offer ongoing support, appreciation, and praise.

6. a. Explore with Lily Lawson activities that she previously enjoyed. Suggest new ones, within her interests and capabilities.

   b. Contract with Mrs. Lawson that she will begin one productive, creative project within 2 weeks that she will complete within a specified period of time.

7. a. Regularly evaluate with Mrs. Lawson and family members progress in Mrs. Lawson's resolution of her grief.

   b. Review with Mrs. Lawson and family members activities in which Mrs. Lawson is involved, her feelings about her achievements and assumption of role related responsibilities.

   c. Provide encouragement.

Family Nursing Care Plan for Closeness Human Need: *Belonging*

Family nursing diagnosis	Due to or related to	As evidenced by	Goal/expected behaviors
Disturbed family closeness needs: belonging Potential for diminished belonging for family members	*Due to multiple causes*—Mrs. Lawson: relocation, loss of spouse, rejection by Jackie and her friends	Sudden death of husband 6 years ago, leaving a familiar neighborhood, household, friends, and neighbors. Moving to her daughter's home, a 20-minute drive from previous home	Family members foster relationships that maximize feelings of belonging • Mrs. Lawson verbalizes that she does not feel socially isolated, that she belongs, by 3 weeks
		Possible feeling of being "unwelcome" in the established household of her daughter and son-in-law initially	
		The abrupt leaving by one of Jackie's friends on first seeing Mrs. Lawson	
		The hasty departure of Jackie's other friends fol-	

(continued)

Belonging (continued)

Family nursing diagnosis	Due to or related to	As evidenced by	Goal/expected behaviors
		lowing Mrs. Lawson's turning up the television set and sitting close to watch them play	
		Jackie leaving to go to her room, slamming the door	
		Resultant potential for loneliness and withdrawal	
	Joseph Boulder—early forced retirement, chronic illness	Early retirement due to disabilities of coronary artery disease and angina	• Joseph Boulder verbalizes that he does not feel socially isolated, that he belongs, by 3 weeks
		Lack of contact with co-workers and colleagues at work	
		Feeling bored by retirement	
	Jackie—potential for deprivation of peer group support	Jackie's friends' apparent displeasure about constant presence of Jackie's grandmother. Hasty departure of Jackie's friends	• Jackie verbalizes satisfactory peer group contact by 3 weeks

Nursing Strategies with Frequencies

1. a. Evaluate Mrs. Lawson's grief process. Assist her to resolve her grief. See Nursing Diagnosis: Potential for Disturbed Self-esteem strategies 4a through d.

   b. Assist Mrs. Lawson to explore and identify possible perceptions of social isolation and lack of belonging.

   c. Encourage physical closeness (touch) within the family. See Human Need for Sexual Integrity.

   d. Encourage Mrs. Lawson to nurture relationships that increase her feelings of belonging. Assist family members to work out times and strategies to involve Mrs. Lawson with the family and friends and neighbors.

   e. Suggest Mrs. Lawson prepare a special breakfast for the family each Sunday morning and lunch twice a week for Mary, Joseph, and herself.

    f. Encourage Jackie and her friends to include Mrs. Lawson in their conversation for at least 5 minutes on the days they visit.

    g. Encourage Mrs. Lawson to make at least one telephone contact with a former neighbor or old friend each week. Help her to arrange a visit to an old friend at least once a month. Perhaps her daughter could drive her there and her friend or neighbor could drive her back.

2. **a.** Explore with Joseph Boulder possible feelings of social isolation or lack of belonging since his retirement.

    b. Suggest that he contact former co-workers and colleagues with whom he was friendly and arrange for lunch together.

    c. Encourage outside activities. See Nursing Diagnosis: Potential for Disturbed Self-esteem, nursing strategies 1a through c, 2a through d, and 3.

3. **a.** Explore with all family members options available to Jackie to maintain peer group contact. Suggest the exploration of community youth group activities.

    b. Also see Human Need for Territoriality—Nursing Diagnosis: Decrease in Personal Space, nursing strategies 3 and 4; and Human Need for Autonomy, Choice—Nursing Diagnosis: Potential for Excessive Independence for Jackie, nursing strategies 3a and b.

    c. Provide opportunity for Jackie and her friends to learn about Mrs. Lawson and her human needs as well as benefits that might accrue to them in learning and caring about an aged person.

    d. Explore with Jackie on an ongoing basis her satisfaction with her peer group relationships.

Family Nursing Care Plan for Closeness Human Need: *Sexual Integrity*

Family nursing diagnosis	Due to or related to	As evidenced by	Goal/expected behaviors
Disturbed family closeness needs: sexual integrity: intimacy Potential for decline in intimacy (Mary and Joseph Boulder)	*Pathologic*—chronic illness of Joseph Boulder *Situational*—Recent changes in family unit and family processes	Joseph Boulder's coronary artery disease—angina, limited physical capabilities. Possible fear of exerting self related to these Addition of a new family member (Lily Lawson). Added responsibility of caring for Mary Boulder's	Family members experience enhanced intimacy in 3 weeks • Mary and Joseph Boulder plan private time together on a daily basis by 2 weeks • Immediately plan a few days away together to be taken within the next 6 weeks

(continued)

Sexual Integrity (continued)

Family nursing diagnosis	Due to or related to	As evidenced by	Goal/expected behaviors
		chronically ill mother and need for ongoing surveillance	• Verbalize mutual satisfaction with their private times together by 3 weeks
		Probably less privacy. Recent forced retirement. Fewer opportunities to spend time away together	
Probable lack of intimacy for Lily Lawson	*Personal/situational*—Living situation and advancing age	Lived alone since the sudden death of her husband 6 years ago. Withdrawal from activities previously enjoyed. Now living with daughter's family	• Mrs. Lily Lawson experiences intimacy in daily living as a family member by 2 weeks • Family members participate in meeting the intimacy needs of Lily Lawson within 2 weeks
		Incomplete data base	

Nursing Strategies with Frequencies

1. **a.** Assist Mary and Joseph Boulder to plan private time together on a daily basis. Explore daily activities, schedules, and assist them to identify a suitable time and place that can be structured into their daily routine (examples: a daily walk alone together, coffee alone together in the morning, private uninterrupted time in their room daily).
   b. Encourage meaningful communication during these times.
2. **a.** See nursing strategies for Human Need for Rest and Leisure.
   b. Encourage the Boulders to arrange a caretaker for Mrs. Lawson and Jackie, such as the Boulder's older children for their occasional short trips.
3. Elicit feedback from Mary and Joseph Boulder concerning their satisfaction with their intimate times together.
4. **a.** Assist Mrs. Lawson to explore and verbalize her feelings regarding touch, hugging, and need for intimacy.
   b. Further assess sensory losses.
   c. Explain to family members that aging carries with it many losses, one of them being loss of physical contact. Further explain the human need for sexual integrity and intimacy.
   d. Encourage physical closeness (touch) toward Mrs. Lawson on a daily basis in the form of touch, hugging, and kissing.

e. Facilitate social contacts outside the family, as well, through senior center, contact with old friends, etc.

5. Reinforce all of the above with the family members. They may just have to be made aware of the need for physical closeness and will probably initiate it on their own.

Family Nursing Care Plan for Freedom Human Need: *Freedom from Pain*

Family nursing diagnosis	Due to or related to	As evidenced by	Goal/expected behaviors
Disturbed family freedom needs: freedom from pain Chest pain (Joseph Boulder)	*Pathophysiologic—*Coronary artery disease and intermittent episodes of angina	History of angina Past history of heart attack Takes nitroglycerine as needed Restricts his activity Incomplete data base	Client experiences freedom from episodes of angina-induced pain ▪ Identifies factors/activities that precipitate or aggravate pain by 1 week ▪ Identifies techniques that alleviate the pain experience by 1 week ▪ Utilizes effective methods for coping with the pain experience by 1 month

Nursing Strategies with Frequencies

1. a. Within 1 week, assess the angina further with Joseph Boulder.

- Review the history of his heart condition.
- Review medications taken.
- Elicit information about pain characteristics: frequency of episodes, duration of attack, effect of nitroglycerine, how long and how many tablets it takes to get relief, side effects of medication, radiation patterns of the pain.
- His own reaction to the pain and reaction of family members.

b. Assess Joseph and Mary Boulder's knowledge about coronary artery disease and angina. Determine knowledge deficits and initiate appropriate teaching.

c. Identify precipitating/aggravating factors such as exertion, overeating, stress, fatigue, other specific activities by careful history.

2. a. Review with client the proper use of nitroglycerine tablets.

    b. Check with cardiologist about possible use of the transdermal nitroglycerine patch for Joseph Boulder.

    c. Review other techniques of pain relief that he has used in the past and evaluate their effectiveness (examples: rest, preferred position for rest, pain medication).

3. a. At 2 weeks, begin to discuss methods of modifying client's lifestyle to control risk factors, aggravating factors. Include family members.

- Discuss possible benefits of weight loss.
- Institute a progressive exercise program with approval of cardiologist.
- Control stress, teach stress management techniques: progressive relaxation, guided imagery, behavior modification.

    b. Teach family members to identify the precipitating factors of angina, to understand medications that Joseph Boulder is taking. Teach Joseph and family members the signs and symptoms that indicate advancing disease.

    c. On an ongoing basis, review with client status of the angina and strategies he and family members use to alleviate/cope with the pain.

Family Nursing Care Plan for Freedom Human Need: *Territoriality*

Family nursing diagnosis	Due to or related to	As evidenced by	Goal/expected behaviors
Disturbed family freedom needs: territoriality Decrease in personal space for family members	*Multifactorial—* • Age • Chronic illness • Altered routines, activities, and general living patterns	Mrs. Lawson's inability to maintain own home; now required to live with daughter's family. As a result, she may be experiencing some loss of identity, may feel like "guest" living in the home of another after long years of maintaining own household Disapproval of the presence of Mrs. Lawson by Jackie and friends in space Jackie considered her "territory." Intrusion by Mrs. Lawson implied by the reaction of Jackie's friends: one abruptly leaving upon seeing Mrs. Lawson. The	Family members clarify, share, and restore territorial space and privacy for each other within 1 month • Family members establish a new home territoriality for Mrs. Lawson within the next 2 weeks • Mrs. Lawson refers to daughter's home as "her home" in 1 month • Jackie and her friends are able to use the den after school by themselves twice a week

(continued)

Territoriality (continued)

Family nursing diagnosis	Due to or related to	As evidenced by	Goal/expected behaviors
		others leaving when Mrs. Lawson turned up the volume on the television and sat close to watch their game Jackie's seemingly angry response, slamming den door as she went to her room The addition of Mrs. Lawson to the family and retirement of Joseph Boulder Mary Boulder had the entire home and most of the day to herself and her own interests and activities prior to Joseph's retirement and the move of her mother. Now she has little time for herself. Her territory is being shared at all times with her husband and mother. Curtailed her participation in out-of-home activities, Altar Society and Choir. Joseph Boulder, now home all the time, no current outside activities. Feeling "bored" with retirement. Data base incomplete	and her bedroom at least once a week starting next week • Jackie expresses satisfaction with new arrangements after 2 weeks • All family members establish a shared time and place for social exchange at least 4 times a week • Mary and Joseph Boulder individually arrange a daily time and place where each can be alone if desired, within 2 weeks • Family members demonstrate a spirit of cooperation and respect for space and privacy of other members in 2 weeks by specific actions such as: a. Mrs. Lawson cares for all household plants and propagates new ones, some to go in Jackie's room b. Mrs. Boulder is willing to share the kitchen as a social space with Mrs. Lawson and Joseph c. Mary and Joseph have the use of the den exclusively for themselves after 10 P.M. every evening. • Mary Boulder resumes at least one of her former activities outside the home, which involves participation at least twice a week, within 1 month

6. **a.** Encourage Mary and Joseph Boulder to look at a typical day and identify times and places where each of them can be alone to rest or engage in an enjoyed activity (examples: workshop in garage or basement for Joseph Boulder, own bedroom at specific times during day, kitchen, visit a friend or neighbor).
   b. Encourage them to specifically plan their private time and personal space needs.
   c. Encourage Mary Boulder to take advantage of all those times available through the day for herself. Suggest she consider planning a leisurely breakfast for herself at least once a week.

7. **a.** Assist family members to implement these specific actions and encourage them to suggest others.
   b. Provide positive reinforcement for all family members (praise, approval) as they demonstrate group cooperation and respect for space and privacy of others.

8. **a.** Explore with Mrs. Boulder her feelings/desires about resuming former outside activities (guilt, perceived obligation to husband and mother, etc.).
   b. Encourage her participation in church activities, which she has stated mean much to her—Ladies Altar Society and Choir.

Family Nursing Care Plan for Freedom Human Need: *Self-Control, Self-Determination, Responsibility*

Family nursing diagnosis	Due to or related to	As evidenced by	Goal/expected behaviors
Disturbed family freedom needs: self-control, self-determination, responsibility	*Developmental and situational factors*—Loss of independence for Lily Lawson and Joseph Boulder	Mrs. Lawson's age, pathologic and psychological constraints imposed by chronic illness—diabetes mellitus	Family members establish individually appropriate levels of personal control in 1 month
Diminished personal control for family members		Inability to maintain herself in her own home. Need to reside with daughter's family because she can no longer care for herself	• Lily Lawson reports performing all her own activities of daily living (ADL) and most health related tasks within 1 month • Is responsible for selected designat-

(continued)

Nursing Strategies with Frequencies

1. **a.** At next visit, discuss the change in territorial space brought by having a new family member, or the return of former mer bers during holidays and summers, including use of comm rooms, bath facilities, sleeping space.

   b. Assist all family members in clarifying, arranging, and assistin to meet territorial needs of Mrs. Lawson and the redistribution territorial space without depriving space needs of othe members.

   c. Suggest the use of Mrs. Lawson's own furnishings, wall cover ings, television for her bedroom.

2. **a.** Encourage other family members to help to make Mrs. Lawson feel at home. Refer to her bedroom as "her room" (not guest room or someone's "old" room), and the household as "her home."

   b. Encourage Mrs. Lawson to be responsible for caring for her own room and assist with other household activities as previously arranged.

   c. Encourage Mrs. Lawson to invite a friend or former neighbor to visit her in her new home within 3 weeks.

   d. Use all above strategies to meet this goal.

3. Assist family members to negotiate for Jackie to be able to use the den after school twice a week uninterrupted to socialize with her friends. Assist to arrange that Jackie can use her own room on at least one other day per week.

4. **a.** Involve Jackie maximally in the above arrangements. Emphasize importance of Jackie's input and feedback regarding the situation.

   b. Stress to parents that Jackie is at an age where her input must be seen as valuable and her involvement in some democratic family process is important.

5. **a.** Encourage Mrs. Lawson to assist with meal preparation in the kitchen. Recommend this as a private time for exchange between mother and daughter and a time to enhance their relationship as adults.

   b. Encourage family members to eat dinner together as a group at least four times a week and to spend several hours per week together in the den after dinner to foster family discussions and problem solving, to increase communication about territorial and privacy needs among members.

Self-Control, Self-Determination, Responsibility (continued)

Family nursing diagnosis	Due to or related to	As evidenced by	Goal/expected behaviors
		Financial constraints of a fixed income	ed household tasks within 1 month
		Potential for Mrs. Lawson to feel she is burdensome to daughter and son-in-law	• Engages in at least one activity that she formerly enjoyed within 3 weeks
		Diminished visual and auditory acuity	
	Pathologic and psychological affronts—coronary artery disease, chronic illness of Joseph Boulder	*Joseph Boulder*—Constraints imposed by chronic illness	• Joseph Boulder maintains and expands management of household maintenance, budget, and planned family activities within 1 month
	Social/economic affronts—early retirement (forced) of Joseph Boulder	Early retirement from job and related loss of control, determination, and responsibility. Loss of regular contact with colleagues at work	• Mary Boulder resumes at least one of her former activities outside the home within 1 month
	Possible excess responsibility for Mary Boulder	*Mary Boulder*—Increased responsibility associated with care of mother and husband's retirement and chronic illness	• Begins health maintenance activities by having a complete health evaluation by a qualified health care provider (nurse practitioner or physician) by 1 month
	Health maintenance deficit for Mrs. Boulder	Curtailment of out-of-home activities	
		Personal neglect of her own health care requirements for past 10 years	• Jackie demonstrates sensitivity to Mrs. Lawson's need to participate in family activities within 2 weeks
		Jackie—Possible perceived loss of some control within the family	
		Some demonstrated lack of personal control demonstrated by her behavior toward her grandmother	• All family members express satisfaction with individual levels of responsibility and personal control within 1 month
		Data base incomplete	

Nursing Strategies with Frequencies

1. a. Within 2 weeks, assess Mrs. Lawson's self-care abilities/deficits. With Mrs. Lawson and Mary Boulder, review Mrs. Lawson's abilities to perform activities of daily living (ADL). Assess how she managed prior to moving in with her daughter's family.

  b. Observe her performance of selected ADLs and health-related tasks (drawing up insulin, administering it, foot care, etc.).

  c. Assess Mrs. Lawson's health beliefs, especially regarding her diabetes mellitus. Briefly assess her locus of control (LOC) (internal versus external).

  Internal: Seeks to change own behaviors or environment to adjust to problems.

  External: Expects others or outside factors, such as fate, luck, to solve problems.

  Based on this determination, determine the impact of the loss of independence. (Those with internal LOC will experience more profound feelings of powerlessness in this kind of situation than persons with external LOC.)

  Gear strategies for increasing her participation in her care toward the determined locus of control.

  Encourage Mrs. Lawson to perform her activities of daily living and to perform her own health-related tasks as menu planning, insulin administration, and urine testing for ketone.

  d. Teach Mrs. Lawson how to monitor blood glucose levels and encourage her independence in this as much as is possible.

  e. Support family members effort to encourage Mrs. Lawson to assume more self-control and responsibility.

2. See Nursing Diagnosis: Potential for Disturbed Self-esteem, nursing strategies 5a through c, 6a and b, and 7a through c.

3. See item 2 above. Facilitate Mrs. Lawson's resumption of activities she formerly enjoyed.

4. a. Within 2 weeks, assess Joseph Boulder's feelings regarding loss of power, personal control within the family. Evaluate the impact this has had on him.

  b. Briefly assess his LOC to help evaluate the impact of loss of control; if severe, could lead to depression.

  c. Encourage Joseph Boulder to continue and expand his management of household maintenance, budgetary activities, spokesman for the family which he handled prior to his retirement. Also validate the importance of participating in activities outside the home.

5. a. Within 2 weeks, assess the impact of these recent family changes, increased responsibility and curtailment of outside activities on Mrs. Boulder. Help her to explore and express her feelings about them.

    b. Assist her to feel that she can "let-go" of some of these responsibilities, by delegating, asking for assistance from other family members and community resources.

    c. Encourage her to resume at least one of her former activities outside the home and begin making arrangements right away.

6. a. Assess Mary Boulder's health beliefs and LOC. Assist her to verbalize her reasons for lack of preventive care/health supervision for so long. Use nonjudgmental communication.

    b. Take a complete health history and perform a brief screening examination in the home, emphasizing vital signs, cardiac examination, breast examination, and refer for complete evaluation.

    c. By the above assessment and strategies implemented earlier, determine: knowledge of disease and preventive activities (cancer warning signs, arthritis warning signs, effects of obesity, dental care); appropriate screening procedures for age and gender; risk factors for selected illnesses; nutritional status (done earlier); exercise practices (done earlier); safety awareness and practices; stress management; and social support networks.

    d. Promote positive health behaviors by providing specific information about screening procedures for age-related risks and health alterations. Explain procedure, rationale, and recommended frequency.

Procedure	Frequency
Blood pressure check	Annually
Cancer checkup	Annually
Mammogram	Annually[a]
Stool guaiac	Annually
Self-breast examination	Monthly
Pap smear	Every 2–3 years[a]
Immunizations—especially pneumococcal and influenza	Annually[a]
Glaucoma check	Every 3–5 years
Sigmoidoscopy	Every 4 years if negative
Complete physical examination with laboratory evaluation	Every 3–5 years[a]

[a]Or as recommended.

    e. After referral, check with Mrs. Boulder at next visit as to when appointment is scheduled. Follow-up on this regularly.

   f. Reinforce health maintenance activities on a regular basis.
 7. a. Assist Jackie to understand and be sensitive to Mrs. Lawson's need to participate in family activities and to be able to exert some control for herself in the new household within 2 weeks.
   b. Assist Jackie to see the impact of her behavior on her grandmother and to assume responsibility for her actions. Support that she impose self-control related to those behaviors that might be interpreted by Mrs. Lawson as rejection.
 8. Meet with family members in 1 month to review above goal and strategies and evaluate whether they have been effective in decreasing perceived powerlessness.

Family Nursing Care Plan for Freedom Human Need: *Autonomy, Choice*

Family nursing diagnosis	Due to or related to	As evidenced by	Goal/expected behaviors
Disturbed family freedom needs: autonomy, choice Potential for excessive autonomy (independence) for Jackie	*Developmental and situational factors—* • Youngest child • Older parents • Adolescence • Changed family situation	Jackie is the youngest child and only one at home now, resulting in limited demands on her to share herself and her possessions. Limited competition for parents' attention Jackie is in her middle adolescence, a time when peer group contact and acceptance are extremely important, while the need and desire for parental limits and guidance also exist Jackie's friends exhibited apparent displeasure at Jackie's home situation after school and unwillingness to spend time there for lack of privacy and fear of intrusion	Jackie experiences an appropriate level of autonomy (independence) for a 15-year-old girl • Jackie effectively exercises autonomy and choice within the household as determined/negotiated by entire family group, within 1 month • Effectively exercises responsible autonomous choice with peers in selected school or social circumstances within 1 month • Verbalizes satisfaction with arrangement to spend time at home after school with friends or at the home of a friend in a "safe" environment by 1 month

(continued)

Autonomy, Choice (continued)

Family nursing diagnosis	Due to or related to	As evidenced by	Goal/expected behaviors
		Possibly, Jackie may make up lost time with her peer group outside the home, removed from the limits imposed within the home by her parents and the relatively safe environment of the home.	
		Nursing diagnoses related to lack of privacy, belonging, to love and be loved support the potential for excess autonomy	

Nursing Strategies with Frequencies

1. **a.** Within the next 2 weeks, discuss with family members Jackie's need for autonomy, choice, and the fulfillment of this need within the structure of the household and within the limits set based on her age and role within the family.

   b. Explore with Jackie's parents if this is a concern to them.

   c. Explain adolescent needs for autonomy, privacy, structure, law and limits, and the requisite of peer group identification. Emphasize the middle adolescent's needs and desires for caring, limit setting, and guidance.

   d. Also see Human Need for Territoriality— Nursing Diagnosis: Decrease in Personal Space, nursing strategies 3 and 4a and b.

2. Assist Jackie to outline all the areas with peers and in selected social and school settings where opportunity for autonomy and choice prevail. Explore with Jackie the impact on others when she exerts autonomy and the impact on her of other's implementation of autonomy, choice. Encourage open communication and discussion among family members.

3. **a.** Encourage Jackie to talk with her girl friends about the possibility of going to their homes on a rotating basis on the days that Jackie is not able to have them at her home.

   b. Between the arrangements made for Jackie at the Boulder home and the arrangements made with her girl friends, evaluate with Jackie her satisfaction with them.

NURSING CARE PLAN FOR THE COMMUNITY
Developed by Virginia Smith

Introduction: The Community of Milford, Clay County, as Client

The provision of health care in rural areas is both a national and an international problem. Even nations with national health insurance schemes have difficulty in providing adequate, acceptable, and accessible medical and health care services. With the advent of Medicare and Medicaid in the United States, it became apparent from studying the number of persons that sought care from nurses and physicians and the number of visits made that the rural poor have been subsidizing health and medical care of the urban poor.

Major problems for rural citizens include:

1. Accidents, especially from heavy farm equipment
2. Exposure to dust, pollen, and a variety of chemicals, e.g., insecticides, pesticides, rodenticides, fertilizers
3. Exposure to animal diseases that may be transmissible to humans, e.g., anthrax, rabies, and tularemia
4. Inaccessibility to health care
5. Physician/client ratio much less than in urban centers and physician's age usually higher
6. Influx of migrant workers during harvest season having multiple health problems emanating from poor nutrition, lack of sanitation, low immunization levels, history of no prior health care or lack of continuity of health care, which encompasses maternal and child care, diagnosis, and treatment of acute and chronic illnesses.

Client Situation:

Milford is a small, rural community in Clay County in a southeastern state of the United States, which had decreased in population from 1082 in 1970 to 840 by 1980. The outmigration was composed primarily of young male adults, which increased the mean age of the community from 28 to 35. Adults from 18 to 65 years of age had completed an average of 10 years of school in 1980, an increase from the average of 7 years in 1970. The birth rate has been gradually decreasing and is lower than the state rate. Major causes of death are comparable to those of the state but the order differs with the accident and infant death rate being higher than that of the state.

In addition, deaths were reported from measles and diphtheria in children from 2 to 12 years of age. The population over 65 years of age has increased from 15 to 22 percent.

Farming is the principal occupation; dairies and feed crops predominate. There are 72 farms; 64 of these are small: 35 to 100 acres and farmed by the owner. Eight farms consist of 100 to 300 acres but are owned by large corporations as tax write-offs, being farmed by tenant farmers. The land consists of low rolling hills and the Elk River forms the southern boundary.

Educational and health services, with the exception of a small elementary school, are located in Ruanna, the county seat of Clay County (population 3000, located 45 miles from Milford). There is a 60-bed community hospital, a private group practice of three family physicians and an adult nurse practitioner, one dentist, and the Clay County Health Department where one public health nurse provides community health nursing services to the residents of Milford 2 days per week. The nearest secondary hospital is 160 miles away; the nearest tertiary hospital is 415 miles distant.

Several weeks ago, city government officials from a summer resort city on the coast presented to the Clay County Board of Supervisors a proposal that the resort city finance the building of a large reservoir from which Milford could then purchase water from the county. This proposal, if accepted and approved, would have a direct effect on Milford as 20 of the small farms and 1 large farm (one-third of the land area) would be flooded and become part of the reservoir. The citizens of Milford are very upset about this proposal.

Milford has access to one public health nurse, Mary Arnold, employed by Clay County Health Department. She is married to one of the farmers in Milford and has lived in the community for 14 years. She is a baccalaureate nursing graduate from one of the state universities and, as part of her educational preparation, had prepared a written assignment based on the results of her investigation of a community health problem. Since she was employed by the health department she began collecting data on health indicators for the population of Milford, using the knowledge gained from her previous investigative community health assignment. She collected data from statistical sources, environmental sanitarians, social workers, the public health nursing supervisor and health director, family physicians, and used her own knowledge as a resident of Milford. For several years she had served as a volunteer to teach health subjects for the 4-H Club, had performed vision and hearing screening in the elementary school, and is now serving on an ad hoc committee of the county government to determine the need for a skilled nursing home in Clay County.

The community nursing care plan depicts the health needs of the community of Milford as identified by Mary Arnold based on data collected utilizing the nursing process and the human need theory framework.

Community Nursing Care Plan for Survival Human Need: *Air*

Community nursing diagnosis	Due to or related to	As evidenced by	Goal/expected behaviors
Altered pattern in survival need fulfillment: Disturbed pattern of aeration	Environmental affronts: pollutants, dust, pollens, chemicals	Increase in physical symptoms of allergic rhinitis, asthma, chronic obstructive pulmonary disease (COPD) and resultant increase in purchase of over-the-counter medications, use of home remedies, and visits to physicians Stated exposure to dust, pollens and chemicals by Milford citizens	Citizens report decreased exposure to air pollutants with subsequent decrease in symptoms and incidence of diseases of respiratory system within 1 year

Nursing Strategies with Frequencies

1. Share statistical data: allergic rhinitis, COPD, asthma, pneumonia with nursing supervisor. Seek assistance of nursing supervisor to arrange conference with public health director requesting that he contact family physicians, Occupational Safety and Health Administration (OSHA) for preventive measures, e.g., change to less toxic chemicals, improved method of handling and storage of farm chemicals, availability and use of protective clothing and face masks.
2. Establish a health education program to minimize danger to the respiratory system from exposure to pollutants, dust, pollens, and chemicals.

Community Nursing Care Plan for Survival Human Need: *Nutrition*

Community nursing diagnosis	Due to or related to	As provided by	Goal/expected behaviors
Altered survival need fulfillment: Disturbed intake of nutrients and calories, particularly fats and salt	Chronic functional farm role structure resulting in persistent hard labor, impact of weather Pathologic affronts of hypertension, congestive heart disease, stroke	Higher than expected mortality and morbidity from heart disease and vascular lesions of the central nervous system	Citizens experience improved eating patterns reflecting control of hypertension with its potential for heart disease and stroke within 2 years
			• Reduction in percentage of Milford citizens with hypertension within 2 years.
			• Reduction in morbidity and mortality from stroke, heart attack, and congestive heart disease in 2 years
			• Eighty percent of the population of Milford with blood pressure over 140/90 are rendered medical treatment for hypertension in 6 months.
			• Known hypertensive persons symptom-free with prescribed medication and dietary control

Nursing Strategies with Frequencies

1. Teach pro-heart nutrition at all age levels: at well-baby clinics, consumer education, at supermarkets; school lunch program, etc., focusing on lowering sodium and fat intake.
2. Distribute consumer nutrition aids obtained from farm extension office. Prepare supplementary nutritional information from data based on survey of nutritional practices in Milford.
3. Installation of electronic blood pressure monitoring device at the Milford Bank.
4. Conduct classes on weight control, relaxation, how to quit smoking, effective exercising for adolescents, young and older adults.

5. Establish a screening service for hypertension at minimal cost to test the total population of Milford with reliable interpretation, advice, and follow-up.
6. Seek volunteers from the farm families to learn how to take blood pressure and to participate in the screening process.
7. Continue monitoring of known hypertensive persons to ensure their continuance with adequate treatment for control.

Community Nursing Care Plan for Survival Human Need: *Safety*

Community nursing diagnosis	Due to or related to	As evidenced by	Goal/expected behaviors
Alteration in survival need fulfillment: Diminished safety	Intermittent situational occurrence of rural occupation and associated hazards Educational and informational deficits of Milford citizens	Higher than expected rate of accidents from heavy farm equipment	Citizens report increase safety within 6 months • Improve competency of equipment operators within 6 months • Statistical decrease in number of accidents from heavy farm equipment within 1 year

Nursing Strategies with Frequencies

1. Contact the farm extension agent and secure cooperation in joint planning for a farm safety program in which farm equipment manufacturers will provide demonstration and practice sessions for farmers, their wives and children using and servicing heavy farm equipment. Timing—selected winter weekends.
2. Conduct a survey of local farmers and their families for additional safety programs they deem necessary. Initiate plans with farm extension agent and farmer representatives.

Community Nursing Care Plan for Closeness Human Need: *Confidence*

Community nursing diagnosis	Due to or related to	As evidenced by	Goal/expected behaviors
Altered pattern in provision for closeness need fulfillment: Loss of confidence in health care system when pregnant	Inaccessibility of medical therapies Externally induced educational and informational deficits	Failure to seek prenatal care until late in second or early third trimester	Citizens report increase confidence in health and nursing care through early and continued use during pregnancy within 1 year

(continued)

Confidence (continued)

Community nursing diagnosis	Due to or related to	As evidenced by	Goal/expected behaviors
(particularly tenant farmers' wives)		Higher than expected (in comparison to state) risk of low birth weight infants in tenant farmer population	• Establish nursing clinic to provide maternity care and periodic medical care for tenant farm women and their families within 3 months • Identify and correct deficits in the quantity, quality, and availability of medical therapy within 1 year • Seventy-five percent of pregnant wives of tenant farmers will seek prenatal care in the first trimester within 1 year • Decline in rate of low birth weight infants in the tenant farm families within 2 years

Nursing Strategies with Frequencies

1. Determine interest and acceptance of nursing clinic by prospective clients. Arrange a meeting in one of the prospective clients' homes, showing a film on anatomy and physiology of pregnancy, describing services, and answering questions.
2. After obtaining positive results, secure final approval of nursing supervisor and public health director to establish a nursing clinic in Milford. Establish liaison with family physicians to provide periodic medical care for expectant clients.
3. Arrange with local church to provide space for the nursing clinic, and for volunteer baby sitting.
4. Using the American Public Health Association guide to maternity care, plan content of periodic examination and instruction by the nurse.
5. Arrange for referral of identified high-risk mothers for delivery in secondary or tertiary hospitals with costs paid by state funds.
6. Conduct the nursing clinic, meeting for 3 hours one afternoon per month. Provide home follow-up when indicated.

Community Nursing Care Plan for Closeness Human Needs: *To Love and Be Loved, Tenderness*

Community nursing diagnosis	Due to or related to	As evidenced by	Goal/expected behaviors
Alteration of closeness need fulfillment: Lack of love and tenderness for infants and toddlers demonstrated by tenant farm parents	Chronic social and economic affronts inherent in tenant farming Educational and informational deficits regarding child rearing	Growth and development delays in language, motor, and personal–social skills	Citizens show increased external demonstration of love and tenderness to infants and toddlers by parents and significant others. • Evidence of improvement in growth and development delays in 80 percent of infants and toddlers within 6 months. • Eliminate growth and development delays in 50 to 60 percent of infants and toddlers in 1 year

Nursing Strategies with Frequencies

1. Plan for nursing clinic to provide monthly well-child clinic supplemented by home visits.
2. Establish baseline measurement data of growth and development delays using the Denver Developmental Test, lack of environmental stimulation in the home using Caldwell inventory, and nutritional deficits by checking diet history and hematocrit.
3. Provide classes and individual counseling on child's need for love, tenderness, communication, stimulation, and proper nutrition so that normal growth and development can occur. Provide individual counseling about each deficit making recommendations about correction using Washington Guide suggestions.
4. Avoid inflicting guilt or blame on parents, thus decreasing their ability to demonstrate love and tenderness.

Community Nursing Care Plan for Closeness Human Need: *Sexual Integrity*

Community nursing diagnosis	Due to or related to	As evidenced by	Goal/expected behaviors
Alteraton of closeness need fulfill-	Externally induced, cultural	Lack of sex education in schools and	Citizens show decreased preoccu-

(continued)

Sexual Integrity (continued)

Community nursing diagnosis	Due to or related to	As evidenced by	Goal/expected behaviors
ment: Preoccupation with sexual dimension	imposition regarding sexual practice, religious impacts, and educational and informational deficits inherent in the belief that sex education is immoral and, if offered in the school, will result in promiscuity	many homes Increase in illegitimate births, teenage pregnancies, genital herpes, and abortions	pation with sexual dimension within 2 years • Decrease in rate of illegitimate births, teenage pregnancy, genital herpes, and abortions in 1 to 2 years • Demonstrate 50 percent of the families that provide sex education for their children in the home in 1 to 2 years

Nursing Strategies with Frequencies

1. Work with mothers, including fathers whenever and as often as possible, instructing them about sexuality and sex education so that they can instruct children in the home.
2. The above instruction should allay their fears about the immorality of this instruction taught in schools, and prepare them to fulfill their stated belief that sex instruction should be taught in the home. Providing parents, and subsequently their children, with information on human sexuality, may lessen excessive preoccupation with sex and immorality.
3. Provide informational resource materials, pamphlets, etc., as needed and requested.

Community Nursing Care Plan for Freedom Human Need: *Territoriality*

Community nursing diagnosis	Due to or related to	As evidenced by	Goal/expected behaviors
Alteration in freedom need fulfillment: Threatened invasion of territory	Potential political impact and imposition if Clay County officials accept the reservoir proposal from the coastal resort city	One-third of Milford land or 20 small farms and one large farm would be flooded by water if proposed reservoir is approved and built	Citizens experience removal of threat to fulfillment of Milford's territoriality in 6 months

(continued)

Territoriality (continued)

Community nursing diagnosis	Due to or related to	As evidenced by	Goal/expected behaviors
			• Clay County officials will reject proposal within 6 months or revise it to either use less land area or select an alternative unpopulated site within 1 year

Nursing Strategies with Frequencies

1. Participate in and encourage recruitment of all Milford citizens to attend citizens' protest meetings.

2. Communicate concern to County Board of Supervisors, state and local congressmen, and to the Farm Bureau regarding loss of Milford farm territory. Share names, addresses, and phone numbers of legislators and Farm Bureau personnel with Milford citizens.

3. Ask corporation owning large farm to exert influence.

4. Encourage use of alternative unpopulated site for reservoir. Identify and plot selected sites on map and distribute widely.

Community Nursing Care Plan for Freedom Human Needs: *Self-Control, Self-Determination, Responsibility*

Community nursing diagnosis	Due to or related to	As evidenced by	Goal/expected behaviors
Alteration in freedom need fulfillment: Diminished responsibility, self-determination, self-control	Chronic physiologic miscalculation and/or nonacceptance regarding immunizations, particularly measles, DPT, tetanus	Recent deaths from measles and diphtheria in the Milford community High rate of absenteeism from elementary school in spring due to measles Frequent farm injuries necessitate administration of tetanus toxoid and keeping immunizations up-to-date	Assume responsibility by parents for having infants immunized at recommended times within 1 year • No deaths from preventable communicable diseases in 1 year

(continued)

Self-Control, Self-Determination, Responsibility (continued)

Community nursing diagnosis	Due to or related to	As evidenced by	Goal/expected behaviors
			• Eighty percent fewer cases of measles within 1 year • Seventy-five percent of farmers who need a tetanus booster will have complied in 1 year • Elementary school enforce state regulation requiring evidence of immunization prior to attending school

Nursing Strategies with Frequencies

1. Publicize the need for immunization of infants emphasizing complications of each communicable disease. Arrange talks on radio, health column in local paper, distribute pamphlets in local and county grocery stores.

2. Administer immunizations in new well-child clinic.

3. Make communicable disease prevention part of every home visit.

4. Ask public health director's cooperation in enforcing state regulation as regards immunization in school.

NURSING CARE PLAN FOR WOMAN WITH ALZHEIMER'S DISEASE
Developed by Margaret Miller and Jeannette Theriauet

Client Data

The client is a 52-year-old, married woman. Her medical diagnosis is middle stage Alzheimer's disease. Her spouse (husband) is the responsible caregiver in the home setting. There are no children.

Nursing Care Plan for Human Need: *Acceptance of Self and Others*

Nursing diagnosis	Due to or related to	As evidenced by	Goal/expected behaviors
Disturbed patterns of expression and fulfillment of need for acceptance Potential lack of acceptance by family members	Progressive degenerative process of Alzheimer's disease and resultant memory loss, confusion, inappropriate behavior Personality changes that may be misunderstood by family members	Personality changes Emotional liability Irritability with one's own forgetfulness Defensiveness or embarrassment Excuses made for forgetfulness or inappropriate behavior Sadness Depression Family denial Frustration Anger Bewilderment Guilt	Family and client demonstrate increased acceptance during scheduled sessions • A specific professional health provider is available to family and client • Client is less defensive and experiences acceptance by self and family as expressed by client and family member within 2 weeks • Family members are more accepting of the client's behavior; changes are attributed to the disorder; effective ways of interpreting the meaning of the behavior are established as identified by family • Family members make use of social support groups provided by health care professionals • Evidence of reaching out to relatives and neighbors by family members and by client through telephone calls, letters, visits, and verbal expressions

(continued)

Acceptance of Self and Others (continued)

Nursing diagnosis	Due to or related to	As evidenced by	Goal/expected behaviors
			• A measure of control is evident by client in activities of daily living (ADL), decision-making. Spouse verbalizes positive comments about self and spouse within 2 weeks

Nursing Strategies with Frequencies

1. Provide the client and family members with specific information about the nature and course of Alzheimer's disease.

2. Assess the client's perception of self prior to onset of disorder; explore client's feelings and attitudes about present condition, the meanings attached to an irreversible dementia, decreased independence.

3. Explore the attitudes of family members.

4. Explore and evaluate coping mechanisms of client and family members.

5. Clarify misconceptions concerning Alzheimer's disease. Review the possible changes that might occur, such as angry outbursts, foul language, inappropriate behavior, and family is able to identify meaning of behavior within 2 weeks.

6. Allow the family to verbalize feelings including guilt, depression, and bitterness. Assist family to work through feelings of hurt, embarrassment, or bewilderment. Assist family in seeing beyond the client's behavior, to understand its significance, to be able to confront the client within 1 month.

7. Provide the family with specific information on available services within the community and initiate some reaching out within 2 weeks.

8. Assure the family and the client of continued assistance to help them deal with problems as much as possible.

9. Stress the importance of providing help to the client as needed while allowing as much autonomy as possible.

10. Explore appropriate approaches in care of the client, stressing patience and gentleness. Discuss the importance of nonverbal communication as the client may be more sensitive to the manner expressed than to the meaning of words.
11. Emphasize by word and action with the client and the family the fact that the disorder does not diminish the client's worth as a human being and family member.
12. Provide family with lists of resources available (day care, respite care, support groups, legal and financial assistance).
13. Recognize with sensitivity the potential role reversal and responsibilities for the spouse in the future.
14. Provide the following readings for the family:

   - Cohen, D., & Eisendorfer, C. *Loss of self: A family resource for the care of Alzheimer's disease and related disorders.* New York: Norton Press, 1986.
   - Horne, J. *Caregiving: Helping an aging loved one.* Washington, D.C.: AARP Books (1909 K Street, Washington D.C. 20049), 1986.
   - Leroux, C. *Coping and caring: Living with Alzheimer's disease.* Washington, D.C., AARP Books, 1986.
   - Mace, N. & Robins, P. *The 36-hour day: A family guide to caring for persons with Alzheimer's disease, related dementing illnesses and memory loss in later life.* Baltimore: Johns Hopkins University Press, 1981.

Nursing Care Plan for Human Need: *Activity*

Nursing diagnosis	Due to or related to	As evidenced by	Goal/expected behaviors
Disturbed patterns of activity Potential hyperactivity Insufficient activity	Progressive degenerative process of Alzheimer's disease Destruction of neurons in the cerebral cortex particularly the frontal, parietal, and temporal lobes	Repetitive motion Twitching Excessive fidgeting Restlessness Apraxia Constant agitated pacing Gait imbalance Wandering behavior Lack of coordination and/or disequilibrium interfere with self-care	Client will maintain useful mobililty, exercise as much as possible, appropriate to the client's level of fitness • Family develops an activity schedule • Revisions made according to client's status

(continued)

Activity (continued)

Nursing diagnosis	Due to or related to	As evidenced by	Goal/expected behaviors
		Later stages: tremors, jerks, flexion of lower extremities	• Client exhibits less restlessness and fidgeting • Client shows no evidence of physical injury • Client displays reduced pacing and increased calmness within 2 weeks

Nursing Strategies with Frequencies

1. Assess activity pattern of the family and the client, and assist in developing a specific 24-hour pattern of activities, planning one specific activity at a time.
2. Establish a regular, predictable, and simple routine for meals, exercise, bedtime, and other activities within 1 week.
3. Accompany on walks as often as possible and at least BID (twice a day). Avoid client isolation.
4. Provide noncomplex activities—vacuuming or raking leaves, bouncing a ball outside. Provide repetitive and purposeful motion that can help reduce the incessant restlessness within 2 weeks.
5. Encourage activity in sports, shopping, and helping around the home.
6. Direct the client's attention and keep occupied at a task.
7. Provide television viewing of shows with uncomplicated plots.
8. Schedule outings with neighbors or relatives on a regular basis.
9. As physical mobility becomes increasingly impaired, assist family in providing passive and active range of motion exercises.
10. Assist family to manage a wheelchair if and when necessary.
11. Demonstrate physical care to family caregivers as the client needs increase.
12. In later stages, as the client's condition deteriorates and physical mobility becomes markedly impaired, encourage use of alternating pressure mattress or flotation mattress.
13. Turn the client from side to side every 2 hours.
14. Demonstrate to family how to assist the client out of bed at least three times a day. Sit with the client and maintain feet elevation.
15. Provide periodic playing of soft, soothing music.

Nursing Care Plan for Human Need: *Adaptation to Manage Stress*

Nursing diagnosis	Due to or related to	As evidenced by	Goal/expected behaviors
Diminished ability of the client to manage stress	Inability to interpret complex stimuli and impaired adaptive ability resulting from the pathologic changes throughout the cerebral cortex and in the hippocampus	Overreacting or catastrophic reactions Previous simple tasks become too difficult Sensory overload Withdrawal in social contact	Family manages stress and client exhibits fewer episodes of agitation, anger, and stubborness within 1 month, as client feels less threatened by environment and decreasing cognitive abilities
Diminished ability of the family to manage stress	Increased family responsibilities, such as financial and household, and the time consuming care of the client	Episodes of anger, frustration, expressions of grief	• Reduce incidence of situational crises for client and spouse within 2 weeks • Determine time period that client can remain unattended before exhibiting anxiety • Family members able to arrange time for themselves, for church activities, and for maintaining interpersonal relationship with other people, within 2 months

Nursing Strategies with Frequencies

Client

1. Make home visit to understand the client's home environment and assist the family in eliminating physical barriers and maximizing independence of the client.
2. Provide a quiet soothing environment—uncomplicated wallpaper in bedroom, quiet background music.
3. Use a gentle, kind, patient approach in interaction with the client. Respond in a calm, quiet, unhurried manner.
4. If the client resists activities, wait awhile then come back in a few minutes; the client may forget her objection.
5. Emphasize the importance of routine to counteract the sense of chaos. Establish a daily routine pattern of activities.
6. Present the client with simple alternatives to ease decision-making; "yes" or "no" questions are easier than open-ended ones. Speak slowly and distinctly.

7. Identify the client's particular abilities and impairments with family members; gain insight into the impact of Alzheimer's disease on the client's functioning; this may help the family deal more effectively with problems as they arise.
8. Avoid new or strange situations.
9. Avoid large groups; encourage participation in small group activities with the family.
10. Assist with clothing choices and/or dressing. Use clothes that can be put on and taken off easily.
11. Orient the client to person, place, time. Have clocks and calendars in view.
12. Keep familiar objects in same places.
13. Write down names and often used telephone numbers.
14. Discuss the client's withdrawal from demanding tasks.

Family

1. Provide family members with telephone numbers and referrals to community support groups, to help them work through grief, to learn, and to search for new coping skills.
2. Provide assurance of support for the family throughout the client's illness.
3. Refer the family to the appropriate services for legal and financial matters.
4. Assist the family members in a planned schedule that will allow caregivers opportunities for a quiet time each day.
5. Encourage involvement in other interests.
6. Emphasize the need for family members to be patient with themselves.
7. If appropriate, involve the support of church group members.
8. Obtain booklet: "Managing the Person with Intellectual Loss at Home," 785 Mamaroneck Avenue, White Plains, New York 10165.
9. Obtain telephone answering machine to eliminate stress of answering the telephone experienced by client.
10. Promote client relaxation.

Nursing Care Plan for Human Need: *Air*

Nursing diagnosis	Due to or related to	As evidenced by	Goal/expected behaviors
Potential disturbance in aeration pattern	Inattention when eating or drinking that may lead to aspiration	Choking Wheezing Gasping for breath	Client will be protected from obstructive or impaired aeration as evidenced by clear airway within 12 hours

(continued)

Air (continued)

Nursing diagnosis	Due to or related to	As evidenced by	Goal/expected behaviors
	Limited movement of the muscles of the tongue and pharynx Dysphagia Hyperorality Explore objects compulsively with mouth	Disinterest in use of facial, tongue, and pharyngeal muscles for mastication Apparent discomfort on swallowing Inappropriate use of oral muscles Apparent discomfort on breathing (dyspnea)	• Family knows the importance of air for the client and what hazards can interfere with provision of air • Family can identify specific actions to take in event of interference with air for client, by the end of 1 week

Nursing Strategies with Frequencies

1. Assist the family in accommodating the home routine to the client's need for air.
2. Teach the family basic first aid in the event of choking (Heimlich's maneuver).
3. Cut food into bite-size pieces to avoid choking.
4. Provide a safe environment. Keep objects, such as silverware, matches, small objects, medicines, out of reach of the client.
5. Check the client frequently each night. Provide a room that allows for careful observation.
6. Ensure someone in attendance throughout each meal to assist the client in eating/drinking.
7. Remind the client to chew and swallow when she forgets to do that; repeat this as many times as necessary at each meal.
8. Minimize offensive odors in environment.
9. Maintain healthy temperature and humidity in home.
10. Reduce dust, aerosol sprays.
11. Maintain quiet, calm environment to avoid agitation; avoid feeding/eating if overstimulated.

Nursing Care Plan for Human Need: *Appreciation, Attention*

Nursing diagnosis	Due to or related to	As evidenced by	Goal/expected behaviors
Potential for lack of or diminished appreciation and attention	Increased demands on others placed by the client as the disease progresses	Client's seeming lack of awareness of surroundings and family Indifference Apathy	Client experiences feeling of increased attention and appreciation

(continued)

Appreciation, Attention *(continued)*

Nursing diagnosis	Due to or related to	As evidenced by	Goal/expected behaviors
Disturbed pattern of expressing fulfillment of appreciation and attention	Inability of client to show appreciation for caregivers' effort Diminished cerebral functioning of the sensory association areas of the brain responsible for interpreting visual, auditory, and somatic stimuli	Family frustration when they do not know if care-giving efforts are being perceived. Anger, guilt, depression Progressive memory loss, aphasia, agraphia, "mirror sign" Inability to show appreciation for caregivers' efforts	Family members will have outside support groups to assist in meeting appreciation and attention needs. This requires continual reevaluation

Nursing Strategies with Frequencies

1. Encourage the client's statements about positive, caring traits of family/spouse.
2. Assess the type, amount, and quality of attention client receives from family and friends.
3. Encourage family members to express appreciation for the client's efforts to care for self.
4. Assist in the communication process between the spouse and the client by encouraging attention to nonverbal messages. Use smiles, touch, body language to suggest affection/support.
5. Provide referral to social workers and community support groups. Assure family of continued support.
6. Encourage families to build and maintain their social support system. Emphasize the value of shared responsibility, visitors, and respites; these correlate with successful care-giving outcomes.
7. Actively listen to the client's viewpoints and perceptions of the past.
8. Provide the family a contact with the Alzheimer's disease and related disorders association (ADRDA), as a support group.
9. Explore with the family their feelings of frustration and anger; help them to understand the causes and encourage removal of guilt; encourage the acquisition of rewards and recognition outside the immediate relationship with the client.

Nursing Care Plan for Human Need: *Autonomy, Choice*

Nursing diagnosis	Due to or related to	As evidenced by	Goal/expected behaviors
Diminished autonomy, choice:	Progressive degenerative process of	Inability to perform activities of	Client assumes responsibility for

(continued)

Autonomy, Choice (continued)

Nursing diagnosis	Due to or related to	As evidenced by	Goal/expected behaviors
• For client • For family	Alzheimer's disease	daily living, bathing, dressing	own care as much as physically possible. Abilities vary as disease progresses
	Resultant impaired cognitive abilities	Impaired decision making ability	
	Demands on emotion, time, and finances in caring for client	Constant demands being made on the family by the client's behavioral changes	• Family members seek fulfillment for their need for autonomy and choice as evidenced by involvement in outside interests, by questioning and evaluating advice provided for them
	Cerebral deterioration caused by neurofibrillary tangles affecting dorsalis medialis of the brain	Aphasia	
		Agnosia	
		Apraxia	
		Agraphia	
		Impaired ability to express needs	• Client responds to instructions • Client understands spoken words and repeats instructions

Nursing Strategies with Frequencies

1. Allow the client to do as much as she can for herself but provide assistance when needed.
2. Provide simple, one-sentence instructions when assisting the client in her endeavors.
3. Explore with the family ways that the client's autonomy can be maximized; support family members' efforts to allow autonomy of the client.
4. Plan daily activity schedule incorporating the client's (present or previous) preferences. Plan will be developed within 2 weeks.
5. Provide emotional support to family members including decisions concerning nursing home placement when home care becomes too burdensome. Encourage the family to seek professional caregiver as soon as concerns arise.
6. Refer the family to professional and social community services and family support groups.
7. Promote ongoing support of the client in effort to achieve authentic expression of thoughts, needs.
8. Offer the client simple choices (no more than two options) in ADL activites, once each day, e.g., choice of food at meals, television show selection and music selection.

9. Repeat same phrase as often as necessary if the client does not understand it initially.

Nursing Care Plan for Human Need: *Beauty, Aesthetic Experiences*

Nursing diagnosis	Due to or related to	As evidenced by	Goal/expected behaviors
Disturbance in pattern of expression and fulfillment of beauty and aesthetic experiences	Progressive degenerative process of Alzheimer's disease	Impaired ability to understand or express language Decreased cognitive abilities	Client enjoys aesthetic experiences as evidenced by facial expression • Is interested in looking at photographs or pictures, and in taking long walks • Enjoys listening to music as evidenced by increased duration of time client is able to listen; pleasant facial responses, and when possible, verbal confirmation of pleasure
	Neuronal reduction and damage to posterior portion of temporal lobe	Withdrawal Aphasia Agnosia Mirror sign Poor personal hygiene	• Recognizes a favorite dress that has a brightly colored pattern • Schedules weekly hair styling

Nursing Strategies with Frequencies

1. Encourage the family to take the client for frequent walks, preferably to a park, three times each week.
2. Review with the family the activities, hobbies, and aesthetic interests of the client; incorporate these activities into daily schedule with the family and the client when feasible.
3. Share enjoyment of daily experiences by commenting about such things as a beautiful sunset, a piece of classical music, a poem the client may have enjoyed in the past.
4. Assist the client in caring for a flower garden; encourage her and the family to keep fresh flowers in the house daily.
5. Share photographs or colored illustrated books with client; discuss the illustrations with her.

6. Make favorite articles of clothing available to the client each morning; while dressing, encourage selection of appropriate and matched items.
7. Compliment the client on appearance when hair is styled.

Nursing Care Plan for Human Need: *Belonging*

Nursing diagnosis	Due to or related to	As evidenced by	Goal/expected behaviors
Disturbed patterns nonverbal expressions of belonging	Cerebral deterioration of Wernicke's area, posttemporal lobe and Broca's speech area	Unusual/inappropriate behavior; aphasia; lip smacking; hypermetamorphosis; hoarding food and belongings; tapping of fingers, feet Physical clinging to caregivers	Client and spouse verbalize feelings of increased belonging within 2 weeks • Has reduced hyperactivity (unsual/inappropriate) at the rate of one activity per week
Disturbed patterns of verbal expressions of belonging		Inability to verbalize belongingness	• Family members (spouse) say there is some feeling of belonging while giving care to client • Responds to caregiver with smiles and pleasant facial expressions

Nursing Strategies with Frequencies

1. Show the client mementos of the past that represent belonging, such as old letters or photo albums; plan this as a weekly activity.
2. Explore with the spouse any past events that might be recalled by the client; discuss these in conversation while caring for the client.
3. Include children in activities with the client for limited times.
4. Observe the client's reaction.
5. Contract with friends, family acquaintances, neighbors to volunteer with visiting the client/spouse for regular sessions on a weekly basis.
6. Discuss feelings of isolation commonly experienced by the spouse.
7. Encourage family involvement with diverse persons and activities when away from the client.
8. Verbalize sensitivity to spouse's role and situation.
9. Assist the client to perform simple tasks, such as winding a ball of yarn, dusting, or stacking books, to make her feel useful.

10. Obtain head phones for the spouse and the client to encourage relaxation, distraction, and relief from incessant verbalization by the client.

11. Direct the client to a specific new task when behaviors become repetitive.

12. Encourage the client's involvement with family activities using format for activity care plan that has been jointly developed and revised biweekly.

13. Maintain contact with relatives and neighbors by visiting, telephoning on a weekly basis.

14. Have client assist with any household activities she is capable of performing—assist with daily cleaning, vacuuming, dusting.

15. Express appreciation for all positive efforts the client makes and all goals accomplished.

16. Be gentle, supportive, and patient in interactions with the client; express affection through caring words, touch, concerned expressions, and warm conversations.

17. Provide professional and emotional support of family members. Encourage their participation in support groups within the community and with church groups as appropriate.

18. Schedule community contacts at least every other week.

Nursing Care Plan for Human Need: *Challenge*

Nursing diagnosis	Due to or related to	As evidenced by	Goal/expected behaviors
Potential for experiencing excessive challenge	Impact on the client of debilitating aspects of the disease	The constant demands both physically and financially of caring for client with Alzheimer's disease	Family successfully employs coping strategies to meet challenges as evidenced by:
	Impact on the family of debilitating aspects of the disease	Role changes among family members	• Verbalizations • Continued involvement in social activities
	Reduction in cognition resulting from the disease process	Social isolation of client and caregiver	• Sufficient rest, as they perceive it, within 2 weeks
		Hesitancy to perform the ordinary activities of daily living	• Client shows increased confidence in performing ADL activity; a change toward the positive within 6 weeks
		Frustration, anger, agitation when a challenge is perceived as excessive	• Identify activities consistent with the tolerance and ability of the client

(continued)

Challenge (continued)

Nursing diagnosis	Due to or related to	As evidenced by	Goal/expected behaviors
			• Communication becomes effective for the client; understands at least one message a day • Frustration, agitation reduced to no more than three incidents per week

Nursing Strategies with Frequencies

1. Encourage family members to build and fortify their social support systems; request them to specify each week the systems that will be tapped.
2. Advise the family to share their responsibilities with other willing persons; encourage them to ask for help from relatives, friends, neighbors, church associates. Assist in setting up weekly schedule.
3. Refer to appropriate services for legal and financial planning considerations.
4. Keep the family informed of the appropriate help available when support or resources are needed.
5. Encourage the family to schedule regular and emergency respite from the 24-hour care demands. Provide information about home-helpers, day care, or institutional respite care. Discuss with the spouse the result of his exploration of resources and the arrangements made for assistance. Review the plan weekly.
6. Provide structure and regularity in activities to reduce complexity of physical activity.
7. Provide on-going assessment to determine the client's level of tolerance; adjust/terminate activity when cues from the client suggest fatigue or frustration.
8. Use simple phrases and uncomplicated sentences when communicating.
9. Increase the use of touch, body language, and facial expressions for improved communication.
10. Minimize environmental stimulation that increases the client's anxiety.
11. Assist the client with ADL activities; give step by step instructions; maintain an uncluttered home environment to limit the number of options from which the client must choose.
12. Label objects that are used regularly by the client.

13. Encourage simple tasks/distractions for the client that are easily accomplished.

14. Provide names and addresses of resources for spouse:

- Alzheimer's Disease and Related Disorders Association (ADRDA)
  70 East Lake Street
  Chicago, Illinois 60601
- National Institute on Aging
  Information Center/ALZ
  2209 Distribution Circle
  Silver Spring, Maryland 20910

Nursing Care Plan for Human Need: *Conceptualization, Rationality, Problem Solving*

Nursing diagnosis	Due to or related to	As evidenced by	Goal/expected behaviors
Impaired ability to conceptualize, rationalize, and/or problem solve	Progressive degenerative process of Alzheimer's disease Degeneration of cerebral function	Inability to make decisions Short-term memory loss Inability to recall home address, telephone number Cannot identify season of the year Decreased verbalization Increased use of facial grimaces	Client is able to participate in simple decision making • Knows time to eat each day • Responds appropriately to messages and directions within 1 week • Increases ability to conceptualize, rationalize, and problem solve as identified in regular weekly assessments • Increases attempts to identify environmental factors (e.g., time of day, season of year, etc.) and achievement of correct identification within 2 months • Reduces facial grimacing to no more than 3 to 4 episodes a day by the end of 1 month

Nursing Strategies with Frequencies

1. Assist the family in their care strategies to adjust to changes in the client's cognitive capabilities.
2. Use short words and sentences; use slow distinct speech and wait for the client's response.
3. Ask short, simple questions; if necessary to repeat, ask exactly in the same way.
4. Minimize choices offered to the client such as in choice of meals, activities, choice of wardrobe. Involve the client in as much decision making as possible (without causing confusion) especially in ADL.
5. Provide reminders by verbal descriptions, use of posters, calendars, clocks.
6. Encourage the client's response to pointed questions, allowing adequate time for response.
7. Eliminate distractors (television, radio) while talking with the client.
8. Place yourself in face-to-face position so the client can see your lips and facial expression when talking with her.
9. Speak with the client in clear, well-modulated tone of voice.
10. Schedule at least one session each day when the client is given a simple problem to solve (e.g., Where are your shoes?).
11. Assist the client to conceptualize by explaining sounds and sights (e.g., that is the breeze blowing the curtains; that sound is the wind blowing through the trees). Seek opportunities to clarify these environmental factors with the client at least daily.
12. Provide topics of conversation and recreational activities for the client to occupy time hence reduce the tendency to indulge in grimacing.

Nursing Care Plan for Human Need: *Confidence*

Nursing diagnosis	Due to or related to	As evidenced by	Goal/expected behaviors
Diminished confidence	Change in roles for the client	Family expresses concern and guilt when providing care for the client	Family experiences confidence within 2 weeks, in their ability to care for the client at home. Requires ongoing evaluation and frequent adjustments as condition changes
Disturbed pattern of fulfillment of confidence	The demanding care that is necessary for the client	Withdrawal from usual tasks, such as cooking, driving, managing finances	
	Neurofibrillary tangles in the limbic system or "seat of emotions"		

(continued)

Confidence (continued)

Nursing diagnosis	Due to or related to	As evidenced by	Goal/expected behaviors
			• Helps client to realize satisfaction when unable to be involved in tasks she usually completed

Nursing Strategies with Frequencies

1. Assure the family of continuing professional support during the course of the client's illness.
2. Demonstrate to the family the necessary assistance for the client when performing activities of daily living, on a daily basis early in the care-giving period.
3. Allow the family to discuss care problems, review strategies used, and offer the family suggestions if adjustments or encouragment are needed.
4. Provide the family with information and/or referrals to appropriate community help services.
5. Support the family in their decisions for institutional placement if and when necessary, advising on appropriate facilities, and emphasizing the importance of continual family involvement.
6. Provide the client with alternative activities that she can complete confidently (e.g., dust furniture, dry dishes). Do these three to four times per week.
7. Encourage the client to purchase small toilet items from gift shop, under supervision. Have the client transact such a purchase three times a week.

Nursing Care Plan for Human Need: *Elimination*

Nursing diagnosis	Due to or related to	As evidenced by	Goal/expected behaviors
Disturbed patterns of fecal elimination	Sensory motor impairment	Decreased ability to retain large amounts of urine	Client maintains normal patterns of bowel and bladder elimination within 3 weeks
Disturbed patterns of urinary elimination	Neuronal damage effecting the prefrontal and posterior portions of temporal lobes	Urinary incontinence especially at night	• Client's dignity is maintained by accomplishing urination and defecation in a timely manner and at appropriate
	Decreased mobility associated with Alzheimer's disease	Defecation in inappropriate places (closets, dresser drawers)	

(continued)

Elimination (continued)

Nursing diagnosis	Due to or related to	As evidenced by	Goal/expected behaviors
		Inability to locate bathroom and walk to facility	sites within 3 months • Client adjusts to a routine elimination schedule within 6 weeks

Nursing Strategies with Frequencies

1. Provide and encourage a high fiber diet to help maintain bowel regularity.
2. Observe daily for signs of constipation such as reduced appetite, abdominal distention, and lethargy.
3. Monitor frequency of bowel movements to establish pattern of regularity and deviations from routine and record daily.
4. Identify daily patterns of elimination. Develop a toileting schedule for client with family.
5. Establish a regular toilet routine; take to the bathroom every 2 to 4 hours as determined by assessed need. Adjust to less frequent toileting at night (every 3 to 5 hours).
6. Limit fluid intake to one to two glasses of liquids after evening meal and one to two glasses during the night.
7. Use adult incontinence pads, Depend, or Chux as needed.
8. Provide or assist with perineal care after each toileting.
9. Provide for privacy when voiding and defecating.
10. Facilitate handwashing; have all toilet articles within easy reach and in appropriate, standard place.
11. Place a commode at the client's bedside. Offer a bedpan every 2 hours or assist to commode every 2 hours.
12. Provide an easy access to the bathroom that is marked and lighted clearly.
13. Install holding bars near the toilet to support the client when sitting and/or rising for toileting.
14. Adjust dietary intake to provide vegetables, fruits, other high fiber foods for meals and snacks.

Nursing Care Plan for Human Need: *Fluid and Electrolyte*

Nursing diagnosis	Due to or related to	As evidenced by	Goal/expected behaviors
Potential disturbance in fluid intake patterns	Progressive degenerative process of Alzheimer's disease	Thirst Dehydration Low urine output	Client establishes adequate hydration within 2 days

(continued)

Fluid and Electrolyte (continued)

Nursing diagnosis	Due to or related to	As evidenced by	Goal/expected behaviors
	Neurofibrillary tangles affecting the supraoptic nuclei in the preoptic area of the hypothalamus (thirst center).	Concentrated urine Poor skin turgor Inability to judge temperature of food/fluids Forgetfulness Does not remember to drink fluids	as evidenced by moist, intact tongue, oral mucosa • Adequate hydration maintained every day as evidenced by patterns of normal thirst, improved skin turgor • Offering fluids (at least 8 ounces) to client regularly—hourly during the day; when awake during the night (at least 2 to 3 times each night)

Nursing Strategies with Frequencies

1. Record intake and output for the client every 24-hour period: quantity and type of fluid. Encourage the client to drink citrus juices, milk, cranberry juice, if permitted.
2. Check daily status of skin turgor, oral mucosa, and tongue for dryness, integrity of tissue. Note degree of thirst experienced by the client.
3. Note concentration of urine and identify changes from greater to lesser concentration.
4. Check weight daily at same time each day.
5. Observe temperature of fluids to prevent the client from burning self by drinking fluids when they are too warm.

Nursing Care Plan for Human Need: *Freedom from Pain*

Nursing diagnosis	Due to or related to	As evidenced by	Goal/expected behaviors
Diminished pain sensation Potential inability to express pain or describe its presence Inability to express relief of pain	Decreased pain sensation that occurs with aging Deterioration of cortical areas involved in memory, language, and motor functions that	Decreased sensitivity to hot and cold food and fluids Decreased sensitivity to temperature of bath water Facial grimaces	Client is free from pain and injury. • Measures to promote safe environment have been identified and measures implemented within 24 hours

(continued)

Freedom from Pain (continued)

Nursing diagnosis	Due to or related to	As evidenced by	Goal/expected behaviors
	control coordination of speech patterns Aphasia	Guarding the area of discomfort Inability to speak	• Client effectively communicates discomfort, pain. • Family is interpreting meaning of client's communication within one week; is an ongoing process. • Signals, cues, sign language messages are understood by caregivers and by family. • Family promotes comfort; freedom from pain.

Nursing Strategies with Frequencies

1. Discuss the care of the client with family members. Include the client in care planning as much as possible.
2. Identify behaviors of the client and the care measures and responses family members take. Assist in identifying meaning of the client's behavior and nonverbal cues.
3. Instruct the family to be alert for physical signs of illness, facial grimaces, physical guarding of areas that may be painful, peripheral edema, skin breakdown, or abrasions.
4. Identify increased restlessness, deterioration in behavior, moaning or shouting as evidences of discomfort.
5. Maintain mobility by regular activity, at least every 2 hours, according to physical ability of the client.
6. Assess the client daily, at least, to determine potential sources of discomfort such as tight shoes, ill-fitting clothing, vital signs outside normal range, etc.

Nursing Care Plan for Human Need: *Humor*

Nursing diagnosis	Due to or related to	As evidenced by	Goal/expected behaviors
Disturbed patterns in expression of humor Inability to appreciate humor	Progressive degenerative process of Alzheimer's disease	Sadness; absence of laughter Appearance of depression	Client responds to activities with young children with happy facial expression and laughter

(continued)

Humor (continued)

Nursing diagnosis	Due to or related to	As evidenced by	Goal/expected behaviors
	Cerebral dysfunction as a result of increased aluminum deposits	Seldom seen smiling Lack of pleasant response to efforts of others to elicit smile or chuckle	• Attention is focused and held by enjoyable activities and conversation • Family becomes involved in support group to assist them in using cognitive restructuring as a coping mechanism. They teach one another how to use humor and practical tips; family verbalizes the help of the support groups to maintain a sense of humor

Nursing Strategies with Frequencies

1. Encourage the family to bring children to visit the client; urge activities with the children.
2. Encourage visits to parks, zoos. Encourage participation in happy group activity where laughter occurs.
3. Have the client partake in simple dancing activities.
4. Provide television programs with humor for the client to view.
5. Continue to encourage family participation in support groups.
6. Support and interpret reaction of the family when the client responds with inappropriate laughter, or no response.
7. Encourage laughter to be experienced by the client, the family, and caregivers. Laughter is contagious whether or not stimulated by a humorous incident.

Nursing Care Plan for Human Need: *Interchange of Gases*

Nursing diagnosis	Due to or related to	As evidenced by	Goal/expected behaviors
Potential disturbance in alveolar gas exchange	Progressive degenerative process of Alzheimer's disease Decreased mobility Potential infection Potential aspiration pneumonia	Rapid deterioration in respiratory health Frequent or persistent chest colds Limited stamina in walking any distance	Client maintains adequate alveolar gas exchange • Deep breathing can be accomplished with ease • Fewer chest colds are experienced

(continued)

Interchange of Gases (continued)

Nursing diagnosis	Due to or related to	As evidenced by	Goal/expected behaviors
	Decreased respiratory excursion Shallow respirations	Rapid respirations on limited exertion	• Longer distances can be covered with no pulmonary distress. Distances increased at least the length of the corridor each day • Physical activities, within client's ability, carried out on a daily basis, with activities increased as respiratory health permits

Nursing Strategies with Frequencies

1. Emphasize the importance of follow-up physical, neurologic, psychiatric, and psychological assessment to monitor changes in the client's status.
2. Enforce the safety measures identified in the Nursing Strategies with Frequencies for Human Need for Air.
3. Encourage activity prescribed in the plan to meet activity and exercise needs.
4. Teach the family to identify the symptoms that warn of impending pulmonary problems, e.g. cough, fever, delerium, cyanotic nails/lips, fatigue.
5. Provide list of resource persons (name, telephone number) the family can call upon for help when respiratory problems are suspected.
6. Direct the family to maintain regular log of daily parameters to be reviewed by professional: pulse and respiration rates, energy level, facial color.

Nursing Care Plan for Human Need: *Nutrition*

Nursing diagnosis	Due to or related to	As evidenced by	Goal/expected behaviors
Disturbed nutritional patterns Potential/actual increased nutritional intake or decreased nutritional intake	Progressive degenerative nature of Alzheimer's disease Deterioration of the lateral hypothalamus	Forgets to eat meals Inattention at meals Refusal to eat Loss of table manners	Client maintains optimal nutritional status as evidenced by weight stability (weigh every other day) • Client eats well-balanced meal

(continued)

Nutrition (continued)

Nursing diagnosis	Due to or related to	As evidenced by	Goal/expected behaviors
	Neuronal damage to motor skill transmission	Inability to use knife and fork Eats an excessive amount of food periodically Plays with food; eats with fingers	with calorie specification for patient's age, weight, and body build • Energy level remains normal; requires continued evaluation • Initial expectation for balanced meals and calorie provision is achieved within 1 week

Nursing Strategies with Frequencies

1. Provide well-balanced meals appropriate to the client's eating abilities. If the client is unable to manage fork or knife, prepare finger foods.
2. If the client is hyperactive, plan a high calorie diet with enough fluids during the day to prevent dehydration. Offer fluids between meals and at night.
3. Limit the amount of food choices placed in front of the client at one time; too many options may confuse the client.
4. Prepare foods that are easy for the client to handle and deliver to mouth, and foods the client is able to swallow.
5. Eat at the same time and same place for each meal.
6. Use plastic dishes and utensils. Remove unnecessary cutlery and condiments. Utensils with large handles are helpful.
7. Control temperature of foods to prevent burning mouth; keep foods warm enough to be palatable.
8. Cut food into bite-size pieces; avoid foods that may cause choking (e.g., fish with bones).
9. Assist the family with meal planning and provision of daily caloric intake.
10. Make the client and the family aware of the availability of meals on wheels.
11. Teach the family basic first aid in the event of choking (Heimlich maneuver).
12. Observe for dysphagia.
13. Assist the client to sit upright for meals to avoid aspiration or regurgitation.
14. Avoid routine use of TV dinners or other prepared foods that are high in salt and low in vitamins and roughage.

15. Provide a smock for the client to wear (instead of a bib) to collect food bits that are dropped.
16. Fill glass/cup about 1/2 or 3/4 full to avoid spilling; a feeding cup may facilitate drinking.
17. Encourage the client to chew food and to swallow when the client forgets to do so.
18. Assess dental health and status of dentures when mastication becomes a problem.
19. Eliminate distractions at mealtime to ensure full attention to eating.

Nursing Care Plan for Human Need: *Effective Perception of Reality*

Nursing diagnosis	Due to or related to	As evidenced by	Goal/expected behaviors
Disturbed patterns of the perception of reality	Pathologic changes throughout the cerebral cortex	Inability to recognize and interpret complex sensory stimuli	Client recognizes daily orientation to time, place, persons, and events
Inappropriate perceptions of reality	Progressive cerebral degeneration associated with Alzheimer's disease	Inability to recall addresses, names of family members	• False accusations and statements by the client discontinue within 6 weeks.
Distorted perceptions of reality		Confusion	• Client's perceptions more accurately reflect reality within 2 months
		Disorientation	
		Accusations that are false	
		Factual data statements that are incorrect	

Nursing Strategies with Frequencies

1. Plan for the client a structured environment with regular routines.
2. Maintain pleasant, orderly surroundings.
3. Approach the client in an open, friendly, and relaxed manner.
4. Look directly at the client when addressing her.
5. Use short simple word sentences: (e.g., are you cold? are you hungry? here are your slippers).
6. Ask one question at a time.
7. Accompany verbal communications with facial expressions, gestures, body language.
8. Physical expressions of care are encouraged (gentle touch, supporting the client's arm).
9. Keep personal items in the same and easily accessible places; provide clocks, calendars, pictures of family/client environment.
10. Support the spouse in his efforts to understand and tolerate the client's emotional outbursts and false accusations.

11. Rearrange the client's care schedule if agitation occurs at the time care activities are planned.
12. Encourage the spouse not to support fabricated stories of the client; stress the need to state factual truths of reality.
13. Help the spouse to differentiate the evident behaviors of Alzheimer's disease from those of mental illness.

Nursing Care Plan for Human Need: *Personal Recognition, Esteem, Respect*

Nursing diagnosis	Due to or related to	As evidenced by	Goal/expected behaviors
Disturbed patterns of experiencing personal recognition, respect Potential for experiencing diminished esteem	Inability to realize personal recognition Perceived obstacles to daily problem solving Memory impairment Devalued perception of self-esteem and self-respect Deterioration of the sensory centers in the brain	Verbal expressions that reflect poor self-esteem: "I'm no good any more," "Nobody likes me" Irritability Sadness Depression Agitation Withdrawal Listlessness Paranoia and false ideas	Client verbalizes a positive view of self at least once each week • Less irritability evidenced in group encounters with client in the first month • Presents a cheerful attitude, is less sad, within 2 weeks • Client willingly participates in social encounters at least once within the first month

Nursing Strategies with Frequencies

1. Identify the kind and frequency of interactions the client has maintained with family and friends to establish a baseline.
2. Assess the client's perception of self.
3. Specify the views about the client's perceptions that are held by the spouse.
4. Create a photo album of the client's past life and review it with the client twice a week.
5. Show tenderness, concern, and affection in all interactions with the client; encourage positive, warm approaches among all family and caregivers.
6. Maintain social contacts of the client and the spouse; continue to attend religious services together at least weekly. Limit number of persons in any one conversation with the client.
7. Guide the client into avenues of activity where she can succeed at least daily.
8. Give compliments, words of praise, for each success.

9. Schedule elimination schedule to avoid incontinence.
10. Support the client in carrying out as many self-care activities as possible. Limit to three to four activities per day to avoid fatigue, frustration.

Nursing Care Plan for Human Need: *Protection from Excessive Fear, Anxiety, Chaos*

Nursing diagnosis	Due to or related to	As evidenced by	Goal/expected behaviors
Potential for increased fear Evidence of anxiety Diminished protection from chaos	Impaired cognition and intellectual abilities Altered chemical balance in the brain Neuronal damage due to Alzheimer's disease	Agitation Outbursts of rage Withdrawal Paranoia Anxiety over simple task performance Distorted perception of environmental reality Emotional outbursts when confronted with multiple stimuli	Client is free from fear; anxiety is reduced within 4 weeks as evidenced by calmer attitude, cheerfulness, decreased agitation • Client responds to deliberate, kind approach by a more receptive manner within 2 weeks

Nursing Strategies with Frequencies

1. Assess with the family the potential strategies for providing a non-threatening, quiet, safe environment. Implement these within 1 week.
2. Approach the client in a gentle, unhurried manner; reassure verbally and by touch.
3. Assist the client in doing simple tasks and activities to prevent overwhelming the client.
4. Provide the family with education and counseling regarding Alzheimer's disease; provide the appropriate community resources.
5. Reassure the client about provision of safety by showing her the safe, familiar environment.
6. Encourage the client's protection by recognizing the family and familiar caregivers.
7. Remove stimuli that agitate the client; assess and evaluate effect of calm environment so this can be reinforced.
8. React to the client's outbursts with gentleness and calmness.
9. Demonstrate reality for the client through use of touch, sight, and detailed explanations, repeated several times a day.

Nursing Care Plan for Human Need: *Rest and Leisure*

Nursing diagnosis	Due to or related to	As evidenced by	Goal/expected behaviors
Disturbance in patterns of expressing fulfillment of rest/leisure	Chronic illness of client with Alzheimer's disease	Loss of ability to concentrate attention for a reasonable period of time	Family members specify leisure activities for the client within 1 month
Potential loss of leisure time for family members	Reduced cognitive and sensory abilities	Loss of ability to remember sequences in activities	• A list of four to six leisure activities are scheduled within 1 month.
		Loss of ability to see multifacets of any one situation; unable to see humor in everyday life	• Leisure activities include the family and the client • Family members verbalize the recognition of the need for leisure for the client and for themselves • The client's attention span increases to a 5-minute interval within 1 month • At least one response to a situation of humor is elicited from the client in 6 weeks • Client relaxes and apparently enjoys one short (15 minutes) musical program in 3 weeks

Nursing Strategies with Frequencies

1. Explore the client's preferred leisure activities with family members.
2. Encourage the family to plan specific times for the client's leisure activities; schedule at least one activity daily (e.g., reading).
3. Assess daily the client's ability to participate in rest/leisure activities to which she was accustomed. Adapt activities to present level of functioning (e.g., piano playing).
4. Support the spouse caregiver in scheduling leisure activities for himself; encourage some event at least once each week (e.g., dancing).
5. Assist the spouse to contact respite care agency for assistance with client when the spouse is away, whether for a short or prolonged period of time.

6. Discourage a period of inactivity to force rest.
7. Provide visual, sensory, auditory sources of beauty and aesthetics (flowers, incense, music).

Nursing Care Plan for Human Need: *Safety*

Nursing diagnosis	Due to or related to	As evidenced by	Goal/expected behaviors
Potential physical injury	Progressive degenerative process of Alzheimer's disease Destruction of neurons in the cerebral cortex particularly in frontal, parietal, and temporal lobes	Lack of muscle co-ordination Frequent falls Wandering behaviors Becoming lost Restless, especially at night Time and place disorientation Inappropriate use of eating utensils	Client is protected from physical harm; measures initiated within 2 days ▪ All hazards to safety in client's environment are removed immediately (scissors; metal/silver eating utensils, glass dishes; throw rugs, loose telephone wires, etc.) ▪ Night wandering is reduced

Nursing Strategies with Frequencies

1. Assess the client daily to identify bruises, cuts, abrasions.
2. Assess the client's environment and eliminate physical hazards; maximize independence of the client in her environment.
3. Reduce unnecessary stimuli (i.e., noise, sudden or excessive movements, light).
4. Reduce confused night wandering by having lights (appropriate) at night.
5. Provide for careful observation of the client over 24-hour period.
6. Remove clutter.
7. Make an ID bracelet for the client; include client name, address, nature of the disease, and telephone number.
8. Remove scatter rugs.
9. Install handrails and grab bars in bathroom.
10. Use shades or drapes to diminish shadows on windows.
11. Secure windows, doors; use dead bolt locks that require a key to open.
12. Close off the kitchen, stairways, or any other potentially dangerous site.

13. Remove from the client's environment such hazards as scissors, matches, knives, sharp tools, and electrical appliances.
14. Lock medications in a medicine cabinet.
15. Secure edges of all carpets with double-edged adhesive.
16. Assist with walking if gait is too unsteady for independent ambulation.
17. Provide shoes or slippers with rubber backing to prevent slipping.
18. Reduce water temperature in hot water heater.
19. Maintain calm, quiet atmosphere to discourage restlessness.
20. Monitor walking indoors and outdoors to prevent falls; explain time and place repeatedly to the client to provide orientation.

Nursing Care Plan for Human Need: *Self-Control, Self-Determination, Responsibility*

Nursing diagnosis	Due to or related to	As evidenced by	Goal/expected behaviors
Disturbed patterns of self-control Diminished opportunities for self-determination Irresponsibility for self and others	Progressive pathologic changes of Alzheimer's disease Reduced cognitive capability as a result of the pathologic process	Increased dependency on family members for decision-making, meeting needs for survival Wandering behaviors Inability to perform ADLs (cooking, eating, dressing) Disinterest in finances Inability to complete simple tasks	Client makes decisions about clothing to wear each day, when to obtain fluids • Client obtains fluids to drink three times a day • Wandering is reduced to those hours when client is fatigued (late P.M.) • Client is selecting her own clothing at least twice a week

Nursing Strategies with Frequencies

1. Recognize the spouse's responsibility in decision-making; support his role in this, four to six times per week in initial stages of client illness.
2. Provide opportunity for the client to choose clothing and food daily.
3. Communicate (by the spouse) to the client the financial matters they usually shared; spouse assumes initiative on a monthly schedule.
4. Discourage activities that induce fatigue, hence encourage wandering and agitation.
5. Assess the client's performance levels daily.

Nursing Care Plan for Human Need: *Sensory Integrity*

Nursing diagnosis	Due to or related to	As evidenced by	Goal/expected behaviors
Sensory overload	Pathologic changes throughout the cerebral cortex and the hypocampus Cerebral pathology limits the ability to filter out excessive stimuli	Increased anxiety Irritability Confusion Withdrawal Agitation Stubbornness Aggression	Client experiences reduced sensory overload, evidenced by less irritability, cheerfulness within 3 weeks • Client accepts caregiver's ministrations daily with reduced combativeness within 2 weeks • Client becomes more compliant with response to care in 1 to 2 weeks • Client evidences reduced anxiety in 2 weeks

Nursing Strategies with Frequencies

1. Maintain a quiet, safe environment for the client emphasizing calm, consistency; for example, plain wallpaper, no clutter, soft music.
2. Assess with the family the client's personality, particular abilities and impairments.
3. Establish a specific daily routine for ADL for the client and administer care at a regular time daily.
4. When talking to the client keep sentences simple, give instructions or ask questions one at a time. Give time for the client to respond. Limit decision-making complexities so the client does not feel overwhelmed.
5. Keep calendar, clock in the client's room. Keep the client's personal items within reach and always in the same place.
6. Avoid use of physical restraints.
7. Explain the presence of any new person, item, or event in the client's environment.
8. Avoid displays of annoyance or impatience with the client.

Nursing Care Plan for Human Need: *Sexual Integrity*

Nursing diagnosis	Due to or related to	As evidenced by	Goal/expected behaviors
Potential decline in intimacy between client and spouse	Progressive degenerative process of	Client occasionally forgets name of spouse	Client experiences caring, love, and understanding *(continued)*

Sexual Integrity (continued)

Nursing diagnosis	Due to or related to	As evidenced by	Goal/expected behaviors
	Alzheimer's disease Neuronal damage blocking self-control	Client generally unaware of surroundings Public disrobing related to client's forgetfullness Client is inattentive to spouse when being caressed Fidgeting with button closures on clothing	from significant others through touch, gentleness, and patience; usual patterns of affection evident within 2 months • Spouse can interpret client behaviors of affection and caring. Joins a support group within 6 months • Spouse is able to verbalize needs of client and himself within 4 months

Nursing Strategies with Frequencies

1. Discuss with the spouse the reasons for the exhibitionism that is common among Alzheimer's patients, and is often related to forgetfulness. Potential reason may be inability to locate a bathroom—the client may indicate the need to void by removing clothes in inappropriate places.
2. Explain to the spouse that the client experiences sexual needs in spite of Alzheimer's disease.
3. Encourage display of affection and caring.
4. Explore ways the client may be expressing the need for affection such as patting the spouse or family member, or clinging to a pet.
5. Encourage the spouse to join a support group that will provide a form of replacement for the former confidant, particularly a network of caregivers who are in similar situations.
6. Provide clothing with no button or zipper closure available to the client.
7. Provide distractions for the client when there is evidence of inappropriate behavior (go for a walk, play soft music, work a jigsaw puzzle with her).

Nursing Care Plan for Human Need: *Skin Integrity*

Nursing diagnosis	Due to or related to	As evidenced by	Goal/expected behaviors
Potential disruption in skin integrity	Lack of muscle coordination and impaired mobility	Frequent falls Changes in gait (unsteady)	Client's skin remains intact

(continued)

Skin Integrity (continued)

Nursing diagnosis	Due to or related to	As evidenced by	Goal/expected behaviors
Interruption in skin integrity	due to Alzheimer's disease Potential for injury to skin surfaces Fragile skin due to age	Restlessness at night Immobility in later stages of Alzheimer's disease Abrasions/bruises evidenced on occasion Insensitivity to temperature of food, drinks, environment	• Turns in bed with little or no assistance • Responds happily to daily physical activity • Smiles when lotion applied to skin surfaces

Nursing Strategies with Frequencies

1. Provide a safe environment; include all listed measures for Human Need for Safety.
2. Involve the client in daily physical exercise as tolerated.
3. As condition deteriorates, assist the client in repositioning every 2 hours to prevent pressure sores.
4. Use flotation or alternating pressure mattress.
5. Keep the client's legs elevated when sitting.
6. Perform active range of motion exercises twice each day.
7. Perform passive range of motion daily.
8. Use bath oils and mild soaps; apply skin lotion liberally to dry areas of skin.
9. Assess daily for bruises, blisters, abrasions.
10. Provide comfortable, well-fitted clothing and shoes.
11. Keep skin clean, dry, and protected from urine and feces (if incontinent).
12. Suggest resources for obtaining necessary supplies (Medicare, bulk purchases, etc.) within available means.
13. Direct family/caregivers to report any changes in skin to nurse/physician.

Nursing Care Plan for Human Need: Sleep

Nursing diagnosis	Due to or related to	As evidenced by	Goal/expected behaviors
Disturbance in sleep patterns	Pathology in the reticular activating	Client is restless at night; wanders;	Client experiences 5 to 6 hours of un-

(continued)

Sleep (continued)

Nursing diagnosis	Due to or related to	As evidenced by	Goal/expected behaviors
Potential sleep deprivation	system resulting from Alzheimer's disease Confusion as an outcome of the disease process	shows signs of fatigue; often yawns, is listless Family experiences fatigue	interrupted sleep evidenced by normal daytime energy level. This normal sleeping pattern developed by the end of 3 weeks • Family members have a schedule "on-call" hours so that each member gets 6 hours of uninterrupted sleep at least every other night • Schedule is prepared and put into effect within 48 hours • Plan is developed to implement a sleep/wake schedule that simulates client's and family's usual pattern within 1 week

Nursing Strategies with Frequencies

1. Encourage the client to stay awake during the day. Limit length of naptime ($\frac{1}{2}$ hour) if such is needed.
2. Allow the client to "wind down" in early evening but keep active during the day.
3. Provide a quiet environment for sleep and use "non-busy" patterns in the client's room (wallpaper, bedspread, curtains).
4. Keep small night light on to lessen anxiety.
5. Keep drapes drawn or shades down to prevent shadows in the windows and room.
6. If the client awakens during the night and becomes confused or agitated reorient her in a soft, soothing manner to avoid precipitating agitation.
7. Provide family members with a list of resources (day care, respite care, family support groups).
8. Encourage family members to rotate surveillance of the client so as not to exhaust the care providers who also require sleep.

9. If a sedative is required, observe the client for increased confusion and other side effects of the sedative.
10. Try different methods to help induce sleep at night:

   - Warm bath before bedtime.
   - Back rub.
   - Glass of warm milk.
   - Quiet background music.
   - Small toy animal to cling to.
   - Limit fluids at bedtime.
   - Eliminate noise.
   - Adjust room temperature.

11. Schedule specific time to retire and maintain that schedule each night.

Nursing Care Plan for Human Need: *Spiritual Integrity*

Nursing diagnosis	Due to or related to	As evidenced by	Goal/expected behaviors
Disturbed patterns of expressing spiritual integrity	Progression and ramifications of Alzheimer's disease that cause reduced cognitive abilities	Blaming God for punishing family and/or client Anger that God would allow this to happen Guilt feelings about blaming God and being angry with Him	Family verbalizes that spiritual integrity is maintained within 2 weeks • Verbalizes belief that God is not punishing family and/or client, within 1 month • Actions of prayer and other religious customs are resumed in daily activities within 1 month • Response to references about a Supreme Deity are met with warmth and receptivity

Nursing Strategies with Frequencies

1. Explore the spiritual health of the client and the family; assess the significance of religious practices to the client and the family.
2. Allow ventilation of guilt feelings and anger the family or the client may feel as a result of having Alzheimer's disease. Support the family and the client with an accepting nonjudgmental attitude.

3. Explore with the family spiritual support systems available to the family and encourage their use.
4. Assist the family to identify ways that resource persons can assist their meeting the client's spiritual needs.
5. Incorporate customary rites and/or relics that suggest spirituality at least daily with the client.
6. Ensure consistency of religious and/or spiritual activities among caregivers (e.g., same grace at meals, same bedtime prayers).
7. Regularity and repetitive nature of activities stimulate more positive response from the client.

Nursing Care Plan for Human Need: *Structure, Law, Limits*

Nursing diagnosis	Due to or related to	As evidenced by	Goal/expected behaviors
Disturbed patterns of structure and limits Diminished respect for law	Neuronal degeneration resulting from Alzheimer's disease	Difficulty in completing ADL activity Aphasia "Mirror sign"	Client experiences structure to minimize a feeling of being overwhelmed or confused; optimal function within a structured environment within 1 month
			• Family maintains outside interests and social interactions as evidenced by verbalization in 2 weeks • Client completes at least one ADL each day (e.g., feeding self, tying shoes, buttoning blouse) • Client recognizes the violation of others' territory (e.g., entering another person's room) • Client complies with observance of meal time at least three times a week

Nursing Strategies with Frequencies

1. Assist the family in planning a daily schedule that will best meet the requisites of both the client and the family.

2. Encourage the family to allow the client as much leeway as possible and assist only when needed; permit ambulation and freedom with limits.
3. Involve the client in decision-making as much as possible; for example, help her select which foods to eat first.
4. Maintain social contacts with neighbors and relatives; encourage weekly socialization.
5. Guide the client in donning attire each day.
6. Redirect ambulation route away from others' rooms; attach a marker (ribbon, photo, etc.) to the client's door to help her recognize her own room.
7. Write note and attach to the client's clock for meal time reminder.
8. Establish routine and reinforce directions at each meal hour for 1 week. Instruct the client to assume responsibility for getting to meals on time during the second week.

Nursing Care Plan for Human Need: *Tenderness*

Nursing diagnosis	Due to or related to	As evidenced by	Goal/expected behaviors
Disturbance in pattern of expressing tenderness Disturbed pattern of accepting tenderness	Impaired cognitive and intellectual abilities Changes in personality Neuronal damage of the Wernicke's area and the limbic system of the cerebrum ("the seat of the emotions")	Sadness Visible depression Occasional withdrawal Clinging to family members or caregivers Periodic evidence of excessive touching of children and pets Marked evidence of seeking touch from family or caregivers	Client's closeness and tenderness requirements are met by having someone with her at all times. ▪ Client's need for tenderness is addressed at least daily in the care plan; someone visits client for at least 5 minutes daily. ▪ At least one additional strategy each day is included in the client's daily care

Nursing Strategies with Frequencies

1. Explore with the family the client life-style patterns of interaction and types of social relationships prior to the disorder.
2. Encourage the use of touch, a supporting arm around the shoulder, a kind, gentle manner in all interactions with the client.
3. Assess daily the behaviors of the client; explore with the family the meanings of specific behaviors that may express the need for closeness.

4. Schedule personal interactions with the client at those intervals when personal care is not being given.

5. During daily walks, travel to areas where younger persons or pets are active; encourage interaction with the client.

6. Provide a stuffed animal for the client to cuddle/touch if the family approves this strategy.

7. Use touch, verbal compliments, smiles to communicate gentleness and tenderness to the client. Encourage reciprocal response.

Nursing Care Plan for Human Need: *Territoriality*

Nursing diagnosis	Due to or related to	As evidenced by	Goal/expected behaviors
Disturbed patterns of territoriality	Pathophysiologic state of Alzheimer's disease with resulting neuronal damage of the temporal lobe of the cerebrum	Anxiety Defensiveness Anger False ideas Hallucinations Suspiciousness Delusions Rage Restlessness Agitation Wandering	Client's personal space is defined and respected by all family members within 3 days • Client accepts allotted space in a cheerful, nondefensive, calm manner within 1 week • Client recognizes the space of other family members within 2 weeks and respects that space of others within 1 month • Anger, rage, and agitation are reduced within 2 to 3 days. Total elimination of these episodes is achieved by the end of 2 months • Anxiety and defensiveness evidenced no oftener than once a month • Hallucinations and delusions are not occurring

Nursing Strategies with Frequencies

1. Identify behavior patterns of the client with the family and define the client's response to closeness with others.

2. Explain the concept of territoriality with the family; assist in planning strategies to provide space for the client.
3. Keep the client's personal effects, favorite pictures, books in her room to maintain a personalized geographic space; place them in same spot always.
4. Though the client may require assistance with ADL, provide as much privacy as possible.
5. Explore the family's needs for space; allow them to discuss their feelings of lack of privacy and the constant demands of the client.
6. Develop coping strategies that include participation in support groups and use of respite care.
7. Define space for the client and space for family members within 24 hours.
8. Communicate space allotment with the client and reinforce repeatedly.
9. Make small and easily "lost" items larger and more visible, e.g., large keyrings.
10. When searching for items the client has hidden, check under mattresses, cushions, in shoes, drawers, etc.; focus on past experience with the client to know where items are hidden. These are especially good cues when searching for lost dentures.
11. Recognize the frustration and anger experienced by the caregivers as a normal reaction.

Nursing Care Plan for Human Need: *To Love and to Be Loved*

Nursing diagnosis	Due to or related to	As evidenced by	Goal/expected behaviors
Diminished ability to love and to be loved	Stigma associated with Alzheimer's disease diagnosis	A feeling of being a burden on family	Client accepts loving gestures from family and significant others and conveys love to others
Disturbance in ability to express love and to receive love	State of aging	Ashamed of forgetfulness	
		Agitation and impatience with self	• Family gives evidence of reaching out to friends by telephone calls or letters within first month
		Flat affect and lack of response to displays of affection from family members	
		Withdrawal from experiences of touching by loved ones	• Client verbalizes affection/love • Client displays gentleness and tenderness in contacts with family

(continued)

To Love and to Be Loved (continued)

Nursing diagnosis	Due to or related to	As evidenced by	Goal/expected behaviors
			• Actions and words of affection are initiated within 3 weeks; gradual increase in number of events is evident • Support groups for spouse include client in appropriate extensions of affection within 1 week

Nursing Strategies with Frequencies

1. Identify the means by which the client and the family members convey love for each other.
2. Encourage family members to use a gentle, patient manner; to caress, hold hands, and use nonverbal cues to convey love and concern.
3. Explore the meaning of love with the client and family members. Assist them in expressing their feelings to each other.
4. Involve relatives and neighbors in supporting family members to communicate affection for client. Suggest telephone calls daily to the client, and a card or note each week to say: "we love you" and "we think of you."

Nursing Care Plan for Human Need: Wholesome Body Image

Nursing diagnosis	Due to or related to	As evidenced by	Goal/expected behaviors
Diminished or reduced body image	Progressive degenerative process of Alzheimer's disease resulting in cerebral cortex damage and faulty sensory interpretation	Despair Grief Anger Hurt "Mirror sign" (inability to recognize one's own reflection in the mirror) Negative or passive reaction to image of self	Client and family accept changes in body image • Adaptation begins within 1 week; requires continual support and reinforcement • Mood becomes more positive eventually; noticeable change for the better is evidenced within 1 month

(continued)

Wholesome Body Image (continued)

Nursing diagnosis	Due to or related to	As evidenced by	Goal/expected behaviors
			• Complete fulfillment is long range • Client excels in selected experiences and realizes positive feelings about self

Nursing Strategies with Frequencies

1. Provide the family with specific information about the nature and course of Alzheimer's disease.
2. Assist a care plan strategy that allows as much client independence as possible in activities where success is usually assured.
3. Involve the client in family activities to demonstrate her importance within the family unit. Reminisce about past accomplishments.
4. Incorporate intervention strategies used in Nursing Care Plan for Human Needs: Acceptance of Self and Others; Personal Recognition, Esteem, Respect.
5. Encourage socialization with relatives, neighbors, and religious groups.
6. Urge the client to talk about feelings of despair, grief, anger to enable caregivers and the family to acquire insight.
7. Initiate positive comments when the client looks attractive and performs well.
8. Encourage the family to regularly extend looks, words, actions that communicate affection for and approval of the client.

Nursing Care Plan for Human Need: *Value System*

Nursing diagnosis	Due to or related to	As evidenced by	Goal/expected behaviors
Disturbance in the recognition and use of a value system	Neuronal damage and cerebral dysfunction leading to progression of the disease process	Sadness Depression of client Lack of animation No reference to values and intangibles in life Absence of reference to values held in the past	Client expresses the wish to remain with family and accepts possibility of institutionalization in the future • Family is able to accept the changes in the client's role as a family member

(continued)

Value System (continued)

Nursing diagnosis	Due to or related to	As evidenced by	Goal/expected behaviors
		Behaviors inconsistent with previously held values	• Verbalizes comfort with decisions about placement in an institutional setting if necessary, as evidenced by verbalization • Caregivers are aware of the client's reliance on specific values; these are incorporated into daily activities

Nursing Strategies with Frequencies

1. Explore the client's and the family's attitudes and values. Client's involvement is dependent on level of intellectual abilities. Base guidance on a thorough understanding of the family's history, expectations, old promises, values.
2. Allow the family to vent crushed expectations, hurt, possible disappointment, and anger about the client's illness.
3. Review the stages of illness with the family to provide some structure for the family's care-giving efforts.
4. Validate with the family the client's previous intellectual attainment, competent performance, and contributions to the family and community; include references to these in daily care to show appreciation and worth of client.
5. Explore with the family information about the client's support systems, quality and depth of relationship with peers, family, friends, and caregiving experiences.
6. Obtain information about and encourage use of community services including the religious affiliations.
7. Support the family in their decision to seek nursing home placement when that becomes necessary.
8. Encourage the family participation in support groups; sharing experiences and helping others may be beneficial.
9. Direct the client's attention to other phenomena when behaviors become inconsistent with known values (demanding, critical).
10. Stimulate memories of the client's past values by maintaining similar/same environment (e.g., furniture placement) and activities (e.g., evening prayers).

NURSING CARE PLAN FOR WOMAN
WITH AIDS-RELATED COMPLEX (ARC)
Developed by Anne Laskin, Cynthia Loiacono,
and Ellen Stammer

Client Data

The client is a 25-year-old childless, caucasian woman whose husband died with the diagnosis of acquired immune deficiency syndrome (AIDS). Within the last month, the client has noticed some fatigue, fever, night sweats, diarrhea, weight loss, skin rashes, and swollen lymph glands. Laboratory findings revealed a positive HTLV-III antibody test; skin test anergy; T4 cells less than 400/mm; T4/T8 ratio less than 1.0; a low white blood cell count, a high sedimentation rate; and ITP. Her diagnosis is AIDS-related complex (ARC).

Description of AIDS

AIDS is the most severe disease state resulting from the virus. Once contracted, the human T-lymphotropic virus type III (HTLV-III) infection is chronic and can be completely asymptomatic or show vague symptoms in the early stages. Carriers can spread the disease through sexual routes; by direct inoculation with contaminated blood products, needles, or syringes; or from mother to newborn in utero and through breast-feeding. Early detection is important to slow the spread of this disease.

The virus enters the body and attaches itself to the T4 lymphocyte because a protein on the surface of the T4 cells serves as a receptor site. The virus then penetrates the T4 cell and sheds its protein covering. The RNA is exposed with its special enzyme called reverse transcriptase that converts the viral RNA into proviral DNA. This is integrated into the host genome. New viral particles are produced by normal cellular transcription and translation. Then the potential for viral production is in place, which leads to cell death. The cumulative destruction of these T4 cells leads to T4 depletion.

The T4 cells induce B-cell antibody production, cytotoxic T-cell response, suppressor T-cell response, and the natural killer cell, as well as other responses of the immunologic process. Because the HTLV-III infection depletes T4 cells, it reduces the body's defense in all the responses that depend on T4 cells.

The HTLV-III virus is also neurotropic and attacks cells in the brain, the spinal cord, and the peripheral nerves where the virus can remain and continuously attack other T-cells and be out of reach of drug therapy.

In the first stage of the disease of HTLV-III virus, the infection may be asymptomatic or produce chronic lymphadenopathy. The T4 cell deficiency is not present. The next progressive stage of the disease is AIDS-related complex or ARC. These clients all demonstrate persistent lymphadenopathy and T4 cell deficiency and show some slowing of T4 cell function. They include defects in delayed hypersensitivity, mucous membrane disease, or dermatologic disease.

ARC has been defined as demonstrating two clinical conditions and two laboratory abnormalities especially a lowered T4 cell count and an inverted helper/suppressor ratio T4 to T8. Clients exhibit chronic fatigue, night sweats fever, weight loss, and unexplained diarrhea.

AIDS is the end stage HTLV-III infection. It includes a life-threatening opportunistic infection or Kaposi's sarcoma, a positive HTLV-III antibody test, and a defect in cell-mediated immunity occurring in a person with no documented cause for that immune deficiency. There are neurologic findings, caused by the virus using the brain as a reservoir, and can cause chronic, progressive neurologic disease.

The incubation period may be from 6 months to 10 years. The transmission depends on the virus being alive and stable in the transferred fluid, and then being transferred and penetrating the host and invading T4 cells. Therefore, casual contact would not predispose to HTLV-III infection.

The long-term effects of this disease are not known but the more that is understood, the more nurses can support, teach, and effectively provide nursing care for these clients.

Nursing Care Plan for Human Need: *Safety*

Nursing diagnosis	Due to or related to	As evidenced by	Goal/expected behaviors
Disturbed pattern in expression of safety	*Pathophysiologic* Impact of diagnosis of AIDS-related complex with potential for AIDS development	Anticipatory fears about her future Expresses fear of inability to deal with safety precautions	Client provides the safest environment possible for self and others at risk for transmission of virus (1 day and ongoing)
	Situational Impact of client continuing to remain at home and attempting to maintain general routine living pattern.	Feels she will be too tired to maintain her usual lifestyle Insists in maintaining her pets at home	• Client understands rationales behind various safety/preventive measures to ensure her own optimal health and to safeguard health of others

(continued)

Safety (continued)

Nursing diagnosis	Due to or related to	As evidenced by	Goal/expected behaviors
	Personal Impact of client's desire to maintain pets within home, increasing potential for infections *Educational* Deficits regarding basic housecleaning chores and minimizing opportunities for transmission of virus to others	Expresses desire to increase knowledge regarding prevention of disease transmission and reduction of risk of illness to self (client) and others	• Maintains her pets with the understanding and practice of necessary safety measures • Can accept available help/resources to assist her with pet care and occasional house work requirements. • States feeling of increased mastery over herself, her illness, and her optimal state of wellbeing

Nursing Strategies with Frequencies

1. Assist the client in developing respiratory safeguards within her environment (1 week and ongoing):

   - Review elements of preventive health care with the client.
   - Assist the client to provide for well-ventilated rooms to decrease risk of airborne disease.
   - Review the need for the client to cover mouth and nose with tissue when coughing and sneezing.
   - Remind/assist the client in assuring that heat/air conditioner filters are cleaned/changed frequently (monthly).
   - Instruct the client to minimize contact with others who are ill with respiratory infections; to ensure that any such contact involves good hygienic practices (covering of mouth and nose when sneezing).
   - Teach the client good handwashing techniques and encourage frequency of this practice.

2. Assist the client in understanding and practicing preventive behaviors regarding body secretions (1 week and ongoing):

   - Instruct the client that her razors, toothbrushes, and personal hygiene items that may come in contact with body secretions must be used by the client only.
   - Client's washcloths and towels, between launderings, should be used only by the client.

- Teach the client good handwashing technique and stress the rationale for its importance.
- Encourage the client to use moisturizing lotions for dry skin to assist in prevention of breaks in skin.
- Instruct the client that any linens soiled with the client's body secretions should be kept in plastic bags until ready for laundering and washed separately.

3. Teach the client appropriate, safe, and preventive laundry techniques (1 week and ongoing). Fill in the client's knowledge deficits:

- Household detergents and cleaning solutions can deactivate the AIDS virus.
- Do not overload washer so as to allow full circulation of detergent.
- For cottons/colorfast materials, use 1 cup per load of detergent and bleach.
- For noncolorfast materials, a detergent and a phenolic disinfectant (Lysol) in warm wash water will not fade material. A second wash and rinse, without the phenolic disinfectant, will remove any remaining chemicals.
- Machine dry at a HIGH setting.

4. Teach the client and persons significant to the client (family) preventive and safety techniques of housecleaning to ensure protection for client, friends, and family (2 weeks and ongoing). Fill in knowledge deficits:

- Common household bleach deactivates HTLV-III virus.
- 1 part bleach to 10 parts water (1:10) solution is sufficient for cleaning the bathroom.
- Full strength is best for disinfecting the toilet bowl.
- Dirty water from cleaning or body secretion spills should be flushed down the toilet.
- Mops and sponges should be soaked for 5 minutes in the 1:10 bleach/water solution.
- Bathroom mops and sponges should be used only in bathroom (not for general house cleaning).
- Another set (sponges and mops) should be kept available for spills/secretions in other areas of the house.

5. Teach the client measures for disease prevention in the kitchen area (1 week and ongoing):

- One sponge should be kept separate to scour the kitchen counters and rinse counters prior to food preparation.

- Food handlers should always use good handwashing techniques before handling food. (Do not wash hands in kitchen sink, as food is rinsed there.)
- Normal kitchen tidying, keeping refrigerator clean, washing floors once a week (and cleaning all spills immediately) can help in preventing the growth of bacteria and defend against infection of client.
- Teach the client that being immunocompromised demands carefulness in eating habits and preparation:
    - Avoid unpasteurized milk products (*Salmonella*).
    - Only eat fruits or vegetables peeled or cooked, as they are often fertilized with manure.
    - Meats must be thoroughy cooked.
- Utensils and dishes may be washed together in hot, soapy water and air dried or run through the dishwasher on the hot water cycle.

6. Provide information concerning pets and why their presence increases the risk for development of infections (1 week and ongoing):

- If a cat is present in the home (toxoplasmosis is spread by cat feces and may attack the client's immunocompromised neurologic system), it is preferable for the client not to clean the litter box. If the client must, the client should wear a mask and gloves when cleaning the litter box.
- Bird cages (droppings spread psittacosis, may lead to pneumonia) are best not cleaned by the client. If the client cleans cage, the client must wear gloves and a mask while cleaning.
- The client must NEVER CLEAN A FISH TANK as the mycobacterium in fish tanks produce devastating respiratory pathology and damage to the liver and spleen.

7. Teach the client safe sexual practices to minimize transmission of HTLV-III virus (1 day/ongoing) (see Nursing Care Plan for Human Need: Sexual Integrity).
8. Teach the client the hazards of recreational drug use relating to AIDS (2 weeks):

- Opiates, alcohol, marijuana act as immunosuppressants, thereby increasing susceptibility to infection.
- Inhaled nitrates may increase the risk of developing Kaposi's sarcoma (especially in homosexual men with AIDS).
- Intravenous drug use (especially if needles are shared) increases the risk of transmission.

9. Instruct the client to receive regular physical evaluations and follow-ups:

   - Physical examination and laboratory work to be done every 6 months even when symptom-free.
   - Instruct the client of the importance of seeking prompt health care whenever any symptoms of illness occur.
   - Instruct the client that she should never donate blood, plasma, body organs, other tissues, and provide the rationale for this.
   - Instruct the client that when she visits the dentist or any health care provider, it is appropriate for her to notify these people of her infection with the HTLV-III virus and explain rational.

10. Follow up on making sure that positive HTLV-III antibody test has been reported to the Public Health Department (cases, not names, are reported for statistical reasons only) (within 1 week).

11. Assist the client in reducing stress as a means to prevent further damage to her immune system (2 weeks to 1 month):

   - Teach the client relaxation exercises.
   - Emphasize importance of quiet times, soothing music and environment, time for relaxation.
   - Discuss/teach biofeedback techniques.
   - Allow the client to verbalize feelings openly; listen attentively; and reassure verbally and nonverbally.
   - Recommend a positive mental attitude on a consistent, habitual basis.
   - Emphasize the importance of recognizing tension within self.
   - Advise that highly emotional situations be avoided as much as possible.
   - Advise occasional respite from responsibilty.
   - Be alert for signs of increased anxiety, depression, and make client aware of these symptoms also.
   - Discuss possible requirement for referral to psychiatric nurse specialist for continued supportive psychotherapeutic intervention.
   - Encourage the client to acknowledge when she requires some assistance from others (occasional housekeeper, yard worker) and suggest ways to obtain assistance.

Nursing Care Plan for Human Need: *Sexual Integrity*

Nursing diagnosis	Due to or related to	As evidenced by	Goal/expected behaviors
Disturbed pattern in expression and	*Pathophysiologic*	Change in patterns of sexual behavior	Client reestablishes optimal level

(continued)

Sexual Integrity (continued)

Nursing diagnosis	Due to or related to	As evidenced by	Goal/expected behaviors
fulfillment of sexual integrity	Diagnosis of ARC with potential for actively transmitting HTLV-III virus to others, and the potential for developing AIDS herself *Situational* Spouse died from AIDS. Contact with AIDS virus may result from sexual contact, contact with blood, or perinatal contact with HTLV-III virus *Psychopathologic/ personal* Internally induced anger/ambivalence toward partner/ contact from whom she contracted AIDS virus Depression Emotional distress Loneliness Grief Guilt *Educational* Potential for incorrect assumptions concerning transmission of AIDS virus due to lack of education regarding AIDS, its transmission and safety precautions *Genetic* Potential for transmitting AIDS virus perinatally or through breast-feeding; Client should avoid pregnancy	Fatigue Depression Avoidance of sexual activity with a significant other Candidal vaginitis Loss of significant sexual other Depression: • Flat affect • Preoccupied • Decreased libido • Emotional lability • Irritability • Insomnia or hypersomnia • Chronic fatigue • Feelings of inadequacy • Decreased productivity • Decreased attention span • Poor concentration Avoidance of intimate, sexual contacts Client's expression of founded and unfounded fears regarding sexual identity Expressed fears of transmitting disease to significant others in a sexual/ intimate relationship Expressed concern regarding future ability to reproduce or nurture a child Expresses awareness of increased burden of responsibility	of sexual fulfillment (within 6 months and ongoing) • Expresses an interest in establishing/reestablishing intimate, close relationship with a significant other (within 6 months and ongoing) • Continually seeks knowledge concerning AIDS, its etiology, and safety and preventive factors (ongoing) • Accepts counseling to work through grief and to assist her in dealing with the losses experienced from AIDS/ARC: Loss related to diagnosis of ARC and resultant disruption of sexual identity; loss of significant sexual partner from AIDS (6 months) • Is free from symptoms of vaginitis (2 weeks) • Understands and practices honest and safe sexual practices (one week and ongoing)

(continued)

Sexual Integrity (continued)

Nursing diagnosis	Due to or related to	As evidenced by	Goal/expected behaviors
	Philosophical/ethical		
	Potential for transmission to others, which calls for responsibility and accountability on part of HTLV-III infected client related to sexual contacts		

Nursing Strategies with Frequencies

1. Assist the client in obtaining educational information pertaining to AIDS, including latest research findings, treatments and medications, transmission, safety, and preventive factors (review weekly).

   - Provide sources of reference to client from library, Red Cross, pamphlets, films, and slides, AIDS support groups, Hot Line numbers.
   - Discuss and review information together, making sure to clarify what the client's understanding of information is and allow the client to ask questions and express her feelings about the information.
   - Provide a neutral, nonjudgmental atmosphere, so that the client may feel free to discuss issues honestly without reservations.
   - Provide positive feedback to the client for her initiative in independently seeking information and for reviewing the information provided.
   - In weekly client/nurse meetings, always include a discussion of the latest information read or reviewed by the client and the nurse.

2. Review with the client and teach the guidelines for safe sexual practices (within 1 week and ongoing).

   - From a communicable disease standpoint, a monogamous partner is the safest.
   - Knowing your partner's state of health and life-style reduces the risk of transmitting/receiving communicable diseases.
   - Avoid sex with persons who are intravenous drug users or who have multiple sexual partners.

- Participate in sex in a clean setting. Body cleanliness is a prelude to enjoyable and safe sex. Never share personal hygiene items such as razors or toothbrushes.
- Deep kissing may transmit the HTLV-III virus and should be avoided. Kissing, as long as client or partner has no open cuts or sores on the lips, mouth, or tongue, has a low risk of transmitting HTVL-III. Present available information on AIDS indicates that it is not transmitted by casual kissing. Be creative with other types of body contact that do not involve exchange of body fluids. Sexual experience is not limited to penile penetration. Cuddling, massaging, and mutual masturbation are safer alternatives.
- Exchanging of body fluids has a high risk of transmitting disease. Oral contact or swallowing semen, urine, stool particles, and menstrual flow increases the risk of transmitting disease and should be completely avoided. Oral sex should be avoided when cuts or sores are present in the mouth.
- Sexual practices involving the rectal mucosa are extremely dangerous. Rimming has a very high risk of transmitting disease, especially in nonmonogamous situations. Fisting is extremely dangerous under any circumstances.
- Lubricants should be water-soluble (not oils or greases). Saliva is a poor lubricant, and it may be loaded with germs. The lubricant should not be in an open container or shared with others. Use one that is packaged in a pump, squeeze, or other closed container that dispenses one application at a time. Use nonperfumed lubricants. Anal intercourse causes tiny tears through which germs from both partners can enter the body. Use of a water-soluble lubricant helps reduce friction and tears and should be used even with a condom. Anal or vaginal douching before or after sex increases the risk of acquiring some infections because it removes normal barriers to infection.
- Present data indicate that the use of quality condoms prevents the spread of most sexually transmitted diseases when used appropriately. Some researchers recommend using a diaphragm in adjunct with water-soluble lubricant (5% nonoxynol-9) as a means of reducing transmission risk.
- Urinating after sex may reduce the risk of acquiring some diseases.
- Reduce or eliminate the use of toxic substances such as alcohol, cigarettes, marijuana, amyl nitrate ("poppers"), and nonprescription drugs. These substances affect judgment and tend to decrease the body's ability to fight off infection.
- Maintain your body's immune system by eating well, exercising, and getting adequate rest. Sex should not be used as your only means of stress reduction. Learn other stress reduction tech-

niques such as self-hypnosis and relaxation techniques.
- Discuss the implications of pregnancy and transmission of virus to the fetus.
3. Assist the client in expressing her feelings openly regarding experienced losses as a result of AIDS and her diagnosis of ARC (within 24 hours of diagnosis confirmation and twice a week ongoing).

- Demonstrate calmness and express empathy toward the client.
- Provide an atmosphere of acceptance to encourage maximum expression of the client's thoughts and feelings.
- Display nurturance and a caring manner toward the client.
- Make consistent and repeated efforts to reach out to the client.
- Build a trusting relationship with the client.
- Encourage emotional release through crying and/or verbalization of feelings. Use expression of feelings through art, writing, or music also. Assist client in becoming more comfortable in expressing both positive and negative feelings.
- Recognize the client's feelings of hostility/anger; help the client to become more aware of those feelings.
- Give support and positive feedback for controlling aggression; assuming responsibility for behaviors and appropriate expression of angry feelings.
- Support a realistic assessment of the situation and refrain from negative criticism.
- Explore with the client reasons for self-criticism.
- Provide professional psychiatric referral if symptoms, such as morbid preoccupation with worthlessness, prolonged and marked functional impairment, marked psychomotor retardation, suicidal ideations, excessive anxiety, or an emotional symptomatology, persist as troublesome for the client or others.
- Assist the client in working through normal stages of grief (3 to 6 months).
- Discourage rumination or stopping in one stage of grief work.
- Discourage the client's avoidance of grief work through various excuses.
- Encourage the expression of feelings in ways the client is comfortable and convey your acceptance of these feelings and means of expression.
- Encourage the client to recall experiences, talk about what was involved in her relationship with the lost objects/person.
- Include in interaction with the client some goals for the future and use mutual goal setting as much as possible.
- Help the client plan for the future with regard to changes made necessary by the losses, at whatever levels the losses affect living arrangements, finances, social activities, vocation, recreation.

4. Assist the client in treatment of vaginitis (candidiasis) and understanding measures to employ in preventing further symptoms (1 week and ongoing).

- Assist in confirming diagnosis. Symptoms may be: vulva is erythematous and edematous; thick, white vaginal discharge (resembles cottage cheese)—although some women may have no symptoms or a thin and watery discharge; satellite lesions spread to groin; sexual partner reporting balanitis or cutaneous lesions on penis.
- Diagnosis may be confirmed by Gram-stained smears of introital or vaginal wall scrapings, microscopic examination of wet mount of vaginal discharge, or culture on Sabouraud's modified agar.
- Treat with Nystatin vaginal suppository bid for 7 to 14 days or Miconazole vaginal cream qd for 7 days (per physician perscription).
- Discuss with the client predisposing factors and means of avoiding a recurrence. Emphasize that if and when the client has a sexual partner, the requirement that partner seeks treatment also, if the client has vaginitis.

Nursing Care Plan for Human Need: *Skin Integrity*

Nursing diagnosis	Due to or related to	As evidenced by	Goal/expected behaviors
Diminished skin integrity	*Pathophysiologic* Diagnosis of ARC with potential for developing AIDS Potential for delayed skin hypersensitivity (i.e., anergy) mucous membrane disease (e.g., hairy leukoplakia, oral candidiasis), and dermatologic disease (e.g., cutaneous herpes simplex/zoster, fungal disease) *Personal/educational* Embarrassment over skin disorders	Night sweats Chronic intermittent susceptibility to oral candidiasis and dermatologic diseases • Macular skin discomfort: Itching Shape: round Size: small Color: light red, purple, or bronze Content: no mass or fluid content Elevation: level with skin Distribution: single or multiple • Papular skin discomfort: Itching	Client maintains optimal level of skin integrity within 2 weeks and ongoing • Uses good hygiene and preventive practices • States the reason for her susceptibility to skin and mucous infections with understanding of preventive procedures • Experiences disorder-free skin and mucous membranes

(continued)

Skin Integrity (continued)

Nursing diagnosis	Due to or related to	As evidenced by	Goal/expected behaviors
		Tenderness	
		White with a black center, or violet color	
		Round or angular	
		Small (less than 5 mm in diameter)	
		Solid	
		Raised above skin	
		Single lesions or in a rash	
		Pimple appearance, flat, or pointed top	
		• Pruritus discomfort:	
		Itching	
		Scratching	
		Restlessness	
		Redness	
		Irritability	
		• Scale skin discomfort:	
		Itching	
		Yellow, silvery	
		Irregular shape	
		Irregular size	
		Horny mass; no fluid content	
		Raised above skin	
		Lighter or darker than normal skin	
		Develops on other lesions, often on knees, elbows, scalp, and trunk	
		• Vesicular skin discomfort:	
		Itching	
		Burning, stinging, neuralgic pain	
		Clear, translucent	

(continued)

Skin Integrity (continued)

Nursing diagnosis	Due to or related to	As evidenced by	Goal/expected behaviors
		Round	
		Small (less 5 mm)	
		Serum or water content	
		Raised above skin	
		Single or multiple, in groups or in chains	
		Hard, horny crusts during healing phase	
		Greater than 5 mm, they are bullae	
		• Avoidance of social contacts:	
		States skin lesions upsetting	

Nursing Strategies with Frequencies

1. Assist the client in control/relief of symptoms of skin disorders (2 weeks and ongoing):

Control itching and relieve pain

- Employ measures that produce vasoconstriction, e.g., cool environment; reduce excess clothing and bedding; tepid, cool baths; apply cool wet dressings.
- Instruct to avoid scratching lesions, rashes
- Treat dryness (xerosis) with lubricating creams or lotions applied after bathing and before drying to enhance hydration.
- Apply prescribed lotions or ointments and teach the client correct methods of application.
- Supply analgesic and antipruritic medication as indicated.
- Instruct the client to refrain from self-medication with salves or lotions that are commercially advertised.

Control/relief for inflammatory lesions

- Apply continuous or intermittent wet dressings to reduce intensity of inflammation.
- Remove crusts and scales before applying topical medications.

- Use topical applications containing corticosteroid medications as indicated.
- Rub topical medications well into skin to enhance penetration.
- Observe lesions periodically for changes in response to therapy.

Control oozing and prevent crust formation

- Instruct as to use of tub baths and wet dressings to loosen exudates and scales.
- Instruct to remove medication with mineral oil before reapplying.
- Instruct in use of mildly astringent solutions to precipitate proteins and decrease oozing.
- Instruct in maintaining a high protein diet if oozing is voluminous and serum loss substantial.
- Administer antibiotics by topical application or by mouth as indicated.

Avoidance of damage to skin

- Teach the client to protect healthy skin from maceration when applying wet dressings.
- Remove moisture from skin by blotting gently and avoiding friction.
- Guard against risk of thermal trauma from excessively hot wet dressings.
- Advise to use sunscreening agents to prevent actinic changes.

Ensure efficacy of topical applications

- Use occlusive dressings as needed to retain medication in constant contact with affected skin.
- Elicit the client's cooperation by having the client perform her own dermatologic treatments.
- Instruct the client clearly and in detail to ensure that treatments are carried out as prescribed.

2. Instruct the client as to importance of excellent hygenic practices and the employment of preventive behaviors in controlling skin disorders (2 weeks and ongoing).

- Encourage avoidance of lack of sleep, overwork, infections, and emotional stress.
- Emphasize keeping hands away from skin disorders except when applying treatments.
- Emphasize using good handwashing techniques before and after treatments of skin disorders.
- Explain the causes of skin health problems.
- Explain the reason for and intended effects of the therapy.

- Instruct to maintain cleanliness of skin and nails.
- Recommend the use of individual towels and washcloths with skin disorders.
- If the client has infectious/infected skin lesions, emphasize use of clean, dry linens, individual towels and washcloths, soiled articles to be discarded or sterilized, use of disposable gloves; review sterile technique.

Nursing Care Plan for Human Need: *Nutrition*

Nursing diagnosis	Due to or related to	As evidenced by	Goal/expected behaviors
Undernutrition	*Pathophysiologic* Impact of diagnosis of ARC with potential for AIDS	Lack of appetite Fatigue and lack of energy for meal preparation Fatigue and lack of energy for grocery shopping Weight loss Oral candidiasis • White plaques on oral mucous membranes, gums and tongue • Cannot be wiped out • No pain • Some difficulty in swallowing • Less vigorous eating • Enteric infections	Client improves nutritional status within 1 month and ongoing • Eats adequately balanced meals including required caloric intake • Articulates physiologic importance of good nutrition to maintain her optimal level of wellness • Prepares weekly nutritional menus incorporating well-balanced foods • Deals with her loss and grief in a positive, growth-producing manner rather than compromising her nutritional status • Regains lost weight and maintains appropriate weight for her height
	Situational Impact of daily time schedule on quality and quantity of time devoted to nutrition.	Irregularity of meal schedules and quality Often neglects meals, skips meals, fast foods/junk food, fad diets	
	Personal Impact of depression, worry, and stress on nutritional habits	Occasional bouts of bulimia versus anorexia Reports feelings of sadness and hopelessness with lack of interest in meal	• Freedom from oral candidiasis

(continued)

Nutrition (continued)

Nursing diagnosis	Due to or related to	As evidenced by	Goal/expected behaviors
		preparation and eating	
		Avoids socialization at meals	

Nursing Strategies with Frequencies

1. Assist the client in understanding the importance of a good, well-balanced nutritional state in minimizing the occurrence of opportunistic infections.

   - Provide pamphlets, books, and literature for review and discussion, pertaining to good nutritional habits and its resultant positive effects on the human body (weekly).
   - Assist the client in completing a nutritional assessment and keeping a detailed weekly log of what foods she eats and the amounts eaten.
   - Assess the availability of food, economic circumstances, transportation to stores, and ability to cook (within 2 weeks).
   - Discuss food likes, dislikes, and cultural preferences.
   - Review client's nutritional assessment (weekly) together and determine positive areas. Discuss means of improving on the weaker nutritional areas.
   - Correlate reported nutritional status with the recommended amounts from basic food groups and also from the Recommended Daily Allowances.
   - Assist the client in developing a weekly menu including well-balanced meals and seek weekly feedback from the client as to how the meals are progressing.
   - Suggest and refer for occasional help with housekeeping, grocery shopping, and meal preparation.
   - Check weight daily—same times, same scale, before breakfast in morning.

2. Encourage socialization during meals (at least twice weekly).

   - Discuss possibility of dining with close friend(s) at least twice weekly.
   - Encourage inviting friend to dinner or dining out with friend(s).
   - Encourage participation in church, civic, clubs potluck dinners.

3. Teach the client meaning of being immunocompromised and her need to use careful judgment in her eating habits.

- Avoid unpasteurized milk products; only eat fruits or vegetables peeled or cooked; and all meats eaten must be thoroughly cooked.

4. In treatment of oral candidiasis, provide for oral administration of Nystatin in suspension three to four times daily until symptom free. Apply over affected surfaces of oral cavity after eating. A 1 to 2 percent aqueous solution of gentian violet may also be swabbed in mouth, but this solution should not be swallowed as it could cause gastric irritation. Teach measures to prevent further development of spread of candidiasis.

   - Careful handwashing techniques.
   - Any object that comes into contact (direct or indirect) with mouth must be clean.

   Refer to dentist for twice a year routine evaluations and inform the client to always inform the dentist of her positive HTLV-III.

   - Initiate a program of oral hygiene so that mouth does not become a breeding place for bacteria (1 month).
   - Cleanse the mouth with nonabrasive soft materials (very soft toothbrush, finger wrapped with a layer of gauze and dipped in a cleaning solution).
   - Use mouthwash of 3 parts saline to 1 part hydrogen peroxide (dilute further if irritating).
   - Avoid commercial mouthwashes that may irritate sensitive tissue.
   - If mouth is sore, avoid spicy, hot, and acid foods and avoid irritating foods and fluids like toast and citrus fruit juices.
   - Suggest serving ice cream, ice milk, popsicles for a refreshing change.
   - Emphasize good mouth hygiene before and after meals.

5. Instruct the client in maintaining an awareness of the psychological issues she is dealing with and their effect on her eating habits (1 month).

   - Emphasize the importance of recognizing tension within oneself and the usual ways of dealing with it. Provide praise for positive means of dealing with tension and encourage problem solving to develop better methods of dealing with negative behaviors.
   - Describe behavior patterns and nutritional habits indicating emotional maturity.
   - Discuss appropriate means of obtaining release from emotional stress.
   - Recommend a positive mental attitude.
   - Recommend group/social interactions during meals.

- Refer to psychiatric nurse specialist if the client's troublesome symptoms persist or worsen.

Nursing Care Plan for Human Need: *Activity*

Nursing diagnosis	Due to or related to	As evidenced by	Goal/expected behaviors
Disturbed pattern in fulfillment of activity	*Pathophysiologic* Diagnosis of ARC with decreased functioning of the immunologic system accompanied by loss of some physical strength *Personal* Sense of powerlessness to alter disease process *Psychopathologic* Impact of losses, guilt, grief, stress as a result of AIDS	Chronic fatigue Complains of lack of energy for shopping, meal preparation, household chores, yard work Avoids all structured exercise programs Decreased tolerance for physical activity Shortness of breath Increase in time spent sleeping Worry about physical ability to maintain job Depression, flat affect; sleep disturbances; crying; poor concentration; narrowing of interests; self-isolation; apathy; hostile; broods and obsessed with diagnosis; lack of involvement in any hobbies or pleasurable activities	Client resumes wholesome activity level within 2 weeks and ongoing - Is involved in some consistent, structured form of physical activity - Shows improved physical recovery index - States that she has more energy than prior to exercise program - Maintains present employment - Has increased energy for more positive, growth directed activities with diminished loss and grief - Is involved in a local AIDS support group - Participates in a pleasurable social activity, at least once weekly

Nursing Strategies with Frequencies

1. Assist the client in organizing and implementing an enjoyable and physiologically safe but effective exercise program (within 2 weeks).

   - Determine the following: What the client's current activities consist of; what her past activities were (before ARC); how the past activities differ from the present ones; if client has any untoward symptoms from exercise; and how long it takes her to recover from strenuous exercise (1 week).
   - Obtain copy of records from recently performed physical assessment; must include family and client history, general physical

examination, resting blood pressure, standard 12-lead electrocardiogram, and blood lipid level measurements. If not available, perform or arrange necessary tests for assessment (1 week).

- Review all medications the client is taking. Check for contraindications to exercise and for those having a depressing effect (1 week).
- Obtain results and arrange for exercise stress test (Master two-step, bicycle ergometer, treadmill) or Harvard step test, to determine endurance, physiologic reserve, and metabolic activity (1 week).
- Assist the client in determining the types of exercise she most enjoys (1 week).
- Assist the client in forming an exercise schedule of participation (frequency of three to five times per week for 20 to 30 minutes each for optimal conditioning program).
- Encourage the client to begin exercises in small amounts (comfortable level) with incremental increases in activity level, duration, and frequency, according to client's tolerance level (within 2 weeks).
- Explore possibility of client's joining an exercise group/club—walking, hiking, swimming, jogging, bicycling—within community and encourage the client's participation (2 weeks).

2. Teach the client the importance of wholesome physical and mental activity in assisting her to achieve her optimal level of functioning (within 2 weeks).

- Provide educational resources (literature, discussions, lectures, classes).
- Provide specific literature pertaining to exercise as an aid in releasing grief, guilt, and stress (1 week and ongoing). Encourage involvement in extracurricular hobbies and pleasurable activities (within 1 week and review weekly ongoing).
- Provide catalogues/listings of classes within the community and review with the client to assist her in finding classes of interest to her (1 week).
- Provide community recreation center schedules, listings of events, and classes for the client to consider (1 week). Follow up on the client's actions.
- Refer the client to AIDS support groups with addresses and telephone numbers.

Centers for Disease Control: 1-800 447-AIDS (in Atlanta: (404) 329-3534).
National Institute of Allergy and Infectious Diseases: (301) 496-5717.

Public Health Service: Hot line (general information) 1-800 342-AIDS

AIDS Action Council: Federation of AIDS-Related Organizations; 1115½ Independence Ave. SE; Washington, D.C. 20003; (202) 547-3101.

American Association of Physicians for Human Rights: Box 14366; San Francisco, Ca. 94114; (415) 558-9353.

National Association of People with AIDS: Box 65472; Washington, D.C. 20035; (202) 483-7979.

Lambda Legal Defense and Educational Fund: 132 W 43rd St., fifth floor; New York, N.Y. 10036; (212) 944-9488.

National Gay Task Force: 80 Fifth Ave., Suite 1601; New York, N.Y. 10011; (212) 807-6016 or 1-800 221-7044.

National Hemophilia Foundation: Soho Building; 110 Greene St., Room 406; New York, N.Y. 10012; (212) 219-8180.

National Lesbian and Gay Health Foundation: Box 65472; Washington, D.C. 20035; (202) 797-3708.

There are local support groups in most major cities.

- Review and explore with the client activities she used to find pleasurable (e.g., movies, dining out, picnics) and assist the client in arranging one or two pleasurable outings per week (2 weeks, ongoing).
  Follow up by obtaining feedback from the client as to her evaluation and feelings related to participation in various activities.
- Discuss the importance of the client's accepting and providing emotional support in her involvement with others (1 week and ongoing).
- Discuss methods of channeling emotional energy into activity (1 week and ongoing).

3. Assist the client in expressing her feelings openly regarding experienced losses as a result of AIDS, her diagnosis of ARC, and its impact on physical and mental activity (within 24 hours of diagnosis and ongoing).

- Demonstrate calmness and express empathy toward client.
- Provide an atmosphere of acceptance.
- Display nurturance and caring through touch.
- Encourage the expression of the client's feelings and listen attentively.
- Talk with the client and offer feedback of the client's expressed feelings.
- Encourage questions.

- Encourage the client to face anxiety and encourage emotional release through verbalization of feelings and crying. Use expression of feelings through art, writing, or music.
- Touch may be used to convey caring, interest, nurturance, and to establish bonding between the client and the caregiver with the development of trust.
- Provide professional psychiatric referral if symptoms, such as morbid preoccupations with worthlessness, prolonged and marked functional impairment, marked psychomotor retardation, suicidal ideations, excessive anxiety, or any emotional symptomatology, persist as troublesome for the client or others.
- Explore with the client reasons for self-criticism.
- Support a realistic assessment of the situation and refrain from negative criticizing.

Nursing Care Plan for Human Need: *Spiritual Integrity*

Nursing Diagnosis	Due to or related to	As evidenced by	Goal/expected behaviors
Disturbed pattern of spiritual integrity	*Pathophysiologic* Diagnosis of ARC *Psychopathologic, social* Impact of spouse's death from AIDS, and client's diagnosis of ARC resulting in an emotional and spiritual crisis	Client perceives illness as punishment with resultant guilt Client reports "bargaining with God for health and time" Client's questioning God, her religion, and her faith Decreased attendance in Church-related activities Decreased attendance to Bible studies and prayer, and introspective self-awareness Decreased communication and contact with friends from church (spiritual centered activities) Client is hesitant to discuss feelings and anxieties with priest, minister	Client obtains maximum spiritual integrity (6 months) ▪ Is involved in activities reflecting understanding/interest in inner/spiritual dimensions of self and others (3 months) ▪ Is willing to share spiritual/growth experiences as a means of assisting self and significant others in their spiritual growth (3 to 6 months)

(continued)

Spiritual Integrity (continued)

Nursing diagnosis	Due to or related to	As evidenced by	Goal/expected behaviors
		(spiritual counselor)	
		Expresses feelings of lack of fulfillment in life	
		Expresses desire for unity/peace with loved ones	

Nursing Strategies with Frequencies

1. Encourage the expression (written, verbal) and sharing of feelings and knowledge of a spiritual dimension (weekly).
2. Encourage client to define her spiritual values (weekly).
3. Guide the client with/in prayer as expressed. Provide privacy for prayer.
4. Provide desired spiritual/religious articles and provide information about spiritual programs (radio, television, community, and church services) (ongoing).
5. Encourage spiritually uplifting conversation (weekly).
6. Encourage the client to be involved in support groups, classes in church, within the community (weekly).
7. Encourage contact with friends from church and asking for support (emotional and spiritual) from these resources (weekly).
8. Encourage sharing of concerns/feelings with spiritual advisor (ongoing).
9. Assist the client in setting standards of a meaningful existence (weekly).
10. Assist the client in restructuring her life-style to accommodate a more meaningful existence (weekly).
11. Explore reasons for the client's avoiding in-depth feelings (within 1 month and ongoing).
12. Communicate to the client that the nurse is comfortable with the client's discussion of thoughts and feelings about death (within 1 month and ongoing).
13. Emphasize the client's worth as an individual (always).
14. Encourage the client's involvement in helping others and encourage meaningful spiritual activity (within 1 month).
15. Encourage involvement in interactions and activities with family and significant other to achieve spiritual peace and unity (daily).
16. Refer to pastoral counselor as necessary.

Nursing Care Plan for Human Needs: *Conceptualization, Rationality, Problem Solving*

Nursing diagnosis	Due to or related to	As evidenced by	Goal/expected behaviors
Disturbed pattern in conceptualization, rationality, and problem solving	*Pathophysiologic* Diagnosis of ARC Potential for developing AIDS	Fever Fatigue Night sweats Energy loss Muscle weakness Acquiring opportunistic infections	Client utilizes a problem-solving approach with activities of daily living and personal interactions within 1 month • Makes selections in various purchases within 1 week • Demonstrates ability to select clothing to wear each day within 1 week • Begins to demonstrate knowledge of disease process by the manner in which she conducts her activities of daily living • Maintains a balance in activities, diet, rest, and exercise within 1 month • Understands the basis for fever, fatigue, night sweats, energy loss, and muscle weakness within 1 week
	Personal Inability to make personal decisions Lack of ability to make plans	Verbalizes difficulty in making selections at the grocery store Unable to decide what to wear each day Depression	
	Social Loss of ability to initiate communication with others	Verbalizes indecision in activities of daily living Verbalizes inability to talk to others Isolating from others	
	Educational Lack of knowledge concerning the diagnosis of ARC Lack of knowledge of the relationship of nutrition, exercise, and rest to optimum wellness	Verbalizes incorrect answers about the disease Unaware of relationship of activities of daily living (ADL) to maintenance of health	

Nursing Strategies with Frequencies

1. Provide a "walk-through" for the problem-solving approach and ask her to apply this approach to a selection of activities of daily living and personal interactions. Respond to her efforts.
2. Provide a warm, comfortable, cheery environment (immediate and continuous):

   • Accept her the way she is.
   • Listen to what she has to say.
   • Hear what she is saying and what she is NOT saying.
   • Tune in to her body language.

- Give her uninterrupted time.
- Give her feedback and acknowledge her expressed concerns.

3. Provide educational experiences:

  - Provide factual information about ARC and AIDS.
  - Allow her to ask questions.
  - Encourage her to face her fears and anxieties.
  - Provide access to others who have a similar condition. Have them share their feelings and experiences. Have them share how they made decisions about the issues that bothered them.
  - Together identify a plan for activities of daily living.
  - Encourage simple choice selection and decision making.
  - Give positive feedback.

4. Examine relationships between nutrition, rest, and exercise

  - Together make a plan for a balanced day of living.
  - Have her write it down. Make a check off list.
  - Have her call you at the end of each day at a specified time and discuss what she did that day.
  - Give positive feedback.
  - Make further suggestions.

Nursing Care Plan for Human Needs: *Autonomy, Choice*

Nursing diagnosis	Due to or related to	As evidenced by	Goal/expected behaviors
Potential for lack of autonomy, choice	*Pathophysiologic* Diagnosis of ARC Potential for muscle weakness Potential for developing AIDS	Loss of energy Loss of physical strength Verbalizing "Sometimes I just don't think I have the physical strength to get myself dressed in the morning" Acquiring opportunistic infections	Client develops realistic choice-making skills within 6 months • Begins demonstrating ability to verbalize complete thoughts within 1 month. • Verbalizes thoughts that are logical and demonstrates realistic understanding of limitations within 3 months. • Accepts the reality of the diagnosis and is able to work through feelings regarding the diagnosis:
	Intellectual Difficulty in cognitive functioning Experiencing high amount of emotional pain	Verbalizes inability to think clearly Having difficulty making simple decisions affecting activities of daily living Appearance radi-	

(continued)

Autonomy, Choice (continued)

Nursing diagnosis	Due to or related to	As evidenced by	Goal/expected behaviors
		ates sheer terror Face, pale and tense Eyes, wide, clear, pupils dilated Body, erect, tense	Anger: Time 2 months Fear: Time 3 months Self-pity: Time 3 months Negative thinking: Time 6 months
		Restless behavior Sits on edge of chair Squirms in chair, not relaxed Voice high pitched	• Begins feeling identification with self and illness within 2 weeks • Begins to demonstrate knowledge of disease process
		Verbalization: Sentences incomplete. Lots of hesitation in midsentence. Has difficulty in expressing a complete thought.	by the manner in which she conducts her activities of daily living within 3 months
	Experiencing moderate amount of denial	Verbalizes laboratory made a mistake	
	Decreased ability to exercise judgment	Wants another doctor's opinion	
	Lack of knowledge	Exhibits some anger	
	about disease	Plans verbalized are unrealistic	
		Wants to move to another city	
		Verbalizes incorrect information	
		Illustrates untrue myths about disease in conversation	
	Lack of knowledge concerning alternatives	Knowledge of resources unknown	

Nursing Strategies with Frequencies

1. Provide a warm, comfortable, inviting, relaxed atmosphere (immediate and continuous):

   • Accept her the way she is.

- Listen to what she has to say.
- Hear what she is saying and what she is NOT saying.
- Give her uninterrupted time.
- Give her feedback and acknowledge her expressed concerns.

2. Offset informational deficits and self-care limitations:

- Provide information about ARC and AIDS.
- Be factual.
- Allow her to ask questions.
- Allow her to ventilate anger.
- Encourage her to face her fears and anxieties.
- Provide access to others who have a similar condition. Have them share their feelings and experiences. Point out similarities in feelings.
- Explore coping behaviors. Begin with activities of daily living (that is "safe territory" to the psyche). Relate fatigue level and muscle weakness to activities of daily living and the disease process.
- Encourage simple choice selection and decision making.
- Give positive reinforcement for things done well.
- Give positive encouragement for things she can do.
- Emphasize progress.

3. Explore with client how she handled a personal crisis in the past. Have her talk about what she did. Point out similarities.
4. Examine myths surrounding disease of ARC and AIDS. Relate myths to what she is learning in educational program.

- Schedule for individual and group educational program. Self-paced reading materials, group work.

5. Discourage major life-style changes for a minimum of 1 year. Together assess alternatives for future life-style changes.
6. Provide introduction to support groups: Contact group immediately. Arrange for introductions within 5 days.
7. Schedule individual counseling sessions. Refer to psychiatric nurse specialist if necessary.

Nursing Care Plan for Human Need: *Effective Perception of Reality*

Nursing diagnosis	Due to or related to	As evidenced by	Goal/expected behaviors
Disturbed pattern of perception of reality	*Pathophysiologic* Diagnosis of ARC Potential for developing AIDS	Fever Fatigue Loss of energy	Client effectively perceives and interprets sensory stimuli, now and

(continued)

Effective Perception of Reality (continued)

Nursing diagnosis	Due to or related to	As evidenced by	Goal/expected behaviors
	Pathophysiologic	Acquiring opportunistic infections	ongoing
	Personal	Verbalizes reluctance to socialize with others	• Maximizes competency of sense organs
	Isolating		• Uses calendar with large print
		Absence of visitors in the home	• Uses digital clock in radio to remain oriented to time
		Lack of immediate family	• Constructs entertainment around audio versus video experiences, e.g., radio, tapes, within 3 days
	Physical	Verbalizes that the light hurts her eyes	
	Photosensitivity		
	Blurred vision	Squinting in daylight	• Attends support group within 1 week
		Wearing sunglasses in house	• Receives visitors from support group within 2 weeks
		Verbalizes requiring new glasses	• Verifies perception of stimuli with nurse and support group members within 1 week

Nursing Strategies with Frequencies

1. Assess competency of sense organs now and ongoing.
2. Provide a warm, comfortable, relaxed environment for her to validate perception of stimuli:

   - Accept her the way she is.
   - Listen to what she has to say.
   - Hear what she is saying and what she is NOT saying.
   - Tune in to her body language.
   - Give her uninterrupted time.
   - Give her feedback and acknowledge her expressed concerns.

3. Promote sensory comfort measures within 1 day:

   - Use indirect lighting.
   - Use of magnifying glass when reading.
   - Reading materials with large print.
   - Listening to audio tapes (books on tape).

- Listening to soothing but energizing music on radio.
- Use calendar with large print.
- Use clock with large numbers or lighted digital.

4. Support client's efforts to increase social contact within 3 days:

- Arrange for introduction to member of support group within 1 day.
- Contract with her to attend meetings.
- Arrange with support group for daily visitor.
- Encourage use of telephone to talk to member of support group.

Nursing Care Plan for Human Need: *Belonging*

Nursing diagnosis	Due to or related to	As evidenced by	Goal/expected behaviors
Lack of belonging	*Social*	Rejection by family and peers	Client experiences increased belonging within 3 months
	Inability to be accepted by others	Verbalizing fears	
	Stigma of AIDS and ARC	Avoiding painful encounters	• Participates regularly in group
	Fearful of social interactions	Isolating behaviors	• Bonds with members of support group
	Pathophysiologic	Verbalizes loneliness	• Verbalizes that she is not lonely and that she has friends
	AIDS and ARC	Verbalizes inability to make friends	
	Emotional factors	Verbalizes friends have "left me alone"	Face radiant
	Feelings of alienation		Speech energetic and excited
	Feelings of rejection	Verbalizes feelings of rejection	May cry tears of joy but despair will be gone within 3 months
		Verbalizes that she feels she is not worth much as a person	• Uses correct posture and maintains eye contact when talking to another person within 2 months
	Being alone	Depression	
		Slouching posture	
		Not looking at person when talking	• Relates comfortably with other persons with ARC within 2 months
		Weepy-eyed	
		Episodes of crying	

Nursing Strategies with Frequencies

1. Facilitate bonding through introduction to support groups. Contact group immediately. Arrange for introductions within 5 days:

- Call AIDS Hot Line to find support groups.
- Contact AIDS Task Force to find support groups.

- Contact support group and introduce her to member of group. Have group member come to your office and make the introductions. Allow the two to talk and act as small group facilitator. Explore projects that she could work on with the group to ease in and become a part of the group.
- Find clergy of her faith who will be accepting and introduce her within 1 week.
- Obtain feedback from the client within 2 weeks. How many meetings has she participated in. Does she have telephone numbers of people in support group to contact. Has she been able to "reach out" and use the telephone to call someone even on her "good days" when she is feeling better.

2. Explore with the client her past problem-solving behaviors, now and continuous:

- Give positive reinforcement for good past decisions.
- Explore with her how these decisions might work in present situation.

3. Provide an environment conducive to the exploration of belonging:

- Arrange for an uninterrupted scheduled time with client.
- Allow her to ask questions and listen to what she has to say.
- Allow her to ventilate feelings and provide feedback on expressed feelings.
- Encourage her to face her fears and anxieties about AIDS and ARC.
- Provide access to others who have a similar condition. Have them share their feelings and experiences. Have them share their problem-solving approaches. Point out similarities in feelings and coping behaviors, e.g., what she is going through and what this other person has gone through and how it has been managed.
- Share new knowledge about disease as it becomes available.

Nursing Care Plan for Human Needs: *Acceptance of Self and Others, Acceptance by Others*

Nursing diagnosis	Due to or related to	As evidenced by	Goal/expected behaviors
Diminished acceptance of self Potential rejection by others	*Pathophysiologic* Diagnosis of ARC; potential for developing AIDS *Situational occurrence* Husband died with	Crying Sadness Irritable Disheveled clothing Hair unkempt	Client demonstrates acceptance of self in 1 week • Shares feelings about grief, disease, loneliness and fear within 1 day

(continued)

Acceptance of Self and Others, Acceptance by Others (continued)

Nursing diagnosis	Due to or related to	As evidenced by	Goal/expected behaviors
	AIDS	Dour facies	• Asks questions about disease and own weight loss in 1 day
	Personal	Lack of eye contact	
	Weight loss	Poor body habits	
	Night sweats	Disinterested in surroundings	• Begins good hygiene and grooming habits in 1 day
	Under stress due to grief and fear of own death	Restless	• Contacts a local support group within 2 days
		Halitosis and poor dental hygiene	• Meets another client with ARC within 4 days
		States "I guess it's all over now"	• Practices positive thought patterns beginning day 1
		States "What friends I had are lost now"	• Makes small decisions and gradually returns to independency beginning day 1
		States "When my boss finds out I'll be canned"	
		States "I can't decide, you tell me"	• Expresses positive feelings of self in 1 week
		States "I suppose it'll explode inside me and take over"	

Nursing Strategies with Frequencies

1. Display accepting attitudes that create an environment where the client feels personally accepted because acceptance allows for testing reality and the reaction of others:

   - Approach unhurriedly.
   - Reassure verbally.
   - Encourage the expression of feelings.
   - Listen carefully and attentively.
   - Offer feedback to the person's expressed feelings.
   - Communicate your professional sensitivity to the clients' state.
   - Praise the client when appropriate.
   - Avoid forcing the client to change, instead encourage her and accept her adjustment.

2. Allow opportunities for verbalizing feelings about disease state to increase reality perception. Teach client in areas of lack of knowledge: Begin day 1.

3. Encourage client to reflect on what is good about herself at a certain time each day because this will promote positive attitude and behavior.

4. Encourage decision making, being independent, and assuming responsibilities so as to increase self-acceptance, on first day and ongoing.
5. Direct the client toward good grooming and appropriate dress so her appearance will be satisfying to herself and to others.
6. Encourage client *not* to become *obsessed* with obtaining knowledge about the disease as this will encourage negativism.
7. Refer to local support groups, home health agencies, and other referral services such as the Center for Disease Control, toll-free number 1-800-342-AIDS.
8. Find encouragement by talking with another ARC client who does not have AIDS. Nurse will arrange first meeting by day 4.

Nursing Care Plan for Human Need: *Sleep*

Nursing diagnosis	Due to or related to	As evidenced by	Goal/expected behaviors
Sleep deficit	*Pathophysiologic* Diagnosis of ARC; potential for developing AIDS *Situational* Husband died with AIDS	Fatigue Depression Itchy eyes Reddened eyes Irritability Nervousness Yawning Tiredness Short attention span Difficulty deriving support from others Difficulty making decisions or applying intellectual effort Restlessness Stated "My husband died of AIDS and I think I have it too"	Client demonstrates normal sleep pattern within 5 days • Begins keeping log of sleep patterns on first day • Takes short walk if tired in afternoon to prevent sleep on first day • Returns to preillness rituals by day 2 • Goes to sleep and falls asleep in 20 minutes within day 3 • Awakens at normal time feeling refreshed within day 4 • Verbalizes understanding of her sleep requirement and practices by day 4

Nursing Strategies with Frequencies

1. Continual assessment of quality and quantity of client's sleep:

   • Determine characteristics of client's sleep, such as light, normal, deep, or interrupted sleep.

- Determine length of time client sleeps.
- Ask client to keep a log of sleep pattern such as time retires and awakens and any interruptions with the mental preoccupation noted at that time.
- Plan to review this with client on day 2.
- Explain that loss of sleep can threaten health because during sleep, body energy is used for healing and cell restoration.

2. Inform client of recommended minimum hours of sleep:

   - Explain that 7 to 9 hours are recommended for adults as adequate daily sleep as this is essential to the replacement of energy within tissue cells.

3. Inform client that underweight persons require extra sleep:

   - Explain that underweight persons have less energy reserve than those of normal weight and require more energy restoration through extra sleep.

4. Recommend regular sleep schedule:

   - Suggest client make it a habit to go to bed at the same time each night as stable sleep habits promote physical and emotional health.

5. Promote sleep readiness:

   - Encourage client to provide quiet evening activities, reduced caffeine intake, reduced stimuli in her sleep area, proper temperature and noise control, as well as household security such as door locks and a watch dog.

6. Inquire about client's sleep rituals and promote restoration of familiar bedtime rituals within 3 days:

   - Explain that customary rituals promote relaxation.
   - Have client review own rituals for promoting relaxation and comfort such as bathing before sleep, using familiar pillow and blankets, light reading, warm milk, and religious routines.
   - Encourage additions to patterns such as sleeping on left side when ready to sleep, as this causes slowed heart rate, reducing circulation and promoting sleep, as well as always using fresh gowns as cleanliness promotes comfort and relaxation.

7. Teach the client relaxation exercises, such as relaxation of major muscle groups and body parts, starting with feet and working to face and head. Arrange to review in 3 days.

8. Promote wakefulness during the day to allow for normal restful sleep at the client's normal bedtime.

Nursing Care Plan for Human Needs: *Rest, Leisure*

Nursing diagnosis	Due to or related to	As evidenced by	Goal/expected behaviors
Lack of rest and leisure	*Pathophysiologic* Diagnosis of ARC; potential for developing AIDS *Situational* Husband died with AIDS *Psychopathologic* Working through the grief process for husband *Social and economic* Due to husband's death, vacation socially unacceptable and economically impossible	Time needed to care for husband Time spent at home after husband died, sadly Irritability Quiet Responses often inappropriate Tremors of extremities Poor eye contact Withdrawn Sad facies Eyes twitching States "I never feel rested" Does not participate in groups for leisure States "I never go anywhere" States "I shouldn't spend any money on myself"	Client incorporates rest and leisure in life-style on a daily basis • Discusses trips and leisure experiences beginning week 1 • Expresses desire for change of scenery, week 1 • Expresses requirement for and feelings of entitlement for trip within 2 weeks • Asks relative/significant other to join her at the beach for a weekend by end of week 2 • Reports restful pleasure

Nursing Strategies with Frequencies

1. Determine the client's preillness pattern of rest and leisure and use as a baseline for strategy prescription.
2. Suggest that client change her surroundings by taking a pleasure trip or do things to change routines within 1 week to promote temporary freedom from stressful worry.

   - Support emotional healing.
   - Generate new interests to take the place of focus on sadness.

3. Explore available leisure activities with the client, begin on week 1.

   - Must be of client interest.
   - Must be affordable.
   - Must be easily available to facilitate the client's acceptance.

- Must have convenient health care easily available.

4. Encourage planning or spur-of-the-moment trips to facilitate excitement, begin on week 2.
   - Use reduced rates for off-season.
   - Check newspaper ads and magazines for special packages.

5. Encourage the client to verbalize she is entitled to vacation and leisure.
   - Ask the client to share an experience from a previous vacation.
   - Ask her to describe her most desirable vacation dream.
   - Encourage client to see the advantage of leisure and find a middle-ground between most-desired and the available vacations.

6. Instruct client that a carefree distraction will promote the desired restful feeling.

7. Discuss with the client the types of clubs and groups available for leisure.

8. Ask the client to brainstorm a trip for the weekend with an accepting relative/significant other. Praise with excitement and encourage fulfillment; begin on week 2.

9. Ask client to share a report of her trip. Encourage trip to stimulate feelings of calm.

Nursing Care Plan for Human Need: *Elimination*

Nursing diagnosis	Due to or related to	As evidenced by	Goal/expected behaviors
Excessive elimination of stool	*Pathophysiologic* Diagnosis of ARC	Abnominal cramping	Client demonstrates effective elimination within 4 days
	Potential for developing AIDS and cryptosporidiosis or Salmonellosis	Increased frequency of stool	
		Increased bowel sounds	• Monitors pattern of elimination from first day
	Situational Husband died with AIDS	Clinical evidence of malabsorption such as dry skin, dry mouth, irritated eyes	• Develops skill in intake and output balance within 3 days
	Personal Stress and anxiety due to potential for AIDS development	Loose, liquid stools, flatulence	• Responds knowingly to diet/diarrhea relationship within 4 days
		Irritation of perianal area	• Assumes responsibility for sitz baths, anal care, hand washing within 1 day
		Irritability	
		Weight loss	
		Poor skin turgor	

(continued)

Elimination (continued)

Nursing diagnosis	Due to or related to	As evidenced by	Goal/expected behaviors
		States "I can't seem to retain anything I eat" States "I must be very ill because I have diarrhea"	• Develops skill in disinfecting equipment, bathroom, and self by day 2 • Experiences reduced anxiety about diarrhea by attention to nutritional diet and regulating medication within 1 day and ongoing • Resumes normal peristalsis, good skin turgor, and intact mucosa within 3 days • Returns to weight in keeping with age, gender, height within 1 week

Nursing Strategies with Frequencies

1. Continue assessment of bowel elimination. Check character and number of stools, discomfort level, skin and mucosa around anus daily:

   - Have the client keep log of stool elimination with time, amount, and character of stool daily.
   - Record daily weight (same scale, same type clothing, before breakfast).
   - Record daily intake of food and fluids.
   - Inspect anal mucosa and surrounding skin twice a day.

   Analyze recorded data on daily basis. Discuss with client. Adjust instructions, re: bowel elimination based on data as necessary. Refer to physician for medical intervention if warranted.

2. Instruct the client as to nutritional requirement when experiencing diarrhea:

   - Discourage intake of stimulants as they increase peristalsis.
   - Avoid high fiber and residue foods such as vegetables, whole grain cereals and breads, fresh fruit, and spices.
   - Avoid milk or milk products as undigested lactose pulls water into the intestines, and increases the diarrhea.

- Encourage high pectin foods, such as the pulp of apples, pears or ripe bananas that slow peristalsis by the soothing, emollient effect.
- Encourage foods soothing to the intestine such as warm tea, carbonated beverages, clear liquids such as broth, gelatin, or fruit ices, and full liquid foods such as sherbet, noncream soups, thin wheat cereals, rice cereals, gruel, or crackers.
- Respond to the client's questions about diet.

3. Administer antidiarrheal drugs and teach the client to administer after each stool or around the clock as prescribed.
4. Monitor for constipation to prevent impaction.
5. Administer antibiotics as prescribed and instruct the client as to their use—time, dosage, with meals or on empty stomach, side effects.
6. Encourage the client to soak in a sitz bath, dry rectal area carefully, and apply emollient lotions to painful anal tissues daily. Arrange for disinfection of sitz bath (basin, tub, or chair).
7. Encourage client to respond immediately to the elimination reflex and to avoid straining.
8. Instruct client to thoroughly wash hands with hot soapy water with each elimination to avoid spreading disease. Suggest use of a good hand cream to maintain intact skin.
9. Instruct client to disinfect toilet, and any home area contaminated with feces, with a 1:10 dilution of 5.25 percent sodium hypochlorite and water.
10. Inform the client that diarrhea occurs frequently in ARC.
11. Instruct client that soiled clothing should be kept in a plastic bag and washed separately with bleach, or if colored clothing, with lysol to disinfect. Recommend a second rinse to remove chemicals and preserve skin integrity. Mops and sponges used in the bathroom should be cleaned in bleach at a 1:10 dilution and kept separately from cleaning sets for rest of the house.

Self-Study Questions

1. If Kathleen Krampitz, Andrea Gillman, Annemarie Sokol-Velkie, Jonathan Baselton, Monique Morales, Vincent Valentino, Christopher Harrell, the Lawson family, or the Milford Community were your clients, would the nursing care plans you develop for these clients be comparable to those presented? A person with Alzheimer's disease? A person with ARC?
2. Would you have designated the same actual and potential nursing diagnoses?

3. Would you have designated additional actual or potential nursing diagnoses?

4. If you would have designated additional or different obvious or potential nursing diagnoses, what would be the data base to support your judgment?

5. What would you have designated as the priority for the actual and potential nursing diagnoses inherent in the situation?

6. Do you agree with the goal statement and behavioral outcomes for the client and the timing for goal achievement? If you disagree, what would you specify for these?

7. Would you add to, subtract from, or change the existing nursing strategies and their frequency? If yes, in what way? If you have designated additional or different actual or potential nursing diagnoses, what goal expectation(s) would you specify? What strategies would you prescribe to attain goal achievement for the clients?

SUMMARY

The client situations in this chapter are far from inclusive for all types of encounters that can confront nurses. The goal of presenting these client situations is to suggest the variety of age groups, settings, and problem areas the client may present and to reinforce the value of nursing's human need theory as the framework for application of the nursing process. The territory of nursing is the fostering of human need fulfillment for the client, whether as a person, family, or community. The orderly thought processes suggested in the four phases of the nursing process should make it easier for the nurse to fulfill the nursing responsibilities and assist clients in their efforts to achieve human need fulfillment.

AIDS AND ARC BIBLIOGRAPHY

American Hospital Association. *AIDS*. Chicago, Illinois: American Hospital Association, 1986.

Brosnan, S. Our first home care AIDS patient: Maria. *Nursing 86*, 1986. *16*(9), 37–39.

Bremner, M., & Brown, L. Learning to care for clients with AIDS—the practicum controversy. *Nursing and Health Care*, 1986, 7(5), 251–253.

Casper. V. AIDS: A psychosocial perspective. In D.A. Feldman & T.M. Johnson (Eds.), *The social dimensions of AIDS* (pp. 197–209). New York: Praeger, 1986.

Dhundale, K., & Hubbard, P.M. Home care for the AIDS patient: Safety first. *Nursing 86*, 16(9), 1986, 34–36.

Hauer. L., & Paleo, L. *Women and AIDS*. San Francisco, Ca.: San Francisco AIDS Foundation, 1984.

Klug, R.M. AIDS: Beyond the hospital, Part I. *AJN,* 1986, *86*(9), 1015–1028.

Klug, R.M. AIDS: Beyond the hospital, Part II. *AJN,* 1986, *87*(9), 1126–1132.

Luce, J.M. New developments in the acquired immunodeficiency syndrome: Are treatment, prevention and control possible? *Respiratory Care,* 1986, *31,* 113–116.

Lusby, G., & Schietinger, H. *Infection precautions for people with AIDS living in the community.* San Francisco, Ca.: San Francisco Gay Men's Health Crisis, Department of Education, 1984.

Marwick, C. AIDS-associated virus yields data to intensifying scientific study. *JAMA,* 1985, *254*: 2865–2870.

The HTLV-III Information Center. *Working safely in the AIDS environment.* North Chicago, Illinois: Abbott Laboratories Diagnostics Division, 1986.

The HTLV-III Information Center. *The diagnosis and management of patients with HTLV-III-related disease.* North Chicago, Illinois: Abbott Laboratories Diagnostics Division, 1986.

The HTLV-III Information Center. *The etiology and epidemiology of HTLV-III-related disease.* North Chicago, Illinois: Abbott Laboratories Diagnostics Division, 1986.

Turner, J.G., & Williamson, K.M. AIDS: A challenge for contemporary nursing, Part I. *Focus on Critical Care,* 1986, *13*: 53–61.

Turner, J.G., & Williamson, K.M. AIDS: A challenge for contemporary nursing, Part II. *Focus on Critical Care,* 1986, *13*: 41–49.

U.S. Department of Health and Human Services, Public Health Service. *AIDS Fact Sheet,* 1985.

5

The Future of the Nursing Process

In the preceding chapters it was shown that the development and application of the nursing process within nursing's human need theory provide evidence that this process is vital, ongoing, goal directed, and logical. It is not only oriented to the present, but also to the future. This focus implies a continuum, linking the present to the future in a forward thrust.

The future of the nursing process cannot be predicted with certainty unless the events, trends, and changes of tomorrow are known. Speculations and predictions for mankind will have an impact on how, where, by whom, for whom, and when the nursing process will be utilized.

Future projections about nursing can only be made within the context of the predictions about society, for nursing's purpose and viability directly relate to societal needs for health and nursing care. It follows then that nurses should be aware of what futurists, economists, sociologists, historians, researchers, educators, and nurses have to say about future trends and possibilities. Regardless of the type of future for nursing, the nursing process will serve as a viable tool for rendering nursing; flexibility and adaptability both to clients' requirements for health and nursing care and to health care situations and settings are inherent in the use of the nursing process by academically and experientially qualified practitioners of nursing.

What, then, are some of the predictions stemming from society that will impact on nursing? Specifically, what is the future for areas of economics, population, health, and education? In economics, it is predicted that from now to the year 2025, we will witness superindustrialization, agribusiness (large-scale farming entrepreneurs), a stabilized economy after some fluctuations prior to 1990 and to 2025, heavy reliance on science and technology, urban sprawl, increasing affluence, more stress on egalitarianism, a small work force to supply needs, a time of unprecedented opportunity with maximum responsibility, an expanding economy with money less of a concern, and increased leisure time. In relation to population, it is predicted that there will be decreased population growth, small families, increased aged population, increased life span, increasing proportion of women to men, a rising population of nonwhite persons, lowered fertility, and multiworker families; most women will be in the work force (three-fourths of the married women will be working by 1990 and 65 percent of all women over age 16 will be in the work force). For health, it is predicted that there will be a preventive health care focus, curative advances, increased human–machine communication, proliferation of better standards (for health, safety, food, air, and aesthetic landscaping), increased bioengineering and genetic engineering, increased philosophical and ethical considerations in matters of health, increased requirement for long-term care, rising professional autonomy for health care providers other than physicians, nationalization of health care services, and increasing numbers of health maintenance organizations. In the area of education, it is predicted that there will be a rise of multipurpose universities, higher education for all (academic and technical, lifelong education, articulation of education–industry–military, and expansion of preparation of those to serve society), and increased enrollment of women in higher education. Based on the foregoing, the nurse can speculate on the client population, the descriptive variables inherent in the client, the locus of nursing practice, and the focus for nursing care. Nursing's human need theory framework and the nursing process will frame the mode of professional nursing practice and the inherent data base from which decisions that affect the nurse and the client will be made.

Based on the foregoing predictions to the year 2025 and the current state of nursing, a futuristic portrait for nursing may include autonomy for nurse generalists and nurse specialists; an academic degree in nursing as the credential for practice, education for professional nursing post baccalaureate (akin with other professions); increasing work life for the professional nurse; full professionalization for nursing; assumption by professional nurses of the major portion and responsibility for wellness and illness care; practice by professional nurses in a broad range of settings for service to the person, the family, and the community; assumption of the cost of nursing education by a combination of philanthropy, industry, business, and government rather than as a cost of the health care system; and appointment of an all professional nursing staff for health care agencies. Time will tell if these predictions will be realized. Nurses are and will continue to be engaged in planning for a *preferred* future for nursing rather than accept an imposed future or one in which nursing mainly responds to external occurrences. Since the future begins with tomorrow, it is important that nursing specify its future goals now so that strategies and their target dates can be determined to realize these goals. As for the immediate future, what are the major health concerns for the 1990s?

Each person, whether a professional in the health field or a layman, can form a list of anticipated major health problems. It seems clear that among the continuing health problems in the United States are the following: (a) AIDS and AIDS-related complex (ARC)—because AIDS carries a 100 percent mortality rate, fear and stigma are associated with the disease and people who have it. The impact of the AIDS virus on the immune system of its victims leave them vulnerable to a host of infections. The transmission of the virus and the vulnerability of populations are critical health and nursing issues that will require immediate attention and ongoing concerns for the decades ahead. (b) Drugs and alcohol—persons who take drugs, the care of persons who use drugs, and the reasons drugs and alcohol are used are of major concern. What makes a person, regardless of age, turn to drugs? Finding answers to this question as well as coping with the problems created by the users are the major challenges of our time. (c) Pollution—air, water, land; contributing to this problem is that of overpopulation and the poor distribution of population. As more people occupy the earth, the amount of waste increases (liquid, solid, and gaseous). Crowding creates noise pollution; the metabolic processes of increasing numbers of people create more body waste and increased food consumption creates more garbage. Each of these factors contributes to mental and physical health problems.

The rising cost of health care is another of the major problems. It is receiving much thought from many politicians, both candidates and elected officials. The debate about the involvement of the federal government contains vital issues to be resolved: the never-ending questions about the extent to which the federal government should or should not be involved in financing health care, the manner in which the state and federal governments should be responsible or share responsibility, and how they can do this without usurping the responsibility of local governments.

Continuing technical advancement without concomitant development of (or with the lagging development of) the philosophical, ethical, and moral implications of these advances are already presenting problems that may increase in the future. The impact of these developments on human beings and the environment, particularly those relating to genetic engineering, to the supply and distribution of body organs, to biomechanical organs and body parts, and designation of the time of death, are difficult questions to be answered; the term "sobering" may more accurately describe them. The prevention of illness continues to be emphasized as well as the curative and rehabilitative aspects of care.

How do these relate to the nursing process? These are and continue to be among the issues pertinent to nursing and necessary to the nursing process. For example, with emphasis on economics and on providing quality health care for the consumer of health services, a major issue will be the number of personnel needed, the kind of personnel, their training and education, their roles in health care, and their responsibilities. Are enough persons entering the arena of nursing? Can the consumer of nursing expect that academically and experientially qualified nurses will be available to provide nursing care in complex human situations and conditions? in a variety of settings? for clients well or ill?

The United States possesses some of the best health resources in the world. Yet there are some persons in this country whose health is compromised owing to a lack of educational, economical, and personal resources, and health care. There are nations where only 5 percent of the national income goes to 20 percent of its families at the lowest end of the economic ladder, where malnutrition is a major problem, where care and inoculations are unknown. Rectifying these conditions is an ongoing challenge.

The future of the nursing process can be seen from five points of view:

1. Continuing development and refinement of the process within nursing's human need theory.
2. Contribution toward the growth and development of the profession of nursing through its use.
3. The basis for the use of the nursing process in the development of nursing science through the testing of nursing's human need theory—the definitions, the models, the assumptions.
4. Influences on personal and professional growth and the development of users of the nursing process.
5. Improvement of the health status of recipients of the process.

Deliberate use of the nursing process by nursing practitioners will contribute to the refinement of its component elements and the expansion of the utilization of nursing's human need theory. Improved history taking; development of tools to amass data about the client's status of human need fulfillment; more accurate nursing diagnoses; more effective priority setting; improved design of nursing care plans; more astute specifications of goals with expected client behavioral outcomes; more effective recording of observations about the client; more sensible, purposeful, and effective nurse actions; more emphasis on evaluation as well as on the development of tools for evaluation; and better judgment concerning what to communicate to whom, and when to communicate and how; all are goals of the continuing development of the nursing process.

Numerous authors have developed tools and techniques that are incorporated into the nursing process. Continuing development, testing, and refinement of these tools in a variety of health care settings with the nurse and other nursing and health team members are in order. Formulating a theoretical base for shortening the time lag between the discovery of a new method, or of new knowledge, and its incorporation into nursing practice deserves serious attention in the formulation of a theoretical framework for applying the nursing process.

The contribution of the nursing process to growth and development of the profession of nursing is easily evidenced. Because the heart of the nursing practice is the designation and solution of client problems, nursing's human need theory and other theories or scientific materials developed to explain, direct, or influence nursing practice will contribute to the quality of care rendered to the client and hence will advance the profession and sanction its places as designated by society. Well-designed and complete nursing care plans contribute a wealth of data about clients, their problems, solutions to those problems, and the effectiveness of these solutions. Research is inherent in the process. Hunches, observations, and speculations lend themselves to further research and testing. The careful, analytical extraction and testing of data will contribute to the validation of nursing's human need theory. Nursing histories with associated observations, potential and actual nursing diagnoses, and available nursing care plans can be used to develop model care plans for any person in any particular setting, of any particular age, with any particular problem, having certain resources.

In 1926, Bertha Harmer suggested that nurses retain the written care plans they develop for clients and cluster these plans according to a classification of diseases. Her idea was that nurses could then have available to them organized knowledge that would provide a data base about nursing–client care, would enable review for client progress as well as review for adequacy of nurse actions. Harmer stressed ". . . to compare facts presented for the study of a great many cases of the same class, and of different classes, and to select facts common to all cases of the same class; in other words, to formulate principles, to organize knowledge—the process of making knowledge, which is science."[1]

How challenging is this idea in the 1980s? Are there data available to nurses that are not being used as a data base for studying client care?

Can nursing diagnoses clusters substitute for the "classification of diseases" suggested by Harmer and can this proposal made in the 1920s be pursued by the nurse clinician today?

When considering the influence of the nursing process on the nurse's personal and professional growth and development, a few topics can be considered. For example, the nursing process as a process and functional entity should be a major component of continuing education, which would include its present use as well as additional areas for use in a practice setting. The problem solving that results from the nursing process is a fruitful area, replete with a multitude of situations that could be shared with colleagues for their enlightenment and reaction.

The nursing process lends itself to the nurse's own quest for self-improvement. Continuous evaluation of intellectual, interpersonal, and technical skills and perceptual, communicative, and decision-making abilities will reveal strengths and limitations. Interest in enhancing strengths and minimizing limitations gives direction for study and for the selection of programs, workshops, and professional associations and interactions. Increasing accuracy in problem solving and in predicting the impact on client behavior are important factors in experiencing success in nursing practice. The continuing focus on self-improvement results in the better use of self and in improved contribution to citizens. The nursing process, therefore, can be viewed as an effective method to prevent and minimize obsolescence.

The client will benefit most from a nurse who is knowledgeable, confident, creative, and person-family-community-centered. Whether the client's situation demands that wellness be maintained, care be given during acute or chronic illness, or compassionate support rendered if the client is dying, the client will receive the best care the nurse has to offer. The nurse, too, will be stimulated to continue his or her self-development as the feeling of accomplishment from giving one's best is reaped. Inherent in this feeling of success is a realistic appraisal of oneself and the client situation. It involves being able to accept a setback without being unduly crushed, being able to strive forward despite odds, and being convinced that one's contribution is the best that can be given at a particular time.

The client further benefits by active participation in the identification and resolution of problems. It enhances the client's personhood, membership in a family structure, participation in the community, desire to remain a thinking and feeling person whether well or ill, and to maximize the wellness although he or she is afflicted by some disability.

The nursing process contributes to the nurse's feeling of camaraderie with other members of the health team. The nurse values contributions made and enhances the success of the health professionals by sharing his or her perceptions and goals for the client. A nurse's success is, in turn, enhanced by the nurse being open and receptive to suggestions of other nursing and health team members. The nursing process within nursing's human need theory serves as a communication medium for international nursing interactions, associations, and research.

Inherent in each deliberation about the future of the nursing process is the research process. Presently, the requirement for clinical research is generally recognized by practitioners of nursing, and the quantity and quality of clinical nursing research will predictably improve in the next decade. There is a need for a body of facts and a set of probabilities to guide or assess the nursing care of citizens. A clear knowledge of both the differences in the benefits to the client from nursing interventions and the establishment of means to assess the results of varied interventions are based on sound research.

Research plays an important role in the development and refinement of the nursing process, the validation of nursing's human need theory and contributes to the development of nursing science. Sharing the results of research can benefit the nurse and client directly. The nursing process opens the way for research not only into a multitute of problems but also into each component with each of its elements, which is itself a fruitful area for research. For example, the identification of nursing diagnoses may be viewed as first-level theory development as specified by Dickoff et al. and Kritek.[2,3] Nursing diagnoses may be utilized as hypotheses for testing.

Any of the following studies, as well as a multitude of others, can be undertaken with the hope that the results would contribute to the continuing development of the nursing process within nursing's human need theory framework, constitute a nursing science, and contribute to an increase in the caliber of care rendered to citizens:

1. Comparative studies of nursing histories taken by nurses using nursing's human need theory framework.
2. Studies of the utilization of the nursing history and health assessment in formulating judgments about the wellness state and potential and/or actual nursing diagnoses.
3. Studies of the client's reaction to self-completion of the nursing history form based on the 35 human needs, with and without personal interview.
4. Studies to develop and test assessment tools for each of the 35 human needs—considering variables of age, gender, stage of growth and development, culture, etc.
5. Studies of what constitutes the data base to support the making of a nursing diagnosis for the client; comparative studies

contrasting the data base and nursing diagnosis (diagnoses) made by nurses with a baccalaureate, masters, and the doctoral degrees in nursing.

6. Studies of the goal statements with behavioral outcomes made by nurses in varying settings and with different experiences.

7. Studies of whether or not a selected number of nurses, given the same set of data, would make the same nursing diagnoses; if variation, then studies of this variation according to education, experience, and culture of the nurses.

8. Studies to determine why the nurse selects a particular strategy or action for a client to achieve a stated goal with behavioral outcomes.

9. Studies of how different citizens with a similar health problem resolve problems related to human need fulfillment.

10. Studies of varying patterns of problem resolution according to age, gender, geographic location, socioeconomic level, and educational and cultural backgrounds.

11. Studies to analyze the first encounter of the nurse and client in terms of why the client sought out the nurse; studies to determine if the nurse was the first member of the health team to enter the client into the health care system or if the encounter resulted from the client's prior interaction with a physician or other health team member.

12. Studies to define the client's role in the development of the nursing care plan.

13. Studies to determine factors that comprise the rationale for setting priorities for client problems (nursing diagnoses); a study of whether this priority setting is affected by differences in the nurse's education and experience and those of the client; comparative studies of priority setting for client problems, as designated by the nurse and the client; if conflict in priority setting, a study of the factors inherent in the conflict.

14. When eliciting solutions to client problems (nursing diagnoses), studies to determine how to recognize the best solution.

15. Studies to determine factors inherent in the nurse's decision to refer or not refer a client problem to another health care professional or agency.

16. Studies utilizing the nursing diagnosis as an hypothesis within the nursing's human need theoretical framework of human needs to test if nursing intervention makes a difference in offsetting a human need fulfillment alteration.

17. Studies of perceptions and observations about the client that are recorded and shared in contrast to those withheld; analyti-

cal studies of the data withheld and the rationale for withholding them; comparative studies of the nurse's baccalaureate, master's, and doctoral education and experience in contrast to the quantity and quality of data withheld.

18. Studies to determine variations of and common solutions made by nurses in different settings when confronted with a given client problem, a designated number of staff, and selected equipment and supplies.

19. A study of the rationale for delegating actions to be performed by members of the nursing team rather than by one nurse.

20. Studies of the impact of agency policies on the number, kinds, and quality of decisions made by the nurse relative to assessing, planning, implementing, and evaluating nursing care.

21. Studies to develop tools to evaluate the impact of nurse actions on client behavior.

22. Studies to determine the client's role in evaluating the nursing care rendered.

23. Studies of the impact of the client's evaluation on subsequent nurse actions designated to solve problems.

24. Studies of how effectively nurses evaluate nursing care in relation to goal designation and goal achievement.

25. Studies to determine the extent to which nurses transfer or reproduce decisions utilized in one situation to another.

26. Studies of inherent factors in a situation that foster or deter the transfer or reproduction of decisions.

27. Studies to determine why, when, what, and how nurses use research findings and incorporate them into their use of the nursing process.

In addition to these recommended research studies, it is imperative that nurses use the research findings related to human needs and human behavior, and incorporate these into nursing practice.

The basic thrust for the decades ahead will be the increased interest and effort in nursing theory development. Nursing's human need theory will provide the arena for the use of the nursing process, and the human needs framework will further serve as the system for classifying nursing diagnoses. Human need theory will be a viable entity within which the nursing process will be used; it will also serve as an adjunct to nursing theories currently under development. The adaptation and development of the human need theory framework and the nursing process constitute the most complete, usable nursing theory to date. Further, the theoretical framework and process have the substance for continued theory development and can operationalize other nursing theories being developed at the present time by a number of nurse scholars.

Support is increasing for direct access to nursing by the client and for direct payment by private and public third-party payers to qualified nurses for nursing care rendered to clients and their families. Direct payment to qualified nurses is long overdue. Mastery of the use of the nursing process should be the basis for fair payment for nursing services rendered. The nursing process can provide the framework for designation of costs and fees, cost-effective accounting, and for overall accountability for nursing care provided.

Through the use of the nursing process nurses can demonstrate their commitment to (1) care for the aged and terminally ill clients, (2) improve the care and services to well elderly persons, (3) participate actively with health care professionals and parents in planning and meeting the needs of mothers and children, and (4) more fully exercise their advocacy role.

The nursing process can serve as the core for efforts to utilize computer technology both to enhance communication among professional nurses and to maximize and effectively utilize client care data. "The use of computers heralds the need to define the nursing data base needed to assess, plan, implement, and evaluate patient care."[4] Computer information systems presently in use and the speculation regarding the sophistication of systems for the future necessitate that the nurse become knowledgeable about the realities and possibilities of computerized information systems to facilitate client care and nursing research. McCormick discusses the three parts of nursing data available in a fully computerized nursing record, namely, (1) nursing data as observations and procedures done in response to medical orders as nursing's interdependent function; (2) nursing data resulting from the nursing process which includes assessment, actions, and outcome data (the nursing diagnosis is a component of this independent nursing component), and (3) nursing data which exists as an interrelationship between physician-driven nursing documentation and independent nursing process recording.[5] Romano describes the computerized data base developed by the nursing department for the Clinical Center Medical Information System at the National Institutes of Health in Bethesda, Maryland. The model developed reflects interdependent nursing interventions, independent nursing interventions, and the interaction between them. The independent nursing judgments are those which encompass health problems that the nurse has independently identified, influenced, or resolved and those nursing interventions which differ yet complement the medical treatment but are carried out by the nurse. The concepts on which these data were developed encompass the nursing process and human need theory. Human needs are the focus for nursing care and these human needs are organized in categories to provide a systematic method of improving assessment and communication.[6] This model reinforces the utility of the logical, goal-directed nursing process and the viability of the human need theory framework for the use of the nursing process with the outcome of goal-oriented holistic health care for the client. Nursing's human need theory framework and the nursing process will not only be enhanced by the use of computer technology but will increase the use of and value of computer data systems for health and nursing care.

Improvement of the public image of nursing will come about, in part, through the use of the nursing process and the focus on human need fulfillment, for it is in this framework that nurses have the means to explain the practice of nursing. The public understands human needs, their fulfillment, and the results of alterations in need fulfillment. That nurses make a difference in assuring human need fulfillment for the public who are clients of nursing should be propagated widely so that what nurses do and how the public views nursing are congruent. Kalisch and Kalisch are eloquent in their efforts to establish the current state of the public image of the nurse and to determine the "role the news media plays in informing the public of the existence and effectiveness of nursing and building mass consensus for resources to support and advance its services. The manner in which the public thinks of nurses will strongly influence the destiny of nursing and the contribution that nurses can make."[7]

Nursing will be different in the 21st century. Observing the changes and challenges of the 1990s will enable nurses and nursing to be prepared for a new arena of health care delivery in the future.

Based upon the current activities in nursing, the following will probably be addressed in the nursing profession of the future:

- Will the B.S.N. degree be the required entry level for professional nursing? Will there be two levels of nursing? Under what titles?
- Will "new" theoretical–conceptual structures be proposed?
- Will those theoretical–conceptual structures already reported be adjusted or altered based on the results of systematic studies?
- How successful will nurses be in applying the already defined theoretical–conceptual structures?
- Will some or several of the theoretical–conceptual frameworks merge to cluster ideas and concepts into more comprehensive theories?
- Will pluralism be the thrust for nursing theory development?
- Will the science of nursing be enunciated with limited ambiguity?
- How influential will nurses be in the legislative arena?
- Will the voices of nursing make a difference in achieving equitable pay for nursing in various health care settings?

- Will the roles of nursing be clearly identified in the arenas of health maintenance and care during illness?
- Will the Diagnostic Related Groups (DRGs) continue in effect? What will be the future impact on nursing of these DRGs? Will fewer nurses be needed in acute care facilities?
- What will be the position of nursing in long-term care facilities?
- Will nursing be given the power and the authority to function autonomously in the care of the chronically ill?
- Will health care regulations be sufficiently flexible to enable nurses to use professional knowledge to exercise professional judgment in the care of the elderly?
- Will there be enough nurses, in sufficient numbers, with adequate preparation to become successful entrepreneurs and provide health to a selected population of citizens?
- Will ethical dilemmas be resolved through interdisciplinary teams?
- Will nursing have a significant voice in addressing the ethical problems encountered in health care?
- Will the legal dimensions of nursing and health care become more or less complex?
- Will licensure of professional nurses be clarified?
- Will certification of professional nurses in a selected specialty become more widespread; will salaries, status, positions in nursing reflect the education, experience, and professional recognition of the individual nurse?
- How will computers change nursing?
- Will automation of records enable nurses to concentrate on the intellectual and interpersonal aspects of nursing?
- How rapidly will nurses become more efficient through the use of computers?
- How soon will nurses accept the change to computers in various health care settings?
- Will the use of nursing research and systematic clinical studies in nursing make a difference in client care? What difference?
- Will the cost effectiveness of the use of the nursing process be demonstrated? be recognized?
- How rapidly and with what impact will there be full utilization of home health care; hospice care; ambulatory care? What will be the role of the nurse in these settings?
- What will be the role of the nurse in the presence of the advances in noninvasive technologies?
- Will the increase in legal actions and emphasis on malpractice activities change the nurse's relationships with clients? How?

- What will be the image of the nurse in the 21st century? How will it differ from that of earlier years?

Considering the data available to determine the present state of nursing and to project the future for nurses and nursing, it appears that nurses will be intellectually, interpersonally, and technically involved in fostering human need fulfillment for those members of society who are the clients of nursing. The nursing process within nursing's human need theory framework is the key to quality nursing practice for the present and the future.

REFERENCES

1. Harmer, B. *Methods and principles of teaching the principles and practice of nursing.* New York: Macmillan, 1926.
2. Dickoff, J., James, P., & Wiedenbach, E. Theory in a practice discipline: Part I. Practice oriented theory. *Nursing Research*, 1968, *17*, 415–433.
3. Kritek, P. The generation and classification of nursing diagnoses: Toward a theory of nursing. *Image*, 1978, *10*, 33–40.
4. Romano, C. Documentation of nursing practice using a computerized medical information system. In H. G. Heffernan (Ed.). *Proceedings, Fifth Annual Symposium on Computer Applications in Medical Care.* Los Angeles: IEEE Computer Society, 1981, pp. 746–749.
5. McCormick, K. Nursing research using computerized data base. *Ibid*, pp. 749–752.
6. Romano, *op cit.*
7. Kalisch, P., & Kalisch, B. Perspectives on improving nursing's public image. *Nursing and Health Care*, August 1980, *1*(14), 10–15.

Additional References

Naisbitt, J. *Megatrends.* New York, Warner Communications Company, 1984.
Toffler, A. *Previews and premises.* New York, Bantam Books, 1983.

National and International Codes for Nurses

THE CODE FOR NURSES (NATIONAL)*

1. The nurse provides services with respect for human dignity and the uniqueness of the client unrestricted by considerations of social or economic status, personal attributes, or the nature of the health problems.
2. The nurse safeguards the client's right to privacy by judiciously protecting information of a confidential nature.
3. The nurse acts to safeguard the client and the public when health care and safety are affected by the incompetent, unethical, or illegal practice of any person.
4. The nurse assumes responsibility and accountability for individual nursing judgments and actions.
5. The nurse maintains competence in nursing.
6. The nurse exercises informed judgment and uses individual competence and qualifications as criteria in seeking consultation, accepting responsibilities, and delegating nursing activities to others.
7. The nurse participates in activities that contribute to the ongoing development of the profession's body of knowledge.
8. The nurse participates in the profession's efforts to establish, implement and improve standards of nursing.
9. The nurse participates in the profession's efforts to establish and maintain conditions of employment conducive to high quality nursing care.

*Source: American Nurses' Association. (1985). *Code for nurses with interpretive statements.* Kansas City, Mo.: American Nurses' Association.

10. The nurse participates in the profession's effort to protect the public from misinformation and misrepresentation and to maintain the integrity of nursing.
11. The nurse collaborates with members of the health professions and other citizens in promoting community and national efforts to meet the health needs of the public.

THE CODE FOR NURSES (INTERNATIONAL)*

The fundamental responsibility of the nurse is fourfold: to promote health, to prevent illness, to restore health, and to alleviate suffering.

The need for nursing is universal. Inherent in nursing is respect for life, dignity, and rights of man. It is unrestricted by considerations of nationality, race, creed, color, age, sex, politics, or social status.

Nurses render health services to the individual, the family, and the community and coordinate their services with those of related groups.

Nurses and People

The nurse's primary responsibility is to those people who require nursing care. The nurse, in providing care, respects the beliefs, values, and customs of the individual. The nurse holds in confidence personal information and uses judgment in sharing this information.

Nurses and Practice

The nurse carries personal responsibility for nursing practice and for maintaining competence by continual learning. The nurse maintains the highest standards of nursing care possible within the reality of a specific situation. The nurse uses judgment in relation to individual competence when accepting and delegating responsibilities. The nurse, when acting in a professional capacity, should at all times maintain standards of personal conduct that would reflect credit on the profession.

Nurses and Society

The nurse shares with other citizens the responsibility for initiating and supporting action to meet the health and social needs of the public.

Nurses and Co-workers

The nurse sustains a cooperative relationship with co-workers in nursing and other fields. The nurse takes appropriate action to safeguard

---

*International Council of Nurses' Nursing Code approved by the Council of National Representatives (CNR), Mexico, 1973.

the individual when his or her care is endangered by a co-worker or any other person.

Nurses and the Profession

The nurse plays the major role in determining and implementing desirable standards of nursing practice and nursing education. The nurse is active in developing a core of professional knowledge. The nurse, acting through the professional organization, participates in establishing and maintaining equitable social and economic working conditions in nursing.

B

Standards of Nursing Practice*

Standard I. The Collection of Data about the Health Status of the Client/Patient Is Systematic and Continuous. The Data Are Accessible, Communicated, and Recorded

Rationale. Comprehensive care requires complete and ongoing collection of data about the client/patient to determine the nursing care needs of the client/patient. All health status data about the client/patient must be available for all members of the health care team.

Assessment Factors

1. Health status data include growth and development; biophysical status; emotional status; cultural, religious, socioeconomic background; performance of activities of daily living; patterns of coping; interaction patterns; client's/patient's perception of and satisfaction with his or her health status; client/patient health goals; environment (physical, social, emotional, ecological); and available and accessible human and material resources.
2. Data are collected from client/patient, family, significant others; health care personnel; and individuals within the immediate environment and/or the community.
3. Data are obtained by interview; examination; observation; and reading records, reports, etc.

*Reprinted with permission from American Nurses' Association. *Standards of Practice*. Kansas City, Mo.: American Nurses' Association, 1973.

4. There is a format for the collection of data that provides for a systematic collection of data and facilitates the completeness of data collection.
5. Continuous collection of data is evident by frequent updating and recording of changes in health status.
6. The data are accessible on the client/patient records; retrievable from record-keeping systems; and confidential when appropriate.

Standard II. Nursing Diagnoses Are Derived From Health Status Data

Rationale. The health status of the client/patient is the basis for determining the nursing care needs. The data are analyzed and compared to norms when possible.

Assessment Factors

1. The client's/patient's health status is compared to the norm to determine if there is a deviation from the norm and the degree and direction of deviation.
2. The client's/patient's capabilities and limitations are identified.
3. The nursing diagnoses are related to and congruent with the diagnoses of all other professionals caring for the client/patient.

Standard III. The Plan of Nursing Care Includes Goals Derived From the Nursing Diagnoses

Rationale. The determination of the results to be achieved is an essential part of planning care.

Assessment Factors

1. Goals are mutually set with the client/patient and pertinent others. They are congruent with other planned therapies; they are stated in realistic and measurable terms; they are assigned a time period for achievement.
2. Goals are established to maximize functional capabilities and are congruent with growth and development; biophysical status; behavioral patterns; and human and material resources.

Standard IV. The Plan of Nursing Care Includes Priorities and the Prescribed Nursing Approaches or Measures to Achieve the Goals Derived From the Nursing Diagnoses

Rationale. Nursing actions are planned to promote, maintain, and restore the client's/patient's well-being.

Assessment Factors

1. Physiologic measures are planned to manage (prevent or control) specific patient problems and are related to the nursing diagnoses and goals of care, e.g., ADL, use of self-help devices.
2. Psychosocial measures are specific to the client's/patient's nursing care problem and to the nursing care goals, e.g., techniques to control aggression, motivation.
3. Teaching-learning principles are incorporated into the plan of care and objectives for learning stated in behavioral terms, e.g., specification of content for learner's level, reinforcement, readiness.
4. Approaches are planned to provide for a therapeutic environment:
   Physical environmental factors are used to influence the therapeutic environment, e.g., control of noise, control of temperature.
   Psychosocial measures are used to structure the environment for therapeutic ends, e.g., paternal participation in all phases of the maternity experience.
   Group behaviors are used to structure interaction and influence the therapeutic environment, e.g., conformity, ethos, territorial rights, locomotion.
5. Approaches are specified for orientation of the client/patient to new roles and relationships; relevant health (human and material) resources; modifications in plan of nursing care; and relationship of modifications in nursing care plan to the total care plan.
6. The plan of nursing care includes the use of available and appropriate resources:
   Human resources—other health personnel
   Material resources
   Community.
7. The plan includes an ordered sequence of nursing actions.
8. Nursing approaches are planned on the basis of current scientific knowledge.

Standard V. Nursing Actions Provide for Client/Patient Participation in Health Promotion, Maintenance, and Restoration

Rationale. The client/patient and the family are continually involved in nursing care.

Assessment Factors

1. The client/patient and the family are kept informed about current health status; changes in health status; total health care plan; nursing care plan; roles of health care personnel; and health care resources.
2. The client/patient and the family are provided with the information needed to make decisions and choices about promoting, maintaining, and restoring health; seeking and using appropriate health care personnel; and maintaining and using health care resources.

Standard VI. Nursing Actions Assist the Client/Patient to Maximize His or Her Health Capabilities

Rationale. Nursing actions are designed to promote, maintain, and restore health.

Assessment Factors

1. Nursing actions are consistent with the plan of care; are based on scientific principles; are individualized to the specific situation; are used to provide a safe and therapeutic environment; employ teaching-learning opportunities for the client/patient; and include utilization of appropriate resources.
2. Nursing actions are directed by the client's/patient's physical, physiologic, psychological, and social behavior associated with ingestion of food, fluid and nutrients; elimination of body wastes and excesses in fluid; locomotion and exercise; regulatory mechanisms—body heat, metabolism; relating to others; and self-actualization.

Standard VII. The Client's/Patient's Progress or Lack of Progress Toward Goal Achievement Is Determined by the Client/Patient and the Nurse

Rationale. The quality of nursing care depends on comprehensive and intelligent determination of nursing's impact upon the health status of the client/patient. The client/patient is an essential part of this determination.

Assessment Factors

1. Current data about the client/patient are used to measure his or her progress toward goal achievement.
2. Nursing actions are analyzed for their effectiveness in the goal achievement of the client/patient.
3. The client/patient evaluates nursing actions and goal achievement.
4. Provision is made for nursing follow-up of a particular client/patient to determine the long-term effects of nursing care.

Standard VIII. The Client's/Patient's Progress or Lack of Progress Toward Goal Achievement Directs Reassessment, Reordering of Priorities, New Goal Setting, and Revision of the Plan of Nursing Care

Rationale. The nursing process remains the same, but the input of new information may dictate new or revised approaches.

Assessment Factors

1. Reassessment is directed by goal achievement or lack of goal achievement.
2. New priorities and goals are determined and additional nursing approaches are prescribed appropriately.
3. New nursing actions are accurately and appropriately initiated.

C

Selected Observations Made Using Four Senses

The following is a list of observations that can be made by the nurse through the use of the four senses—seeing, hearing, smelling, and touching.

I. OBSERVATIONS MADE BY SEEING

A. The Client

1. **General appearance and visible mood expression.** Male, female, infant, child, adolescent, young adult, middle-aged adult, older adult, aged, estimation of age, age appropriateness, younger appearing, older appearing, clean, unkempt, tall, slim, short, malnourished, obese, plump, wasting, lean, emaciated, well nourished, gigantism, dwarfism, thin, sad, happy, bored, anxious, fearful, eager, alert, flat affect, Down's syndrome, hostile, suspicious, attentive, sleepy, staring, tearful, frowning, inattentive, nervous, depressed, hyperactive, hyperalert, conscious, preoccupied, distressed, jittery, crying, disoriented, clowning, comatose, unconscious, nonresponsive, stuporous, weak, appearing ill
2. **Visible physical factors**
   a. *Head and neck area:* Macrocephalic, microcephalic, normocephalic, goiter, tumors, swelling, infections, tics, fontanels—bulging, pulsating, closed; paralysis, stiffness, congenital malformations, scars, hematoma, moonface, mask of pregnancy
   b. *Hair:* Amount, distribution—male, female, adult, child, normal, sparse, unusual hairiness, complete baldness, bald spots; texture—fine, coarse, brittle, split ends; color—natural, dyed; baldness—scattered, circumscribed, extensive; long, short, straight,

braided, curled, coiffured, bearded, mustache, simply combed, unkempt, oily, lice, ringworm, hair cosmetics and jewelry, hairpieces, wigs, dandruff

c. *Eyes:* Strabismus, tearing, swollen lids, stye, ecchymotic, conjunctiva—shiny, red, moist, smooth, clear, reddened, irritated; restricted or uneven eye movements; eye makeup; shaggy eyebrows, tweezed eyebrows, ptosis of lids—symmetrical, unequal; bulging eyes, slanted eyes, squinting eyes, puffy lids, photophobic eyes, cataracts, blinking, eyeglasses—regular, bifocals, trifocals, sunglasses, reading, tinted, light sensitive; contact lenses, artificial eyes; pupils—regular, irregular, dilated, contracted; blind, twitching, sleeping, squinting

d. *Nose:* Small, pugnosed, enlarged, distorted, draining—mucus, blood, purulent; normal septum, septal deviation; tumors, dilated nares, pinched nares, scabs, crusts, foreign objects

e. *Ears:* Normal, enlarged, small, absent, deformed—congenital, cauliflower; drainage—bloody, purulent, crusting, clotting, waxy; tympanic membrane—glistening, pearly, red, inflamed, ruptured; swelling in front of and/or behind, foreign objects, jewelry—pierced earrings

f. *Lips, mouth, and teeth:* Tongue—smooth, hairy, ulcerated, protruding, tongue-tied, swollen, coated, distorted, lacerated, excised, lesion, short frenulum; lips—moist, parched, fiery red, cracked, lipstick, presence of food, gum, tobacco, toys in mouth; dentures—partial, full; teeth—full dentition, primary, secondary, protruding, missing replaced, missing unreplaced, transplanted, capped, crowned, broken, gold inlay, decayed, loose; stained teeth—tea, coffee, tobacco, drugs; fillings—minimal, copious, crowns, caps, gold; hairlip, cleft palate—repaired, unrepaired; twitching, scars, distorted configuration, malocclusion, chancre, vomiting—projectile; air swallowing, mouth breathing, normal breathing, difficult breathing, drooling; herpes simplex, tumors, swelling, paralysis, lipstick, eating, vomiting, sucking, drinking, yawning, sneezing, sordes, teeth chattering, postnasal drip

g. *Skin:* Clear, full, firm, plump, thin, aged, warm, cold, dirty, crusted, blushing, bruised, cuts, scratches, abrasions, fistulae, ecchymoses, sinuses; elevations—tumors, warts, blisters, boils, carbuncles, abscesses, pimples, pustules, hives, pox, papules; chafed, sunburn, burns, flaking, distribution of fat in and under the skin, facial butterfly lesion, gangrene, necrosis, petechiae, cracks, fissures, peeling, scaly, rashes—circumscribed, profuse, generalized; acne, hemorrhage, scars, keloid, punctures, vaccination scar, venipuncture, venipuncture scars; color—racial, nationality, hereditary; white, yellow, brown, black; pathologic color—jaundice, pallor, too rosy, cyanotic, mottling; goose flesh; infestation—pin worms, lice; drainage—serous, serosanguinous, bloody, mucus, purulent; callouses, corns, bunions, tattoos, hairy, absence of hair, protrusion of veins, network of nestlike veins, attached umbilical cord, healed umbilicus, sweaty, dehydrated; soiled—urine, blood, feces, purulent material, dirt, other substances such as tar, adhesive marks; discolored—gentian violet, potassium permanganate, silver nitrate, tincture of benzoin; presence of powders, pastes, deodorants, jewelry, tumor, hernia, decubitus ulcers, radiation markings, sutures, diaper rash, prickly heat, nails—well groomed, bitten, hangnails, ridges, grooves, absence of nailpolish, artificial, pitting

h. *Posture:* Position; erect, upright, straight without support, unsteady, straight with support—braces, cane, crutches, walker; distorted—kyphosis, lordosis, scoliosis, shoulders curved, stooped, wry neck, wrenched; pacing, rigid, shuffling gait, foot dragging, lame, sitting—legs and feet relaxed, knees crossed, ankles crossed, swinging legs, in chair, on floor, painful, unable to get up from chair or floor, in wheelchair, on edge of bed; dorsal recumbent, side lying, supine, prone, jacknife, opisthotonus, Fowler's, semi-Fowler's, dorsal lithotomy, knee-chest, immobile, mobile; walking—slowly, rapidly, limping; shivering, awkward, kneeling, squatting, jumping, creeping, crawling, running, fainting, sleep walking, convulsing, writhing, unusual position, palsied, shaking chills, stiffness posture of late pregnancy, sleeping soundly, restless; fetal position, immersed in bedclothes, uncovered, still

i. *Extremities:* Extended, paralyzed, flaccid, spastic; absence of portion (fingers, toes) or all of extremity, contractures, clubbing of fingers and toes, foot drop, hand drop, artificial limb, mongoloid palm, asymmetry, extra gluteal fold, wringing hands, tapping feet, kicking, edematous, discolored, crippled, clubfoot, knockknees, varicosities, red and inflamed, hairy; stained extremities—occupational dyes, tar, nicotine; fingernails and toenails—short, manicured, long, dirty, bitten, hangnails, blood blister, cracked, chipped, ridged, pitted, absent; arch supports, corrective shoes, bunions, barefeet, unequal limb length, bow legs, excessive muscle development, minimal muscle development, fissures and cracks between toes and fingers, dislocation, fractures—green stick, compound; gangrene, parts cut out of shoes, bandages, Band Aids, clenched fist, clutching items, clean hands and feet, soiled hands—dirt, blood, body secretions; tremors, trembling, swelling, weak reflexes, exaggerated reflexes, twitching, flapping, picking, pushing, holding, clapping, patting, scratching, touching, frostbitten, left-handed, right-handed, ambidextrous, handshake—firm grip, tense, anxious, loose, too hard, weak, cold, sweating, limp, flaccid, fleeting, hot dry, calloused, unusually soft

j. *Trunk area:* Breathing—rhythmic, arrhythmic, breath-holding, absence of; barrel chest, protruding ribs, absence of rib, scars, tumors, burns, abrasions, lacerations, pulsations, swelling, distortions, fat distribution, discolorations; breasts—developing, mature, child, male, female, enlarged, symmetric, asymmetric, lactating; nipples—normal nonparous, parous, cracked, inverted, bleeding, absence of breast; silicone implantation, surgical alterations; colostomy; gastrostomy, ileostomy; abdomen—flat, protruding, distended, obese, pregnant; scars, striae; back—spina bifida, pilonidal sinus; hemorrhage, incisions, puncture, hernia—umbilical, inguinal, incisional; fetal movements in late pregnancy, intestinal movement, obvious organ enlargement—liver, spleen

k. *Pelvic and genital area:* Male, female, infant, child, adolescent, adult, congenital anomalies, surgical alterations; discharges—normal, pathogenic; tumors, swelling, menstruating, incontinent, infant stool—meconium, yellow, green; bloody urine, urinary dribbling, constipated stool, diarrhea, hemorrhoids, ulcerations, nodules, cysts, cracks, fissures, abscesses, lacerations, abrasions, urine and stool abnormalities—blood (red and tarry), worms, discolored, stones, undigested food; vaginal hemorrhage, bloody show, amniotic fluid, prolapse—uterine, rectal, surgical alterations

3. **Clothing**. Work clothes, fully clad, underclothing, naked, mod clothing, bizarre clothing, summer light clothing, heavy winter clothing—appropriate and inappropriate to climate; heavy socks, multiple pairs of socks, gloves, business dress, uniform, nightwear—pajamas, nightgown; formal evening wear, clean, soiled, wet, buttons and zippers closed, buttons and zippers opened, diaper, bunting, cultural and national variations, religious garb, bedroom slippers, rubbers, boots, masculine clothing, feminine clothing, institutional clothing, personal clothing

4. **Attachments and prostheses.** Jewelry, wedding band, rings, watches, eyeglasses—bifocals, trifocals, sunglasses, tinted glasses; contact lenses, hearing aids, dentures, bridgework, bandages, dressings, slings, colostomy bag, ileostomy bag, pacemaker, artificial limbs, braces, artificial larynx, facial prostheses, catheters—chest, bladder, drains; intubation—gastric, chest, tracheostomy, gastrostomy, intestinal, rectal; dressings—heavy, absorbent, sponges, Band Aid, adhesive butterfly, improvised bandage, ace bandage; support hose, support socks, heel and elbow protectors, restraints, infusions—venous, perito-

neal, dialysis; monitor leads, EEG and EKG lead attachments, blood pressure cuff; crutches, canes, walkers, wheelchair, corrective shoes, urinary bag—internal, external; vaginal pads, tampons, trusses, braces—teeth, extremities, pelvic, back; sutures, casts, compresses, heating pads, hot water bottle

B. External Environment of the Client

1. **Immediate.** Personal possession—wallet, purse, blanket, pictures, luggage, books, newspaper, letters, briefcase, toilet articles, easy chair, denture cup, toys, food, drugs; room—small, large, medium; room location—health care facility, home, school, campus, industry, migrant camp, nursery, clinic, single home, townhouse, high-rise apartment, home for the aged, mobile home, shack, homeless; type of room—bathroom, kitchen, living room, garage; furnishing—type, number, absence of; presence of other persons—parents, husband, wife, children, neighbors, friends, clergy, lawyer, police, other relatives, strangers, co-workers, colleagues, health care personnel, total number of persons

2. **Neighborhood.** Urban, rural, inner city, suburbs, industrial, retirement community, college town, military installation, homeowners, rentals, young adults, river or harbor town, beach, farm, resort, paved, unpaved, lawns, tree-lined streets, absence of shrubbery, successful stores, well-designed store fronts, deteriorated business area, many vacancies, boarded-up store fronts, flowers, shrubs, trees, lawns, dusty, litter, parks, playground; available services within one block or within walking distances—grocery store, supermarket, specialty stores, delicatessen, bakery, laundry and cleaners, bookstore, shoe repair, physician and dentist offices, schools, church, police department, fire department, ambulance service; health care facilities—outpatient and inpatient, public transportation; heavy traffic, light traffic, museums, theaters, liquor stores, cocktail lounges, bars, coffee houses, pool halls, athletic associations, bowling alleys, street lighting, emergency call system, suicide prevention center, lighted hallways, elevators, indoor plumbing, bathroom—individual, shared; refrigerator, disposal of waste—disposals, garbage cans; pets—dogs, cats, other; presence or absence of flies, rodents, mosquitoes, heat, air conditioning, handrailings on stairways, rugs, wooden floors, dirt floors

II. OBSERVATIONS MADE BY HEARING

A. The Client

1. **Voice and speech.** Calm, excited, high pitched, soprano, alto, bass, falsetto, tenor, demanding, verbal messages—expressions of need, problems, hopes, fears, concerns, attitude, pain, verbal expressions

of identification and orientation, complaints and descriptions of pain—local, generalized, sharp, dull, headache, continuing, intermittent, dizziness, nausea, ringing in the ears; expressions of gratitude, disordered thought, disordered verbal content; requests for items, services, people companionship, love, care; soft, inaudible, loud, jargon, crying, laughing, face-to-face conversation, telephone conversation, masculine, feminine, stammering, eructation, hiccough, burping, esophageal speech, unintelligible speech, talkative, strained, whispering, hoarse, stuttering, trembling, tongue-tied, slurred, lisp, gargle, groan, foreign language, snoring, aphasic, singing, grunting, silent, dialect—local, regional, national, vernacular; moaning, muffled, babbling, screeching, gasping

2. **Breathing.** Rhythmic, slow, rapid, shallow, quiet, forced, difficult inhalation, difficult exhalation, deep, stertorous, Cheyne-Stokes, apnea, wheezing, whistling, blowing, diverted through tracheostomy, coughing, sneezing, labored, shallow, vocal vibrations, yawning, gasping, panting, rales, noisy, rattling, sighing, harsh sounds, high-pitched sounds

3. **Heart sounds.** Apex rate—regular beat, irregular beat, tachycardia, bradycardia; murmur, absence of sound, cardiac rub, extra heart sounds; blood pressure—high, low, high diastolic

4. **Abdomen.** Peristalsis—presence of hyperactive, hypoactive, absence of; flatus

B. Environment

1. **Immediate.** Dripping, clicking, sucking, conversation with client and/or in the vicinity of client, traffic, public address system, laughing, absence of sounds; radio, television, phonograph sounds, noises—squeaks, banging, clanging, knocking, dishes, carts, utensils, elevators, stairs

2. **Neighborhood.** Traffic—heavy, light, distressful, ambulance sirens, police sirens, fire engines; trains, airplanes, car horns, animals—dogs, cats, farm animals, birds and wild animals; music—soft, rock and roll, mixed, loud, popular, live, recorded; children's voices, crying, screaming, calling, telephones, knocking, radio and television, phonograph, church bells, industrial sounds, bumping, hammering, sawing, pulling and pushing items and carts

III. OBSERVATIONS MADE BY TOUCHING

A. The Client—body contour, size

1. **Head.** Hair—dry, coarse, soft, fine, baby fine; fontanels—soft, closed, bulging; lumps, swelling; forehead—warm, cold, moist

2. **Skin.** Smooth, clammy, rough, moist, dry, lumps, fat distribution, tumors, warts, moles, abscesses, edema, cold, cool, warm, hot; pul-

sations—regular, irregular, intermittent, strong, forceful, bounding, weak, scarcely perceptible, thready; goose flesh, painful, swelling
3. **Chest.** Expansion and relaxation, masses, painful areas, breast—lumps, engorged, size, scar, tender, absence of; pulses—brachial, carotid, radial, temporal, femoral, pedal, popliteal, facial; enlarged axillary nodes
4. **Abdomen.** Soft, hard, masses, tumors, distended, flat full urinary bladder, gaseous abdomen, painful, localized swelling, herniation, taut, uterine contractions, scars, palpable stool
5. **Dressings.** Wet, dry
6. **Bedding.** Wet, dry, damp, saturated, warm, cold, smooth, rough, torn, size, absent
7. **Muscle.** Tension, relaxation, throbbing, chills, twitching, spasm, convulsing, tremors, tumors, tics, firmness and fit of prostheses

B. Environment

Temperature and humidity of immediate environment, outdoor temperature and humidity; presence or absence of supports and railings, fences, bedsides

IV. OBSERVATIONS MADE BY SMELLING

A. The Client

Perspiration, body odor, foot odor, axillary odor, pubic odor, hair odor—oily, perfumes, hairdressing; breath odor—sweet, alcohol, musty, tobacco, onion, garlic, commercial gargles, fetid, spicy, aromatic, pungent; bodily discharges—feces, urine, vomitus, purulent, necrotic, burned skin, burned or singed hair; use of chemicals—iodoform, liniments, ointments, anesthetics, antiseptics, deodorant, soap; absence of odors, unidentified odors

B. Environment

Food odors—vegetables, fruits, meat, charcoal pit, barbecue, condiments, spices, coffee, restaurant odor, bakery, decaying food; exhaust—traffic, industrial odors, hospital odors, burning leaves, marijuana, gas odors; odor of deodorants—pine oil, lysol, soap, peppermint; laboratory odors—antiseptics, cleaning materials, sprays; flowers; shrubs, hay, mowed lawn, farm odors, animal odors—skunk, dog, cat, horse; absence of odors, unidentified odors

D

Selected Data That Describe Fulfilled Human Needs

SELECTED DATA ABOUT EACH HUMAN NEED

This selection was intended to provide a data base for caregivers to use in the development of care plans and in the implementation of activities that will assist persons to meet their human needs. This selection was not meant to be exhaustive in its application to the human situation. Readers are encouraged to expand the data base, incorporating variables such as age, growth and development level, gender. Furthermore, readers may wish to organize these data according to Objective/Subjective labels for their own use in clinical applications.

1. Human Need for Acceptance of Self and Others, by Others

Maintains good eye contact; can focus on another in conversation and interactions.
States feeling content and satisfied with self.
Verbalizes virtues and faults; strengths and limitations.
Cognitive understanding of and personal comfort with own biorhythms.
Receptiveness to what is new and different about self and others.
States enjoys being with other people, likes people.
States interest in self and self-improvement, own welfare.
Able to share; engage in "give and take."
Animated happy expression when in presence of significant others.
Names a family member or friend who would care for client if needed.
Speaks favorably when speaking of others.

The authors gratefully acknowledge the contributions of Graduate Nursing Students enrolled in Nurse 610, School of Nursing, Old Dominion University, Norfolk, Virginia.

Shares positive valuing and concern for self with others.

Significant others voice positive regard about client.

States membership participation in church, work, profession, and community organizations.

Talks readily about happenings in association with members of church, work, profession, and community groups.

Speaks favorably of participants/members of activities/groups.

Members give positive support to client and relate time spent together.

States solitude appreciated occasionally.

2. Human Need for Activity

Evidence of well-conditioned body.

Well-developed muscles and significant muscle tone.

Ambulates with no obvious difficulty—cardiovascular, respiratory, neurologic, musculoskeletal fitness.

Ambulation without pulse going above 80.

Uses good body mechanics for pushing and lifting.

Aware of hazards of inactivity.

Is gainfully employed; is a homemaker; does volunteer work.

Describes exercise program, including range of daily, weekly activity.

States ability to participate in most activities without any limitations.

States engaging in a physical activity known to stimulate the cardiorespiratory system.

Plans a warm-up and a cool-down period for each exercise session.

States intellect and memory kept active, e.g., reads newspaper, books; does crossword and other puzzles; follows discussion and game shows.

3. Human Need for Adaptation, to Manage Stress

Responsive.

Verbalizes stressors.

Able to delineate personal response to stress—physiologic, psychologic, social factors.

Can verbalize those strategies effective in diminishing stress.

Can verbalize those strategies that increase stress reaction.

Can think logically.

Uses positive statements, terms, adjectives when speaking of self.

Verbalizes expectations for the future.

Vital signs in normal range.

Relaxed muscle tension.

Demonstrates facility with relaxation techniques.

Verbalizes participation in recreational, diversional activities for stress management.

No evidence of defeatist statements.

Expresses behavioral adequacy in initiating and maintaining interpersonal relationships.

Adapts to changing family/significant others situation; work situation.

Demonstrates flexibility in role performance with family members/significant others in times of crisis or in emergency situations.

4. Human Need for Air

States has ease of breathing.

No breathing difficulty on exertion.

Works and lives in an environment with adequate air quality.

Even breathing pattern.

Rate of respiration (resting adult)—12 to 14/minute.

Communicates—talks, laughs without respiratory exertion.

Vital capacity in normal range.

No wheezing, gasping; allergen-free air.

No complaint of obstruction in nasal passages, in trachea, in bronchi.

Breathes through nose—soundlessly.

Attends to ventilation for conditioning air—temperature, humidity, motion, free of harmful agents.

Has an efficient coughing, sneezing mechanism.

Maintains good body position to support adequate chest cage movement.

Refrains from use of restrictive clothing that might interfere with breathing.

Protective mucus in normal texture, consistency, and amount.

Clear lung sounds.

Expansion of the chest about 20 percent greater during inspiration than during expiration.

Total volume for adult is 500 ml, age adjusted.

Adults' anatomic dead space in millimeters is approximately equal to the ideal weight in pounds.

Normal fremitus.

Functional diaphragm; diaphragmatic excursion usually 3 to 5 cm.

5. Human Need for Appreciation, Attention

Delineates one or more significant others and describes their attention.

Describes two or more positive personal qualities.

Shows mementos, gifts given in appreciation.

Family members, significant others express critical notice of client's uniqueness and talents.

Can identify events in which family, friends, co-workers have shown gratitude for time and talents given.

Effective use of touch—hugging, "pat on back," hand holding.

Expression of well-being and contentment.

Recipient of thoughtful gestures by family/significant others, colleagues and co-workers.

Enjoys positive response of significant others.

Receives rewards (compliments, promotions, citations, letters of acknowledgement) for behavior; will freely give examples.

6. Human Need for Autonomy, Choice

Expresses strong commitment to achieve personal and health goals.

Independent.

Insightful.

Can deliberate.

States thoughts and feelings do not imitate what others think client should think and feel.

Statements of client begin with "I am," "I feel," "I do," "I will," "I want."

States a goal and mode to achieve same.

Feels comfortable saying "No" when appropriate as well as "Yes."

Can make a choice from a list of alternatives generated by self and others.

Capable of informed consent.

Can adjust consent form to suit self.

Can imagine and recall past experiences.

Can distinguish between and among independency, interdependency, dependency.

Strives for authenticity of self.

Can choose a goal as well as the behaviors and actions to realize the goal.

Is selective in receiving and expressing information.

Demonstrates authenticity in behavior and its expression.

7. Human Need for Beauty and Aesthetic Experiences

Uses vocabulary with words such as "lovely," color, texture, and design.

Artistic.

Expresses admiration and pleasure for persons, events, things.

Describes use of color, shape, design in personal and home furnishings.

Experience of pleasure.

Well-groomed; coordinated appearance.

Arranges environment in accordance with personal view of beauty and esthetics.

Paintings and floral arrangements in environment.

Sensory organs and their functions intact; responds to stimuli generated by color, form, artistic arrangement, texture.

Responds emotionally with surprise, contentment, satisfaction, pleasure.

8. Human Need for Belonging

Describes place and relationship within family, group of significant others.

Verbalizes feelings of belonging and association with others.

Names friends and associates.

Active member in social, church, professional organizations.

Family/significant others express belonging relating with client.

Expresses a sense of "close knitness."

States "somebody cares about me and I care about them."

Participates in family living.

"I have a sense that the things I do contribute to the family organization," "my group of significant others."

Personal response is positive, empathic, decisive in reaching a conclusion. Knows he or she belongs.

Projects positive family image and association with co-workers, colleagues.

Willingly explains interactions with family/significant others.

Actively participates in family functions and functions of significant groups—church, work, professional.

Received rewards from family for behavior and willingly gives examples.

Participates in work unit.

Identifies verbally and nonverbally with his or her work unit.

Verbally states belonging.

Quality of voice radiates conviction—full, radiates strength, positive.

Participates in most social functions at work especially those involving the work unit.

Cooperative.

9. Human Need for Challenge

Can be aroused intellectually, emotionally to take on a task, to reach a goal.

Can describe personal goal achievements.

Discusses involvement and expectation in hobbies, special projects.

"I really enjoy trying to achieve my goal at work."

"I really enjoy my home, my children."

"I seldom feel tired or bored."

Indicates professional and personal goals are actively being pursued.

Responds positively to challenges.

Raises thought-provoking questions.

Animated when discussing involvement in home, family, work, community, church activities.

Current roles and responsibility commensurate with education.

10. Human Need for Conceptualization, Rationality, Problem Solving

Collects data about a problem related to self and circumstances.

Verbalizes personal role in determining state of health.

Verbalizes efforts to advance knowledge base.

Decided to participate in health and nursing care.

Asks questions.

Can state hypotheses.

Can abstract from data and define a problem.

Can give a variety of meanings and definitions to a word.

Seems comfortable with complexity and unsolved problems.

Able to navigate in social situations.

Capable of orienting self to human situation and environment.

Competent in decision making.

Capable of verbalizing a view of self and the world.

Predictable and logical in actions and reactions.

Seen as a person with intellect who seeks meaning and understanding of self and the environment.

Explains one's behavior in a logical manner.

Seeks an explanation of circumstances and the nurse in matters of health.

Recalls and shares familiar, biological, and social history as it relates to matter of health.

Selects to adapt personal life-style to enhance wellness.

Thinks abstractly and formulates images, ideas, concepts.

Perceives relationships among ideas, images, concepts.

Finds meaning in wellness-oriented behavior and activities.

11. Human Need for Confidence

States feels good about what has been accomplished for self and by self.

States trusts professional nurse and health care personnel.

"I rarely flip-flop between decisions once I have made one."

"I am happy with my way of handling my personal and health affairs."

Verbalizes abilities and capabilities.

Able to make decisions and answer questions with little discomfort and anxiety.

Shows little hesitation when taking action.

Speaks clearly; easily heard; smooth delivery.

Body language of confidence with straight posture and good eye contact.

States belief in own ability to accomplish tasks and goals.

12. Human Need for Elimination

Able to collect and provide urine sample for analysis.

Urine: Color range from pale yellow to amber; pH is 4.3 to 8.0 (6.0 average).

Urinary output for adult in 24-hour period is 1200 to 1500 ml.

Specific gravity is 1.015 to 1.025.

No glucose or ketones.

Protein (albumin) is 0 to up to 8 mg/dl.

Blood is up to 2 red blood cells.

Urinary bladder integrity—voiding comfortable; bladder empties fully; absence of urgency; no incontinence; normal adult bladder capacity of 250 to 350 ml per voiding.

No burning or pain on urination.

Urine production increased during waking hours and decreased during sleep.

Voids 4 to 5 times a day with 250 to 350 ml per voiding.

No discharge from urethra.

Characteristic odor.

No unusual odor—no strong ammonia odor or indications of infection.

Stool—bowel movements at intervals following a normal pattern; range from 2 to 3 times per day to once every 2 days.

Frequency of bowel movements contingent on type of diet as is character of stools.

Normal stool formed, brown in color, soft.

No excessive pain on defecation, either in anus or higher in the bowel.

No evidence of mucus or blood in stool (bright red or dark tarry).

No occult blood in stool.

No parasites.

Requires no laxatives, suppositories, or enemas to have a bowel movement.

13. Human Need for Fluid and Electrolytes

Describes fluid intake adequate for age, body build, and gender.

"My weight has been the same for the past year—up 2 to 3 pounds, down 2 or 3 pounds."

Satiated.

Normal body temperature, pulse rate, blood pressure, respiration.

Moist, glistening mucosa.

No evidence of edema.

Electrolyte values in the range of:

   Bicarbonate (HCO_3) 22 to 26 mEq.

   Calcium (Ca^{2+}) 4.5 to 5.5 mEq.

   Chloride (Cl^-) 96 to 106 mEq.

   Potassium (K^+) 3.5 to 5.5 mEq.

   Magnesium (Mg^{2+}) 1.5 to 2.5 mEq.

   Sodium (Na^+) 137 to 147 mEq.

   Phosphate (PO_4^{2-}) 1.7 to 2.6 mEq.

Central venous pressure in normal range.

Skin fold moves easily and when released returns to former shape.

Intracellular fluid comprises 45 percent of body weight.

Extracellular fluid comprises 15 percent of body weight.

Normal hematocrit value—men, 45 to 52 percent; women, 37 to 48 percent.

Urinary output 1200 to 1500 ml/24-hour period.

Urine specific gravity 1.015 to 1.025.

Urine pH 4.3 to 8.

No muscle cramps or weaknesses.

14. Human Need for Freedom from Pain

States comfort, absence of pain.

Comments that "I'm not a worrier."

Displays ease of movement, relaxed face, hand, legs.

No evidence of medication for pain; no drugs or alcohol.

Speaks without hesitation or breaks in sentences.

Pulse—normal range.

Respirations—regular, normal rate, depth.

Maintains eye contact.

Attentive, alert.

Intact skin, mucous membranes, musculoskeletal structures.

No excessive perspiration; no "sweaty palms" or beads of perspiration on forehead.

Rest, distraction, relaxation effective in relieving discomforts experienced from overdoing in work and play.

No evidence of rubbing body parts or favoring or protecting body areas.

Protective signal of pain or discomfort intact to protect from tissue damage.

No expression of psychic discomfort or pain, e.g., worry, panic.

No evidence of tears, crying.

15. Human Need for Humor

States "I can see the humor in the human situation."
"Life is never boring."
"Things go bad for me if I take myself or my situation too seriously."
Family and significant others label client funny, comical, with good
    sense of humor.
Jokes.
Smiles.
"Light of laughter" in eyes.
Appropriate laughing, chuckling, giggling.
Can see humor in a trying situation.
Lowers tension in relationship with appropriate comic relief, joke
    telling.
Diminishes a tense human situation with comic relief.
Laughs at self; can share humor about self with others.

16. Human Need for Interchange of Gases

Adult hemoglobin in range of 14.5 to 16 g/100 cc blood.
Arterial oxygen saturation at sea level is 95 to 98 percent.
Venous oxygen saturation.
$Paco_2$ is 35 to 42 mm Hg. and $Pvco_2$ is 40.47 mm Hg.
Intracellular Po_2 is lower than the Po_2 of the interstitial fluids: intracel-
    lular Po_2 ranges from 5 to 60 mm Hg.
Intracellular Pco_2 is 46 mm Hg.
Intact neurologic respiratory center and spinal cord.
Skin and mucous membranes pink.
Normal sensorium.
Blood pH is 7.35 to 7.45.
Warm peripheral tissue and adequate capillary refill; strong peripheral
    pulses.
Blood pressure 120/80 or as adjusted for age.
Functional upper respiratory mechanism—nose, throat, epiglottis, lar-
    ynx, trachea, bronchi, alveoli—for pulmonary ventilation.
Functional mechanism for transport and interchange of oxygen and
    carbon dioxide.
No clubbing of fingers.
Alert.
Oriented.

17. Human Need for Nutrition

States "I am no longer hungry after eating a meal with sufficient
    calories."

States "I feel energetic."

Relates normal healing pattern (within confines of health history).

Relates satisfaction with diet—no social, ethnic, or religious conflicts.

States "I am comfortable with my present weight. It is within 10 pounds of the weight listed on the official height/weight charts."

Relates that self and significant person(s) in client's life are free of drug or alcohol problem.

Weight maintained within 15 percent of ideal as listed in height/weight standards of Metropolitan Life Insurance Tables.

Skin clear, supple, without rashes or lesions.

Nails—pink, strong, without ridges or pitting.

Hair shiny and firm.

Client's daily caloric intake will equal daily energy output; accommodates sedentary, light, moderate, vigorous and strenuous activities.

Client eats a variety of foods including those in the four main food groups.

Complete blood count, coagulation time, electrolytes, hemoglobin, hematocrit, cholesterol, triglycerides, blood glucose are within normal limits for age and gender.

Serum calcium and bone density reflects assimilation of calcium particularly for nursing and menopausal women.

Neurologic function intact.

Good muscle tone present.

Skinfold thickness is age appropriate for subcutaneous adipose layer.

Evidence of good dentition.

No involvement in fad or abnormal diet or supplements.

Has access to food sources and financial resources for food purchases.

18. Human Need for Effective Perception of Reality

Knows today's date, day of week.

Presence of orientation cues—calendar, clock.

Performs activities of daily living; capable of self-care.

Adjusts sensory input to maintain homeostasis.

Wears glasses/hearing aids or devices if needed to maintain fully functioning sensory state.

Validates perception of health status by physical and psychosocial examination, laboratory values.

Receptive and accepting of changes accompanying normal aging.

Looks well and verbalizes this.

Able to receive stimuli through senses and make valid judgments about self and environment.

Can make a realistic appraisal about happenings and involvements with others—family, significant other, community. Appraisal verified by these others.

Can appraise state of physical and psychosocial health.

Capable of planning a workload in keeping with energy level and strength.

Aware of potential illness resulting from life-style, family history, heredity.

Selects, organizes, and interprets stimuli into a significant and coherent picture of reality.

Seeks variety and change in stimuli to maintain healthy sensorium.

Remembers past and recent events.

Can determine behavior originating in self from behavior as a response to environmental stimuli.

Able to understand and interpret reality.

Beliefs are congruent with reality.

19. Human Need for Personal Recognition, Esteem, Respect

Expression of self-worth.

Expression of satisfaction with accomplishments.

Verbalizes recognitions by significant persons, groups.

Verbalizes wholesome respect for talents.

Recognition for courage to achieve wellness, offset illness.

Significant others' positive comments about client's effective role function, knowledge, competencies.

Positive personal recognition for achievements related to wellness.

Positive personal recognition for capabilities in handling illness and offsetting same.

Seeks and receives approval from significant others.

Knows the tasks, activities, actions initiated and maintained to feel good about self.

"I deserve the time and effort I put into feeling good about myself, my health state."

Aware of the influences of others' view on self-esteem. Verbalizes the vulnerability of self-esteem to positive and negative appraisal of self by others.

Expects to be addressed by name and to maintain eye contact when participating with health caregivers. Expects to be the primary source for health-related information about self.

Respects and recognizes self as a feeling, thriving, behaving person, unique and valued.

Knows that esteem of self may be reciprocated by others.

20. Human Need for Protection from Excessive Fear, Anxiety, and Chaos

Calm and receptive.
Alert and oriented with normal attention span.
Able to concentrate.
Eye contact direct and not broken off abruptly.
Facial expression relaxed.
Tone of voice with normal pitch, audible and of normal speed.
Upright posture—body movements are relaxed and fluid, coordinated.
Extension of large muscles—sits stretched out and gestures away from the body.
Absence of muscular tension or tremors.
No facial pallor or excessive perspiration.
Skin warm and dry.
Does not startle easily.
Pulse and blood pressure within normal limits.
Respirations easy and regular, without signs of hyperventilation.
Appearance shows good hygiene and grooming.
No evidence of resentment or distrust.
Organized environment.
No complaints of palpitations, heartburn, queasiness or "butterflies in stomach," nausea and vomiting, weight loss or gain, backache, muscular pain or stiffness, urinary frequency.
No complaints of boredom, depression, feelings of worthlessness.
Capable of relating with family, friends, significant others.
Able to conduct personal affairs.
No report of ego-threatening fears.

21. Human Need for Rest and Leisure

Eager, energetic; alert.
Makes references to feeling relaxed.
Has definitive plans for rest and leisure and expresses entitlement to rest and leisure.
Interested in surroundings.
Creates and enjoys pleasurable time.
Describes hobbies and special interests.
States feels relaxed after rest or hobby experience.
Participates in activities for pleasure on a regular basis.
Clear sclera.
Animated and jovial.
Good eye contact and calm facies.
No sign of excessive perspiration or tremors of extremities.
Pulse, respiration, blood pressure within normal limits.

22. Human Need for Safety

"I feel safe where I live and work."
"I feel I can expect a future because I don't take chances with my life, my health."
States has locks, lighting at home.
Lives in a safe environment with no physical hazards.
Expresses knowledge of what is safe and what is not.
Knows how to prevent spread of communicable diseases.
Practices habits of good hygiene—handwashing, etc.
States does not smoke or use drugs.
Regular check of sense organs to assure functioning.
Has a methodology for prevention of unintentional injuries.
Is aware of bodily impact from thermal energy—extremes of heat and cold; from electricity, from radiation, from chemicals, from microbes.
Sees the maintenance of cleanliness of self and environment important for health promotion and safety.
Makes effort to control noise or disturbing sound.
Accounts for the impact of weather on self—body temperature, mood, comfort level, and productivity.
Verifies knowledge of biological defense mechanisms and their integrity.
Cooperates in maintaining sanitation for self, family, community—safety of food, water, adequate waste disposal, protection from vermin, toxins, poisons.
Participates in safety enhancement activities—fire drills, immunizations, home inspection; uses smoke alarms, seat belts.

23. Human Need for Self-control, Self-determination, Responsibility

Not easily diverted from personal goals by stress or obstacles.
Conveys a firmness of purpose.
Accepts accountability for behavior and actions.
Has made a career choice based on interest and ability.
Capable of effective use of time at work; allows time for self, significant others, as well as co-workers and colleagues.
Places high priority on efforts to maintain optimal wellness state for self and for dependent other members.
Verbally assesses self as very motivated, responsible, accountable.
Motivated toward goal achievement without excessive drive or aggression.
States accurate assessment of responsibilities to self and others.
Absence of habits as observed nailbiting, gum cracking, smoking.

Free of addictions/dependencies—drugs, alcohol, gambling, etc.

Projects an image of self that conveys control over self and one's domain.

Capable and comfortable with striving—the time period before goal achievement.

Expresses awareness of personal limits for performance of expectations.

Capable of delegating responsibilities as needed to person(s) best able to assume them.

Recognizes the prevailing support systems enhancing self-control, self-determination, and self-responsibility.

Deals with anxiety-producing situations in calm, interactive fashion or can tentatively walk away and return to handle situation constructively.

Appreciates the use of power inherent in role(s) and within life and health status.

24. Human Need for Self-fulfillment, to Be, to Become

"I am meeting my goals at the present time."

"I am satisfied with my life."

"I find meaning in my life."

Appears happy with self.

Views future positively especially in relation to self.

Is able to steer own course through life.

Recognizes the strengths and limitations of one's self; allows the real self to be revealed in actions.

Relates positive growth and development experiences.

Tolerates ambiguity and complexities in the human experience.

Realizes that not all problems have ready solutions.

Honors time and makes the most of it.

Seeks the experience of fullness of life with joys and sorrows, challenges and accomplishments.

Can identify life's meaning and purpose for self.

Has future-oriented goals.

Views life as a process—offering continuous experience, both positive and negative, that assist one to develop physically, emotionally, socially, psychologically, and spiritually.

25. Human Need for Sensory Integrity

States that eyes cause no problem; "Able to see what is wished to be seen."

States has no headaches with or after reading, doing close work.

States has no problem hearing.

States rarely asks anyone to repeat words or phrases.

States can hear ticking of a watch.

Normal visual acuity as measured by Snellin chart.

Normal visual fields—eye movement, pressure, fundoscopic examination.

Normal physical structure of eye and ear.

No glasses or contact lens or well-fitted glasses or lenses.

Observed reading and watching television with no difficulty or adjustment needed.

Observed ability to distinguish voices, locate direction of sound. Uses normal voice volume.

Identifies whispers and normally voiced words.

States able to distinguish sweet, salty, bitter, and sour tastes.

Taste competency verified by use of solutions (sugar, salt, lemon juice, vinegar) to outer lateral anterior half of tongue.

States no unusual taste sensations present, such as metallic or chemical tastes. No telltale breath odors.

States sense of smell intact. Correctly identifies and distinguishes odors such as coffee, lemon extract.

States has no difficulty breathing through nose.

No evidence of reddened or sore nostrils.

No structural nasal defect.

Voice sounds normal; no sounds of nasal stuffiness.

States able to feel heat, cold, pain.

Able to distinguish among items in touch test—cotton swab, prick of pin. Normal sensation.

States skin functional—no evidence of burning, tingling, numbness of skin or extremities.

Sense of touch functional—skin intact; hands; fingertips; palms of hands functionally intact. No injuries, lesions, abrasions, burns.

States balance steady with no recent falls or loss of balance.

Observed normal posture, gait, and stance.

Good hygiene and grooming to all body areas.

Sense of balance and awareness of position verified on changes of position with eyes closed.

26. Human Need for Sexual Integrity

Relates a satisfying relationship with a significant other involving open communication.

States "I am comfortable with my body; I like who I am."

May relate contentment with sexual life.

Relates satisfaction in gender role.

On physical examination, external organs normal and healthy.

When questioned about sexual history, client may be embarrassed but remains self-assured and confident in answers.

Describes gender role and responsibilities.

Understands that physical, psychological, social, cultural, and spiritual dimensions impact the sexual self.

Demonstrates acceptance and comfortable recognition of self as sexual being.

Awareness that one's maleness or femaleness affects personal and social relationships, one's outlook and expression of self, relationships with others.

Can trust the revelation of self to another person.

Capable of the decisions and choices that lead to continued fulfillment of self as sexual being.

Capable of establishing relationships with significant others, including love relationships.

Comfortable in ascribed roles, those of being male or female, being son or daughter, spouse, parent.

Experiences freedom in refining and expanding vocational role that thwarts traditional gender role expectations and can transcend these expectations.

Vocational role choices reflect interests, aptitude, capabilities, values rather than gender.

Relates values that influence control of self as sexual being and impact of external influences of these values.

Expresses knowledge of congruence between development of self-identity and development of sexual integrity.

Knowledgeable about human reproduction issues—menarche, childbearing, birth control, menopause/climacteric.

Absence of problems related to sexual intercourse.

27. Human Need for Skin Integrity

States bathes daily but every other day in winter.

Uses moisturizers, emollients on skin when dry.

Drinks at least eight glasses of water to keep skin soft.

Keeps out of sun and uses sun screen.

Explains good sensation from all skin areas.

Absence of cuts, bruises, rashes, lesions, burns, areas of inflammation.

Skin color pink; color uniform.

Resilient skin turgor.

Mucous membranes intact and pink in color; are moist.

Nailbeds pink in color; fingernails neatly trimmed, toenails cut straight across.

Bright clear, shiny eyes; no sores at corner of eyelids.

Lips smooth.
Hair shiny, firm; not easily plucked.
Tongue deep red in appearance; not swollen or smooth.
Normal body temperature.
Expression of satisfaction with skin condition.

28. Human Need for Sleep

"I feel awake and refreshed."
"I am ready for the day."
"I had a good night's sleep."
Appears awake and alert to environment.
Experience of REM and NREM sleep in ratio of 1 to 2 hours REM to 7.5 to
     8 hours total sleep.
Falls asleep before 30 minutes of time is passed.
Verbalizes sleep requirements and can describe usual/normal sleep
     pattern.
Describes the consistency of sleep pattern.
Has established presleep rituals that effectively promote sleep.
Sleeps through the night with possibly one awakening. If an awakening
     is experienced, it is short lived.
Sleeps till designated time of awakening.
Has knowledge that stimulants and depressant substances may disturb
     sleep.
Accommodates impact on sleep pattern with changes in work shift pat-
     tern and air travel across time zones.
Facilitates sleep with food and fluids containing the amino acid trypto-
     phan; does not take drugs to induce sleep.
Relates experience of wakefulness during waking hours.
If a nap is required, its timing is such that it does not interfere with night
     time sleep.
Wears clothing for sleep that allows unrestricted movement and ac-
     commodates temperature of environment for sleeping.
Attends to bedding and bed and arranges same for self to promote body
     alignment and safety.
Attends to the environment for sleeping regarding noise control, tem-
     perature, humidity, locks and other security measures.

29. Human Need for Spiritual Integrity

Can state beliefs about a supernatural or divine force influencing
     thoughts, feelings, behavior.
Capable of having faith in an outcome or expectation.
Able to draw on supernatural or divine force for inspiration and support
     in activities of daily living and to enhance self-determination.

Can draw upon rituals, settings, and materials as spiritual or religious symbols to enhance spiritual focus of self.

Able to articulate where and how hope and sources of strength are enhanced.

Aware of relationship between spiritual beliefs and state of wellness and well-being.

Has access to information and resources to maintain spiritual integrity.

Expects that others will afford self the freedom to pursue spiritual experiences.

Can identify persons who comprise personal spiritual/religious support systems.

Relates level of identification with institutionalized religion.

Can articulate circumstance, protocols, persons, environments that engender spiritual pain, anxiety, guilt, alienation, or loss.

Knows the location and manner of contacting spiritual caregivers.

30. Human Need for Structure, Law, Limits

Verbalizes recognition of laws, with or without authority present.

Looks for an environment that is ordered and predictable.

Recognizes the rights of others in interactions with others, in civic, church, family, work affairs.

States role and responsibility for family/significant other(s).

Knows physical limits, endurance for work, play, feelings.

Understands impact of sick role and limits acceptable to family unit and economics for this role.

Relates rules, customs, and practices within family/significant other unit in matters of wellness and illness.

Describes mode to offset needless restrictions of structure and limits in the work place.

Familiar with legislation governing personal and health behavior.

Seeks order in personal, home, and work environments.

Has a sense of the wholesome range for acceptance of uniformity and conformity in life activities.

Uses accepted rules of etiquette in interactions with others and in correspondence.

Displays organized structured behaviors for task completion—activities of daily living—wellness behaviors.

Willing to negotiate rule change(s) if rules are counterproductive or outmoded relative to wellness and illness.

Can set limits on detrimental behavior of self and dependent others.

Meets appointments and commitments.

Can follow prescribed/required health-related regimens (including medications) related to physical or psychological wellness/illness.

31. Human Need to Love and Be Loved

States "I love my family and I know they love me."
States happy and hopeful.
States feels needed.
Has emotional closeness with significant person(s).
Responds to others with consideration and positive regard.
Demonstrates emotional strength.
Close friendships maintained.
Absence of abusive relationship.
Evidence of cuddling, caressing, and cradling of infant and others.
Use of touch to convey love and caring.
Verbal expressions of love, affection to dependent children, family
      members, significant others.
Comfortable with intimate relationship with mate.
States feels loved by others.
Behavior of self contributes to another's welfare and self-fulfillment.
Capable of bonding with infant, family/significant others.
Expresses feelings of hope and continuity.
Responsive to childbearing, child rearing responsibilities.
Contentment with intergenerational involvements.
Experiences companionship, shared interests, and interpersonal
      honesty.
Admiration of the individuality of self and others.
Comfortable with separations within togetherness.

32. Human Need for Tenderness

States rarely lonely; can always count on family and significant others
      to be nurturing.
"I can relax with my friends and family."
Evidence of hugs and pat on back for significant other. Reciprocated by
      significant other.
Listens. Verbalizes sensitivity to feelings of others.
Letters and conversations incorporate tender feelings.
Eye contact with significant persons.
Visits and attentiveness of family, friends, significant others.
Can be sympathetic, empathic.
Vocabulary contains tender words, kind words.
Considerate.
Gentle in manner and in speech behavior.
Feels protective of those most vulnerable—the young, the helpless.
Comfortable in the role of caretaker when required.
Can accept being taken care of when circumstances and health states
      demands this behavior.

33. Human Need for Territoriality

Comfortable with personal space.

Tolerates flexible physical space.

Knows boundary of areas of expertise, skills.

Outlines ideas and can distinguish these ideas from those owned by others.

Claims ownership for personal items and objects.

Verbalizes balance between privacy and community with significant others for presentation of self and satisfaction of affiliation with significant others.

Uses reasonable vigilance to protect territory.

Has a place called home.

Maintains interactional distances commensurate with closeness of relationship.

Invests more energy in areas that have more importance for self. Areas are marked with more personal objects or symbols.

Recognizes role boundaries and understands reactions of self and others to role of intrusion.

Can effectively use public territory, e.g., health care arena.

Defends territory of self against loss, violation, and devaluation.

Capable of physical exclusion when solitude or physical seclusion is desired.

Responsibly gives permission for personal access with limited intrusion required to preserve state of wellness.

34. Human Need for Wholesome Body Image

States actively engaged in appropriate exercise to maintain body health, integrity, form.

States appropriate assessment of image and satisfaction with appearance.

Discusses body image in wholesome, accepting, positive terms.

Neatly groomed.

Makes effort to bring out the best of bodily assets—complimentary clothing, make-up, hairstyle.

Weight congruent with height.

Good posture.

Well-nourished.

Facial expressions are appropriate to verbal responses.

States satisfied with way one looks.

States feels good about self.

Positive response about presentation of self from family, friends, significant others.

Demonstrates knowledge of functioning of body interior as well as body exterior.

Can place "deviations from normal" relating to body form and function as specified by societal forces, such as advertising, in perspective.

Can accommodate bodily changes over time—infancy, childhood, adulthood, aging, pregnancy, climacteric.

Can incorporate biological, psychological, social aspects of body image development and definition.

Cognizant of infuences on body image—group norms for ideal dimensions of body parts, cosmetics, tattooing, dieting, etc.

Aware of body image distortions produced by drugs such as marijuana, hashish, mescaline, lysergic acid.

35. Human Need for Value System

Willing to share what is expected from life.

Expresses what is valued most—people, things, places.

Expresses who and what one would die for, live for.

Value expressions evident from cultural, professional, church, community groups.

Statement of client goals related to wellness or to illness.

Demonstrates a social conscience.

Articulates ethical values and principles.

Has a basis for determining right and wrong actions and responses.

Nursing Diagnoses Specified by Nursing's Human Need Theory and Those Selected for Clinical Trial and Research by NANDA

The data in the following tabular material present the distinguishing characteristics of the nursing diagnoses developed according to Nursing's Human Needs Theory and those developed by NANDA (North American Nursing Diagnosis Association).

	Nursing diagnoses	
Human need	Nursing's human need theory	NANDA[a]
Acceptance of self and others, acceptance by others	Overacceptance of self and others, acceptance by others	Violence (potential for): self-directed or directed at others
	Disturbance in patterns of expression and/or fulfillment of acceptance	
	Rejection of self and others	
	Rejection by others	
Activity	Excessive activity (hyperactivity)	Activity intolerance
		Activity intolerance, potential

(continued)

| Human need | Nursing diagnoses | |
	Nursing's human need theory	NANDA[a]
	Disturbance in patterns of expression and/or fulfillment of activity	Mobility, impaired physical
	Insufficient activity	
Adaptation, to manage stress	Excessive adaptation	Coping, family: potential for growth
	Disturbance in patterns of expression and/or fulfillment of need for adaptation, management of stress	Coping, ineffective family: compromised
		Coping, ineffective family: disabling
	Insufficient adaptation	Coping, ineffective individual
		Adjustment, impaired[b]
		Posttrauma response[b]
Air	Excessive aeration, hyperaeration	Airway clearance, ineffective
	Disturbance in patterns of expression and/or fulfillment for aeration	Breathing pattern, ineffective
	Insufficient aeration	
Appreciation, attention	Excessive appreciation and attention	
	Disturbance in patterns of expression and/or fulfillment of appreciation, attention	
	Lack of appreciation, attention	
Autonomy, choice	Excessive autonomy, choice	Hopelessness[b]
		Neglect, unilateral[b]
	Disturbance in patterns of expression and/or fulfillment of autonomy, choice	Noncompliance (specify)
		Powerlessness
	Lack of autonomy, choice	
Beauty and aesthetic experiences	Preoccupation with beauty and aesthetic experiences	
	Disturbance in patterns of expression and/or fulfillment of beauty and aesthetic experiences	
	Lack of beauty and aesthetic experiences	
Belonging	Excessive belonging	Social isolation
	Disturbance in patterns of expression and/or fulfill-	Social interaction, impaired[b]

(continued)

	Nursing diagnoses	
Human need	**Nursing's human need theory**	**NANDA**[a]
	ment of belonging	
Challenge	Lack of belonging	
	Excessive challenge	
	Disturbance in patterns of expression and/or fulfillment of challenge	
	Lack of challenge	
Conceptualization, rationality, problem solving	Preoccupation with conceptualization, rationality, problem solving	Thought processes, alteration in
	Disturbance in patterns of expression and/or fulfillment of conceptualization, rationality, problem solving	
	Inability to conceptualize, rationalize, problem solve	
Confidence	Overconfidence	
	Disturbance in patterns of expression and/or fulfillment of confidence	
	Lack of confidence	
Elimination (end products of metabolism, toxins, poisons, chemicals, drugs)	Excessive elimination of metabolic end products, nutrients, fluids, chemicals, electrolytes, drugs	Bowel elimination, alteration in: Constipation Diarrhea Incontinence
	Disturbance in patterns of expression and/or fulfillment of elimination of end products, nutrients, fluids, chemicals, electrolytes, toxins, drugs	Incontinence: Functional[b] Reflex[b] Stress[b] Total[b] Urge[b]
	Lack of or diminished elimination of metabolic end products, nutrients, electrolytes, chemicals, toxins, drugs	Urinary elimination, alteration in patterns Urinary retention[b]
Fluid and electrolytes	Excessive hydration and electrolytes	Fluid volume, alteration in: Excess
	Disturbance in patterns of expression and/or fulfillment of fluid hydration, and electrolyte intake	Fluid volume deficit: Actual Potential
	Depletion of fluids and electrolytes	Oral mucous membrane, alteration in

(continued)

Human need	Nursing diagnoses	
	Nursing's human need theory	NANDA[a]
Freedom from pain	Excessive freedom from pain, lack of appropriate pain signals	Comfort, alteration in: Pain Chronic pain[b]
	Disturbance in patterns of expression of pain sensation and/or patterns of relief of pain	
	Inability to experience pain relief	
Humor	Excessive or continuous use of humor, hilarity	
	Disturbance in patterns of expression and/or use of humor	
	Inability to experience humor	
Interchange of gases	Excessive gaseous exchange	Cardiac output, alteration in: Decreased
	Disturbance in patterns of expression and/or fulfillment of gaseous exchange	Gas exchange, impaired
	Insufficient gaseous exchange	Tissue perfusion, alteration in: Cerebral Cardiopulmonary Renal Gastrointestinal Peripheral
		Tissue integrity, impaired[b]
To love and be loved	Excessive expression of love and requirement to be loved	Family process, alteration in
	Disturbance in patterns of expression and/or fulfillment of love need	Grieving: Anticipatory Dysfunctional
	Diminished or lack of ability to love and be loved	Parenting, alteration in: Actual Potential
Nutrition	Excessive nutritional intake	Nutrition, alteration in: Less than body requirements
	Disturbance in patterns of intake of nutrients	More than body requirements
	Insufficient or lack of nutritional intake	Potential for more than body requirements
		Swallowing, impaired[b]
Effective perception of reality	Hypersensitive perception of reality	
	Disturbance in patterns of	

(continued)

	Nursing diagnoses	
Human need	**Nursing's human need theory**	**NANDA[a]**
	expression and/or fulfill-ment of perception of real-ity	
	Ineffective, inaccurate per-ception of reality	
Personal recognition, es-teem, respect	Overrecognition, respect, excessive esteem	Self-concept, self-esteem, role performance, person-al identity
	Disturbance in patterns of expression and/or fulfill-ment of recognition, es-teem, respect	
	Lack of recognition, es-teem, and respect	
Protection from excessive fear, anxiety, and chaos	Excessive fear, anxiety, chaos	Fear
		Anxiety
	Disturbance in patterns of expression and/or fulfill-ment of protection from excessive fear, anxiety, chaos	
	Lack of expression of fear and anxiety, lack of pro-tection	
Rest and leisure	Excessive rest, overuse of leisure	
	Disturbance in patterns of expression and/or fulfill-ment of rest and leisure	
	Restlessness, lack of rest and/or leisure	Diversional activity, deficit
Safety	Excessive thwarting of safety	Body temperature, poten-tial alteration in[b]
	Disturbance in patterns of expression and/or fulfill-ment of safety need	Hyperthermia[b]
		Hypothermia[b]
		Infection, potential for[b]
	Diminished or lack of safety	Injury, potential for: (poisoning, potential for; suffocation, potential for; trauma, potential for)
		Thermoregulation, ineffec-tive[b]
Self-control, self-determi-nation, responsibility	Excessive self-control, self-determination, responsi-bility	Health maintenance, alter-ation in
		Home maintenance man-agement, impaired
	Disturbance in patterns of expression and/or fulfill-	Self-care deficit:

(continued)

Human need	Nursing's human need theory	NANDA[a]
	ment of self-control, self-determination, responsibility	Feeding Bathing/hygiene Dressing/grooming Toileting
	Diminished or lack of self-control, self-determination, responsibility	
Self-fulfillment, to be, to become	Independency, preoccupation with becoming	
	Disturbance in patterns of expression and/or fulfillment of self-fulfillment, becoming	
	Lack of fulfillment of self, of feeling of becoming, prolonged dependency	
Sensory integrity	Sensory overload	Sensory-perceptual alteration: Visual Auditory Kinesthetic Gustatory Tactile Olfactory
	Disturbance in patterns of expression and/or fulfillment of sensory integrity	
	Sensory deprivation	
Sexual integrity	Preoccupation with sexual dimension	Rape trauma syndrome Sexual dysfunction Sexual patterns, altered[b]
	Disturbance in patterns of expression and/or fulfillment of sexual integrity	
	Lack of attention to sexual integrity	
Skin integrity	Preoccupation with maintenance of skin integrity	Skin integrity, impairment of: Actual Potential
	Disturbance in patterns of expression and/or fulfillment of skin integrity	
	Diminished or lack of skin integrity	
Sleep	Excessive sleep	Sleep pattern disturbance
	Disturbance in patterns of expression and/or fulfillment of sleep	
	Insufficient or lack of sleep	
Spiritual integrity	Preoccupation with spiritual dimension	Spiritual distress (distress of the human spirit)
	Disturbance in patterns of expression and/or fulfill-	

(continued)

Human need	Nursing's human need theory	NANDA[a]
	ment of spiritual integrity	
	Diminished or lack of spiritual integrity	
Structure, law, limits	Excessive structure, law, and limits	
	Disturbance in patterns of expression and/or fulfillment of structure, law, and limits	
	Diminished or lack of structure, law, and limits	
Tenderness	Excessive, smothering tenderness	
	Disturbance in patterns of expression and/or fulfillment of tenderness	
	Diminished or lack of tenderness	
Territoriality	Excessive territorial requirement	
	Disturbance in patterns of expression and/or fulfillment of territoriality	
	Diminished or lack of territorial space	
Wholesome body image	Excessive valuation of overall image and/or selected body parts	Self-concept, disturbance in body image
	Disturbance in patterns of expression and/or fulfillment of wholesome body image	
	Diminished or poor body image, unwholesome body image	
Value system	Excessive or rigid application of value system	
	Disturbance in patterns of expression and/or fulfillment of value system	
	Diminished or lack of value system	
		Others:
		Communication, impaired: Verbal

(continued)

Human need	Nursing diagnoses	
	Nursing's human need theory	NANDA[a]
		Growth and development, altered[b]
		Knowledge deficit (specify)

The authors gratefully acknowledge the ideas of Paula Lewis, Assistant Professor of Nursing, and Toni Clark, Adjunct Faculty, of Columbia Union College, Department of Nursing, Takoma Park, Maryland, in preparing these data.

[a]Taken from McLane, A.M. (ed.). *Classification of nursing diagnoses: Proceedings of the 7th conference.* St. Louis: C.V. Mosby, 1987.

[b]Diagnoses accepted in 1986.

Bibliography

BOOKS

Abdellah, F., Beland, I., Martin A., Matheney, R.V. *Patient-centered approaches to nursing*. New York: Macmillan, 1960.

American Nurses' Association. *Standards of nursing practice*. Kansas City, Mo.: American Nurses' Association, 1978.

American Nurses' Association. *The study of credentialing in nursing. A new approach*. Kansas City, Mo.: American Nurses' Association, 1979, p.x.

Atkinson, L.D., & Murray, M.E. *Understanding the nursing process*. New York: Macmillan Publishing Co., 1986.

Bennett, A.M., Foster, P.C., & Wiedenbach, E. In J.B. George (Chairperson), The Nursing Theories Conference Group, *Nursing theories*. Englewood Cliffs, N.J.: Prentice-Hall, 1980 (pp. 138–149).

Bloom, B.S., Hastings, J.T., & Madaus, G.F. *Handbook on formative and summative evaluation of student learning*. New York: McGraw-Hill, 1971.

Bonney, V., & Rothberg, J. *Nursing diagnosis and therapy—An instrument for evaluation and measurement*. New York: The League Exchange, National League for Nursing, 1963.

Brook, R.H. *Quality of care assessment: Comparison of two methods of peer review*. Bethesda, Md.: U.S. Department of Health, Education and Welfare, No. HRA-74-3100, 1973.

Brown, E.L. *Nursing for the future*. New York: Russell Sage Foundation, 1948.

Brown, E.L. *Newer dimensions of patient care* (Parts 1, 2, and 3). New York: Russell Sage Foundation, 1964.

Byrne, M., & Thompson, L. *Key concepts for the study and practice of nursing*, 2nd ed. St. Louis: Mosby, 1978.

Carnevali, D. L. *Nursing care planning—Diagnosis and management*, 3rd ed. Philadelphia: J.B. Lippincott, 1983.

Carlson, J.H., Craft, C.A., & McGuire, A.D. *Nursing diagnosis*. Philadelphia: Saunders, 1982.

Christensen, W.W., & Rupp, P.R. *Computers in nursing management.* Frederick, Md.: Aspen Publishers, Inc., 1986, p. 325.

Combs, A., Richards, A.C., & Richards, F. *Perceptual psychology—A humanistic approach to the study of persons.* New York: Harper & Row, 1976, p. 52.

Committee on Nursing Home Regulation, Institute of Medicine. *Improving the quality of care in nursing homes.* Washington, D.C.: National Academy Press, 1986, p. 415.

Crane, M.D., & Orlando, I.J. In J.B. George (Chairperson), The Nursing Theories Conference Group, *Nursing theories,* Englewood Cliffs, N.J.: Prentice-Hall, 1980, pp. 213–237.

Davidson, S.V.S. (Ed.). *PETO utilization and audit in patient care.* St. Louis: Mosby, 1976.

Doenges, M.E., Jeffries, M.F., & Moorhouse, M.F. *Nursing care plans: Nursing diagnoses in planning patient care.* Philadelphia: F.A. Davis Co., 1984, p. 693.

Duldt, B.W., & Griffin, K. *Theoretical perspective for nursing.* Boston, Little, Brown & Co., 1985, p. 276.

Donabedian, A. *Explorations in quality assessment and monitoring.* Vol. 1. The definition of quality and approaches to its assessment, Ann Arbor, Mich.: Health Administration Press, 1980.

Donabedian, A. *Explorations in quality assessment and monitoring.* Vol. 2. The criteria and standards of quality. Ann Arbor, Mich.: Health Administration Press, 1980.

Fish, S., & Shelly, J.A. *Spiritual care: The nurse's role.* Downers Grove, Ill.: Inter-Varsity Press, 1978.

Frances, G., & Munjas, B. *Manual of social psychologic assessment.* New York: Appleton-Century-Crofts, 1976.

Frankenburg, W.K., & Dodds, J.B. *Denver development screening test manual.* Denver: Ladoca Project and Publishing Foundation, 1970.

Freeman, R.B. (Ed.). *Family coping index* (developed and published by Johns Hopkins School of Hygiene and Public Health and Richmond Instructive Visiting Nurse Association–City Health Department, Nursing Service, Baltimore, Md.) (Richmond-Hopkins Cooperative Nursing Study), 1964.

Froebe, D.J., & Bain, R.J. *Quality assurance programs and controls in nursing.* St. Louis: Mosby, 1976.

Gebbie, K.M. (Ed.). *Summary of the second national conference—Classification of nursing diagnosis.* St. Louis: Clearinghouse-National Group for Classification of Nursing Diagnoses, 1976.

Gebbie, K.M., & Lavin, M.A. *Classification of nursing diagnoses.* Proceedings of the First National Conference. St. Louis: Mosby, 1975.

Gordon, M. *Nursing diagnosis—Process and application,* New York: McGraw-Hill, 1982.

Gowan, M.O. *Administration of college and university programs in nursing, from the viewpoint of nurse education.* Report of the Proceedings of the Workshop on Administration of College Programs in Nursing. Washington, D.C.: The Catholic University of America Press, 1944.

Griffith, J.W., & Christensen, P.J. *Nursing process: Application of theories, frameworks, and models.* St. Louis: C.V. Mosby, 1982.

Grubbs, J. An interpretation of the Johnson behavioral system model for nursing practice. In J.P. Riehl & C. Roy (Eds.), *Conceptual models for nursing practice*, 2nd ed. New York: Appleton-Century-Crofts, 1980, pp. 217–254.

Hardy, M.E. (Ed.). *Theoretical foundations for nursing*. New York: MSS Information Corporation, 1973.

Harmer, B. *Methods and principles of teaching the principles and practice of nursing*. New York: Macmillan, 1926.

Haussmann, R.K.D., Hegyvary, S.T., & Newman, J.F. *Monitoring quality of nursing care, Part II: Assessment and study of correlates*. Bethesda, Md.: U.S. Department of Health, Education, and Welfare, 1976.

Henderson, V. *The nature of nursing*. New York: Macmillan, 1966.

Holzemer, W.L. Computer assisted decision making in the nursing process. *NLN Publication*, 1985, Sept. (41-1985): 51–62.

Hoskins, L.M. The nursing diagnosis. In F.L. Bower (Ed.), *Nursing assessment*. New York: Wiley, 1977.

Hurst, J., & Walker, H.K. (Eds.). *The problem-oriented system*. New York: Medcom, 1972.

Jelinek, R.C., Haussmann, R.K.D., Hegyvary, S.T., & Newman, J. *A methodology for monitoring quality of nursing care*. Bethesda, Md.: U.S. Department of Health, Education, and Welfare, 1974.

Johnson, D.E. The behavioral system model for nursing. In J.P. Riehl & C. Roy (Eds.), *Conceptual models for nursing practice*, 2nd ed. New York: Appleton-Century-Crofts, 1980, pp. 207–216.

Kim, M.J., & Moritz, D.A. (Eds.). *Classification of nursing diagnoses*. Proceedings of the third and fourth national conferences. New York: McGraw-Hill, 1982.

King, I.M. *Toward a theory for nursing*. New York: Wiley, 1971.

King, I.M. *A theory for nursing*. New York: Wiley, 1981.

Klineberg, O. Human needs: A social-psychological approach. In K. Lederer (Ed.), *Human needs*. Cambridge, Mass.: Oelgeschlager, Gunn & Hain, 1980, pp. 19–35.

Lederer, K. *Human needs*. Cambridge, Mass.: Oelgeschlager, Gunn & Hain, 1980.

Levine, M. Trophicognosis: An alternative to nursing diagnosis. In *ANA Regional Clinical Conference*. New York: Appleton-Century-Crofts, 1966, pp. 55–70.

Lewis, L.,Carozza, V.,Carroll, M., Darragh, R., Patrick, M., & Schadt, E. *Defining clinical content, graduate nursing programs, medical-surgical nursing*. Boulder, Co.: Western Interstate Commission for Higher Education, 1967.

Little, D.E., & Carnevali, D.L. *Nursing care planning*, 2nd ed. Philadelphia: Lippincott, 1976.

Mace, N., & Rabins, O.P. *The 36-hour day: A family guide to caring for persons with Alzheimer's disease, related dementing illnesses, and memory loss in later life*. Baltimore, Md.: Johns Hopkins University Press, 1982.

Maryland Appraisal of Patient Progress. Baltimore, Md. Department of Health and Mental Hygiene, Division of Licensing & Certification, 1982.

Maslow, A.H. *Toward a psychology of being*, 2nd ed. Princeton, N.J.: Van Nostrand, 1968.

Maslow, A.H. *Motivation and personality,* 2nd ed. New York: Harper & Row, 1970.

McCaffery, M. *Nursing management of the patient with pain.* Philadelphia: Lippincott, 1972.

McHale, J., & McHale, N. *Basic human needs: A framework for action.* New Brunswick, N.J.: Transaction, 1978.

McKay, R.P. *The process of theory development in nursing.* New York: Teachers College, Columbia University, 1965.

McLane, A.M., & Fehring, R.J. *Nursing diagnosis: A review of the literature.* In M.J. Kim, G.K. McFarland, & A.M. McLane (Eds.), *Classification of nursing diagnoses: Proceedings of the fifth national conference* (525–540), St. Louis: C.V. Mosby, 1984.

Meisenheimer, C.G. *Quality assurance—A complete guide to effective programs.* Frederick, Md., Aspen Publishers, Inc., 1985, p. 312.

Montagu, A. *On being human.* New York: Hawthorn, 1966.

Montagu, A. *The direction of human development.* New York: Hawthorn, 1970.

Montagu, A. *Touching—The human significance of the skin.* New York: Harper & Row, 1971.

National Citizens' Coalition for Nursing Home Reform. *A consumer perspective on quality care: The resident's point of view.* Washington, D.C. (1424 16th St., N.W. 20036), 1985.

National League for Nursing. *Evaluation—The whys and the ways.* New York: The National League for Nursing, 1975.

National League for Nursing. *Quality assurance—A joint venture.* New York: The National League for Nursing, 1975.

National League for Nursing. *Quality assurance—Models for nursing education.* New York: The National League for Nursing, 1976.

Neuman, B. The Betty Neuman health-care systems model: A total person approach to patient problems. In J.P. Riehl & C. Roy (Eds.), *Conceptual models for nursing practice,* 2nd ed. New York: Appleton-Century-Crofts, 1980, pp. 119–134.

Nightingale, F. *Notes on nursing: What it is and what it is not.* A facsimile of the first edition published in 1859. Philadelphia: Lippincott, 1946.

Nursing Development Conference Group. *Concept formalization in nursing—Process and product,* 2nd ed. Boston: Little, Brown, 1979.

Nursing Theories Conference Group. *Nursing theories—The base for professional nursing practice.* Englewood Cliffs, N.J.: Prentice-Hall, 1980.

Orem, D.E. *Nursing: Concepts of practice,* 2nd ed. New York: McGraw-Hill, 1980.

Orlando, I.J. *The dynamic nurse–patient relationship.* New York: Putnam, 1961.

Orlando, I.J. *The discipline and teaching of nursing process.* New York: Putnam, 1972.

Paterson, J.G. The tortuous way toward nursing theory. In *Theory development, what, why, how?* New York: National League for Nursing, 1978.

Paterson, J.G., & Zderad, L.T. *Humanistic nursing.* New York: Wiley, 1976.

Peplau, H.E. *Interpersonal relations in nursing,* New York: Putnam, 1952.

Peplau, H.E. Theory: The professional dimension. In C.M. Norris (Ed.), *Proceedings of the first nursing theory conference,* March 20–21, 1969, Kansas City, Kan.: University of Kansas Medical Center, 1969.

Phaneuf, M.C. *The nursing audit—Profile for excellence*. New York: Appleton-Century-Crofts, 1972.

Phaneuf, M.C. *The nursing audit—Self-regulation in nursing practice*, 2nd ed. New York: Appleton-Century-Crofts, 1976.

Poulin, M. *Configurations of nursing practice, issues in professional nursing practice*. Kansas City, Mo.: American Nurses' Association, 1985.

Riehl, J.P., & Roy C. (Eds.). *Conceptual models for nursing practice* (2nd ed.). New York: Appleton-Century-Crofts, 1980.

Rogers, M.E. *Nursing science: Introduction to the theoretical basis of nursing*. Philadelphia: Davis, 1970.

Rogers, M.E. Nursing—A science of unitary man. In J.P. Riehl & C. Roy (Eds.), *Conceptual models for nursing practice*, 2nd ed. New York: Appleton-Century-Crofts, 1980, pp. 329–337.

Roy, C. *Introduction to nursing: An adaptation model*. Englewood Cliffs, N.J.: Prentice-Hall, 1976.

Roy, C., & Roberts, S.L. *Theory construction in nursing—Adaptation model*. Englewood Cliffs, N.J.: Prentice-Hall, 1981.

Schroeder, P.S., & Maibusch, R.M. *Nursing quality assurance—A unit-based approach*. Frederick, Md.: Aspen Publishers, Inc. 1984.

Solomon, S.B. Quest for Quality. *NLN Public Policy Bulletin*, IV (2), 1986.

Stevens, B.J. *Nursing theory—Analysis, application, evaluation*, 2nd ed. Boston: Little, Brown, 1984.

Toffler, A. *Future shock*. New York: Random House, 1970.

Torres, G., & Yura, H. *Today's conceptual framework: Its relationship to the curriculum development process*. New York: National League for Nursing, 1974.

Torres, G., & Yura, H. The meaning and functions of concepts and theories within education and nursing. In *Faculty-curriculum development*. New York: National League for Nursing, 1975.

Travelbee, J. *Interpersonal aspects of nursing*. Philadelphia: Davis, 1966.

Travelbee, J. *Interpersonal aspects of nursing*, 2nd ed. Philadelphia: Davis, 1971.

Travelbee, J. *Intervention in psychiatric nursing: Process in the one to one relationship*. Philadelphia: Davis, 1969.

Wandelt, M.A., & Agar, J.W. *Quality patient care scale*. New York: Appleton-Century-Crofts, 1974.

Wandelt, M.A., & Stewart, D.S. *Slater nursing competencies rating scales*. New York: Appleton-Century-Crofts, 1975.

Watson, J. *Nursing: Human science and human care: A theory of nursing*. E. Norwalk, Conn.: Appleton-Century-Crofts, 1985.

Wiedenbach, E. *Clinical nursing: A helping art*. New York: Springer, 1964.

Yura, H. Climate to foster utilization of the nursing process. In *Providing a climate for the utilization of nursing personnel*. New York: National League for Nursing, 1975.

Yura, H., Ozimek, D., & Walsh, M.B. *Nursing leadership: Theory and process* (2nd ed.). New York: Appleton-Century-Crofts, 1981.

Yura, H., Torres, G., Chioni, R.M., Frank, E., Lynch, E.A., McKay, R.P., Stanton, M., Carlson, S., O'Leary, H.J., & Kelley, J.A. (Eds.). Faculty-Curriculum Development. New York: National League for Nursing, 1986.

Yura, H., & Walsh, M.B. *Human needs and the nursing process*. New York: Appleton-Century-Crofts, 1978.

Yura, H., & Walsh, M.B. *Human needs 2 and the nursing process*. New York: Appleton-Century-Crofts, 1982.

Yura, H., & Walsh, M.B. *Human needs 3 and the nursing process*. New York: Appleton-Century-Crofts, 1983.

Yurick, A.G., Spier, B.E., Robb, S.S., & Ebert, N.J. *The aged person and the nursing process*. E. Norwalk, Conn.: Appleton-Century-Crofts, 1984, p. 587.

Zderad, L.T. From here-and-now to theory: Reflections on "how." In *Theory development, what, why, how?* New York: National League for Nursing, 1978.

Periodicals

Abdellah, F.G. The nature of nursing science. *Nursing Research*, 1969, *18*, 390–393.

American Nurses' Association. ANA's First Position on Education for Nursing. *American Journal of Nursing*, 1965, *65*, 106–111.

American Nurses' Association. Code for Nurses with Interpretive Statements. Kansas City, Mo., American Nurses' Association, 1985.

American Nurses' Association. New RN examination based on nursing process. *The American Nurse*, 1982, *14*: 1.

Andreoli, K., & Musser, L.A. Computers in nursing care—The state of the art. *Nursing Outlook*, 1985, *33*(1): 16–21.

Aspinall, M.J. Nursing diagnosis—The weak link. *Nursing Outlook*, 1976, *24*: 433–436.

Aspinall, M.J. Use of a decision tree to improve accuracy of diagnosis. *Nursing Research*, 1979, *28*: 182–185.

Avant, K. Nursing diagnosis: Maternal attachment. *Advances in Nursing Science*, 1979, *2*: 45–55.

Block, D. Evaluation of nursing care in terms of process and outcome: Issues in research and quality assurance. *Nursing Research*, 1975, *24*: 256–263.

Billingsley, M.C. The process study. *Nurse Practitioner*, 1986, *11*(1): 53, 56, 68.

Chambers, W. Nursing diagnosis. *American Journal of Nursing*, 1962, *62*: 102–104.

Chinn, P.L., & Jacobs, M.K. A model for theory development in nursing. *Advances in Nursing Science*, 1978, *1*: 1–11.

Cosier, R.A., Alpin, J.C. Intuition and decision-making—Some empirical evidence. *Psychological Reports*. 1982, *51*, 275–281.

Dickoff, J., & James P. A theory of theories: A position paper. *Nursing Research*, 1968, *17*: 203.

Dickoff, J., & James, P. Researching research's role in theory development. *Nursing Research*, 1968, *17*: 204–206.

Dickoff, J. & James, P. Beliefs and values: Bases for curriculum design. *Nursing Research*, 1970, *19*: 415–427.

Dickoff, J., & James, P. A theory of theories: A position paper. Nursing research—tenacity or inquiry. *Nursing Research*, 1975, *24*: 84–88.

Dickoff, J. & James, P. Part II: Designing nursing research—Eight points of encounter. *Nursing Research*, 1975, *24*: 164–176.

Dickoff, J., James, P., & Wiedenbach, E. Theory in a practice discipline, Part I. Practice oriented theory. *Nursing Research*, 1968, *17*: 415–435.

Dickoff, J., James, P. & Wiedenbach, E. Theory in a practice discipline, Part II. Practice oriented research. *Nursing Research*, 1968, *17*: 545–554.

Donabedian, A. Promoting quality through evaluating the process of patient care. *Medical Care*, 1968, *6*: 181–202.

Dossey, B., & Guzzetta, C.E. Nursing diagnosis. *Nursing 81*, 1981, *11*: 34–38.

Durand, M., & Prince, R. Nursing diagnosis: Process and decision. *Nursing Forum*, 1966, *5*: 50–64.

Field, L. The implementation of nursing diagnosis in clinical practice. *Nursing Clinics of North America*, 1979, *14*: 497.

Gebbie, K.M., & Lavin, M.A. Classifying nursing diagnoses. *American Journal of Nursing*, 1974, *74*: 250–253.

Goodwin, J.O., & Edwards, B.S. Developing a computer program to assist the nursing process: Phase I—From systems analysis to an expandable program *Nursing Research*, 1975, *24*: 299–305.

Gordon, M. Assessing activity tolerance. *American Journal of Nursing*, 1976, *76*: 72–75.

Gordon, M. Nursing diagnosis and the diagnostic process. *American Journal of Nursing*, 1976, *76*: 1298–1300.

Gordon, M. The concept of nursing diagnosis. *Nursing Clinics of North America*, 1979, *14*: 491.

Gordon, M. Predictive strategies in diagnostic tasks. *Nursing Research*, 1980, *29*: 39–45.

Gordon, M. Symposium on the implementation of nursing diagnosis. *Nursing Clinics of North America*, 1979, *14*: 483–569.

Gordon, M., & Sweeney, M.A. Methodological problems and issues in identifying and standardizing nursing diagnoses. *Advances in Nursing Science*, 1979, *2*: 1–15.

Gordon, M., Sweeney, M.A., & McKeehan, K. Nursing diagnosis: Looking at its use in the clinical area. *American Journal of Nursing*, 1980, *80*: 672–674.

Guillen, M.A.: The intuitive edge. *Psychology Today*. 1984, *18*, 68–69.

Hall, L.E. Quality of nursing care. Address at meeting of Department of Baccalaureate and Higher Degree Programs of the New Jersey League for Nursing, February 7, 1955, Seton Hall University, Newark, New Jersey. *Public Health News*, June 1955.

Hall, L.E. The Loeb Center for Nursing and Rehabilitation, Montefiore Hospital and Medical Center, Bronx, New York. *International Journal of Nursing Studies*, 1969, *6*: 81–97.

Halloran, E.J. Nursing workload, medical diagnosis, related groups, and nursing diagnosis. *Research in Nursing and Health*, 1985, *8*(4): 421–433.

Hanlon, J.H. Theory and the practice of nursing. *Journal of Continuing Education in Nursing*, 1974, *5*: 12–18.

Hardy, M.E. Theories: Components, development, evaluation. *Nursing Research*, 1974, *23*: 100–107.

Hardy, M.E. Perspectives on nursing theory. *Advances in Nursing Science*, 1978, *1*: 37.

Haussmann, R.K.D., & Hegyvary, S.T. Field testing the nursing quality monitoring methodology: Phase II. *Nursing Research*, 1976, *25*: 324–331.

Henderson, B. Nursing diagnosis: Theory and practice. *Advances in Nursing Science*, 1978, *1*: 75.

Henderson, V. The nature of nursing. *American Journal of Nursing*, 1964, *64*: 62–68.

Henderson, V. Excellence in nursing. *American Journal of Nursing*, 1969, *69*: 2133–2137.

Henderson, V. On nursing care plans and their history. *Nursing Outlook*, 1973, *21*: 378–379.

Henderson, V. The concept of nursing. *Journal of Advanced Nursing*, 1978, *3*: 113–130.

Hilger, E.E. Developing nursing outcome criteria. *Nursing Clinics of North America*, 1974, *9*: 323–330.

Hornung, G.J. Nursing diagnosis—An exercise in judgment. *Nursing Outlook*, 1956, *4*: 29–30.

Johnson, D.E. A philosophy of nursing. *Nursing Outlook*, 1959, *7*: 198–200.

Johnson, D. E. The nature of a science of nursing. *Nursing Outlook*, 1959, *7*: 291–294.

Johnson, D.E. The significance of nursing care. *American Journal of Nursing*, 1961, *61*: 63–66.

Johnson, D.E. Today's action will determine tomorrow's nursing. *Nursing Outlook*, 1965, *13*: 38–41.

Johnson, D.E. Theory in nursing: Borrowed and unique. *Nursing Research*, 1968, *17*: 206–298.

Johnson, D.E. Development of theory: A requisite for nursing as a primary health profession. *Nursing Research*, 1974, *23*: 375.

Jones, P.E. A terminology for nursing diagnoses. *Advances in Nursing Science*, 1979, *2*: 65.

King, I. A conceptual frame of reference for nursing. *Nursing Research*, 1968, *17*: 27–31.

King, L.S. What is a diagnosis? *Journal of the American Medical Association*, 1967, *202*: 154–157.

Komorita, N.I. Nursing diagnosis. *American Journal of Nursing*, 1963, *63*: 83–86.

Kragel, J., Schmidt, V., Shukla, R.K., & Goldsmith, C.E. A system of patient care based on patient needs. *Nursing Outlook*, 1972, *20*: 257–264.

Kreuter, F.R. What is good nursing care? *Nursing Outlook*, 1957, *5*: 302–304.

Kritek, P.B. The generation and classification of nursing diagnoses: Toward a theory of nursing. *Image*, 1978, *10*: 33–40.

Kritek, P.B. Commentary: The development of nursing diagnosis and theory. *Advances in Nursing Science*, 1979, *2*: 73–79.

Kritek, P.B. Nursing diagnosis—Theoretical Foundations. *Occupational Health Nursing*, 1985, *33*(8): 393–396.

Levine, M.E. Adaptation and assessment: A rationale for nursing intervention. *American Journal of Nursing*, 1966, *66*: 2450–2453.

Levine, M.E. The four conservation principles of nursing. *Nursing Forum*, 1967, *6*: 45–59.

Mastal, M. Analysis and expansion of the Roy adaptation model. *Advances in Nursing Science*, 1980, *2*(4): 71–81.

Matthews, C.A., & Gaul, A.L. Nursing diagnosis from the perspective of concept attainment and critical thinking. *Advances in Nursing Science,* 1979, *2*: 17.

McCain, F. Nursing by assessment, not intuition. *American Journal of Nursing,* 1965, *65*: 82–84.

McFarlane, E.A. Nursing theory—The comparison of four theoretical proposals. *Journal of Advanced Nursing,* 1980, *5*: 3–19.

McKay, R. Theories, models, and systems for nursing. *Nursing Research,* 1969, *18*: 393–399.

Meleis, A.I., & Brenner, P. Process or product evaluation? *Nursing Outlook,* 1975, *23*: 303–307.

Miaskowski, C.A. Nursing diagnosis within the context of the nursing process. *Occupational Health Nursing,* 1985, *33*(8): 401–404.

Mortitz, D.A., & Sexton, D.L. Evaluation: A suggested method for appraising quality. *Journal of Nursing Education,* 1980, *9*: 17.

Mundinger, M.O., & Jauron, G.D. Developing a nursing diagnosis. *Nursing Outlook,* 1975, *23*: 94–98.

Nayer, D.D. The ANA position paper. *Imprint,* 1976, *23*: 23ff.

Phaneuf, M.C. A nursing audit method. *Nursing Outlook,* 1964, *12*: 45.

Phaneuf, M.C. The nursing audit for evaluation of patient care. *Nursing Outlook,* 1966, *14*: 51–54.

Popkess, S.A. Diagnosing your patient's strengths. *Nursing 81,* 1981, *11*: 34–37.

Price, M.R. How nursing diagnosis helps focus your care: The patient is starving—But why? *R.N.,* 1979, *42*: 45–48.

Price, M.R. Nursing diagnosis: Making a concept come alive. *American Journal of Nursing,* 1980, *4*: 668–671.

Ramey, I.G. Setting nursing standards and evaluating care. *Journal of Nursing Administration,* 1973, *3*: 27.

Ramey, I.G. Peer review. *American Journal of Nursing,* 1974, *74*: 63–67.

Ridle, J.C. Quality assurance in ambulatory care. *Nursing Clinics of North America,* 1977, *12*: 583–593.

Rogers, M. Euphemisms in nursing's future. *Image,* 1975, *7*: 3–9.

Rothberg, J.S. Why nursing diagnosis? *American Journal of Nursing,* 1967, *67*: 1040–1042.

Roy, C. Adaptation: A conceptual framework for nursing. *Nursing Outlook,* 1970, *18*: 42–45.

Roy, C. Adaptation: A basis for nursing practice. *Nursing Outlook,* 1971, *19*: 254–257.

Roy, C. Adaptation: Implications for curriculum change. *Nursing Outlook,* 1973, *21*: 163–168.

Roy, C. A diagnostic classification system for nursing. *Nursing Outlook,* 1976, *23*(2): 90–94.

Rubin, C.F., Rinaldi, L.A., & Dietz, R.R. Nursing audit—Nurses evaluation nursing. *American Journal of Nursing,* 1972, *72*: 916–921.

Shoemaker, J.K. How nursing diagnosis helps focus your care. *R.N.,* 1979, *42*: 56.

Shoemaker, J.K. Characteristics of a nursing diagnosis. *Occupational Health Nursing,* 1985, *33*(8): 387–389.

Stoll, R.I. Guides for spiritual assessment. *American Journal of Nursing*, 1979, 79: 1574–1577.

Stolte, K. (1986). A complimentary view of nursing diagnosis. *Public Health Nursing, 1986, 3*(1): 23–28.

Stuart, G.W. How professionalized is nursing? *Image*, 1981, 13: 18–23.

Symposium on Nursing Diagnosis. *Nursing Clinics of North America*, 1985, *20*(4): 609–808.

Taylor, J.W. Measuring the outcomes of nursing care. *Nursing Clinics of North America*, 1974, 9: 337–348.

Travelbee, J. What do we mean by rapport? *American Journal of Nursing*, 1963, 63: 70.

Travelbee, J. What's wrong with sympathy? *American Journal of Nursing*, 1964, 64: 68.

Travelbee, J. To find meaning in illness. *Nursing 72*, 1972, 2: 6–8.

Wiedenback, E. The helping art of nursing. *American Journal of Nursing*, 1963, 63: 54–57.

Wiggins, L. Lydia Hall's place in the development of theory in nursing. *Image*, 1980, *12*(1): 10–12.

Wright, C. Computer-aided nursing diagnosis for community health nurses. *Nursing Clinics of North America*, 1985, *20*(3): 487–495.

Zderad, L. Empathetic nursing. *Nursing Clinics of North America*, 1969, 4: 655–662.

Zimmer, M.J. Quality assurance for outcomes of patient care. *Nursing Clinics of North America*, 1974, 9: 305–315.

Zimmer, M.J. Guidelines for development of outcome criteria. *Nursing Clinics of North America*, 1974, 9: 317–321.

Index

S